Oxford Handbook of
Critical Care Nursing

Sheila K. Adam

Head of Nursing
University College London Hospitals
NHS Foundation Trust

Sue Osborne

Independent Consultant

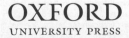

OXFORD
UNIVERSITY PRESS

OXFORD
UNIVERSITY PRESS

WB 300.1

Great Clarendon Street, Oxford OX2 6DP

Oxford University Press is a department of the University of Oxford.
It furthers the University's objective of excellence in research, scholarship,
and education by publishing worldwide in

Oxford New York

Auckland Cape Town Dar es Salaam Hong Kong Karachi
Kuala Lumpur Madrid Melbourne Mexico City Nairobi
New Delhi Shanghai Taipei Toronto

With offices in

Argentina Austria Brazil Chile Czech Republic France Greece
Guatemala Hungary Italy Japan Poland Portugal Singapore
South Korea Switzerland Thailand Turkey Ukraine Vietnam

Oxford is a registered trade mark of Oxford University Press
in the UK and in certain other countries

Published in the United States
by Oxford University Press Inc., New York

© Oxford University Press, 2009

British Library Cataloguing in Publication Data
Data available

Library of Congress Cataloging in Publication Data
Data available

Typeset by Cepha Imaging Private Ltd., Bangalore, India
Printed in China
on acid-free paper through
Asia Pacific Offset

ISBN 978-0-19-921590-4

10 9 8 7 6 5 4 3 2 1

Preface

Critical care nursing is complex, highly skilled, demanding, and very rewarding. It requires knowledge and understanding of the physiology and patho-physiology of all the major organs; the effect of the critical care environment, and critical illness on the individual and their family; the importance of communication and collaboration with colleagues, patient and family; and the ability to intervene with a calm, compassionate, skilled, and knowledgeable manner.

The volume of knowledge and capability required is vast and it is not the intent of this book to cover all of it. Rather we have tried to provide the essence of what could be considered important to the delivery of highly skilled and caring critical care nursing in an easy to access and read format.

The book is intended to be a handy reference guide for nurses who are new to the critical care area, as well as a reminder for those with more experience. This format does not support detailed referencing of an evidence base, but we have referred to 'Further information' where we feel particular articles or books are important to the topic.

Critical care is constantly changing and developing, and although we have tried to reflect current best practice, there will always be variations where 'best' is not absolute. We have therefore reflected best practice as we know it from our own experience.

Sheila K. Adam

Sue Osborne

Acknowledgements

Medical Editors

Mervyn Singer: Professor of Intensive Care Medicine, and Director, Bloomsbury Institute of Intensive Care Medicine, University College, London, UK.

Andrew R. Webb: Medical Director and Consultant Physician, Department of Intensive Care, University College, London.

Chapter Authors

Chapter 13: Neurological care.

Sandra Fairley: Clinical Nurse Specialist, Neurosurgical and Neuromedical Intensive Care, National Hospital for Neurology and Neurosurgery, London, UK.

Prue Hardy: Clinical Governance Nurse, National Hospital for Neurology and Neurosurgery, London, UK.

We are indebted to our medical editors for their constructive criticism, efficiency and advice. Sheila Adam would also like to thank her husband, David Fathers, and children, Florence and Alex. Sue Osborne would like to thank her partner Mervyn and children, Ellie and Joshua. Without our family's patience, encouragement, and enthusiasm this book would not have been possible.

Contents

Detailed contents

Abbreviations and symbols

📖	cross reference
↑	increased
↓	decreased
$A\text{-}aDO_2$	alveolar-arterial oxygen difference
ABC	Airway, Breathing, Circulation
ABG	arterial blood gas
ACE	angiotensin-converting enzyme
ACh	acetylcholine
ACLS	advanced cardiac life support
ACS	abdominal compartment syndrome
ACS	acute coronary syndrome
ACT	activated clotting time
ACTH	adrenocorticotrophic hormone
ADH	antidiuretic hormone
ADP	adenosine diphosphate
AF	atrial fibrillation
AFE	amniotic fluid embolism
AGN	acute glomerulonephritis
AHP	allied health professionals
AIDS	acquired immune deficiency syndrome
ALI	acute lung injury
ALL	acute lymphatic leukaemia
ALT	alaninine aminotransferase
AML	acute myeloid leukaemia
ANCA	anti-nuclear cytoplasmic antibodies
AP	airway pressure
APACHE	acute physiology and chronic health evaluation
APC	antigen-presenting cell
APC	atrial premature contraction (Ch 5)
APTT	activated partial thromboplastin time
ARDS	acute respiratory distress syndrome
ARF	acute renal failure
AST	aspartate transaminase
ATN	acute tubular necrosis
ATP	adenosine triphosphate

AV	atrioventricular
aVF	augmented view foot
aVL	augmented view left
aVR	augmented view right
bd	bis die (twice daily)
BIS™	bispectral index
BiPAP	bilevel positive airway pressure
BNP	brain (B)-type natriuretic peptide
BP	blood pressure
bpm	beats per minute
BSA	body surface area
BSD	brain stem death
C.diff	*Clostridium difficile*
CABG	coronary artery bypass graft
$CaCl_2$	calcium chloride
cAMP	cyclic adenosine monophosphate
CAVH	continuous arteriovenous haemofiltration
CBF	cerebral blood flow
CBV	cerebral blood volume
CCK	cholecystokinin
CCU	critical care unit
CFM	cerebral function monitor
cGMP	cyclic guanosine monophosphate
ChE	cholinesterase
CI	cardiac index
CK	creatinine kinase
CLL	chronic lymphatic leukaemia
CML	chronic myeloid leukaemia
CMV	controlled mandatory ventilation/cytomegalovirus
CNS	central nervous system
CO	cardiac output
COP	capillary oncotic pressure
COPD	chronic obstructive pulmonary disease
CPAP	continuous positive airway pressure
CPK	creatinine phosphokinase
CPP	cerebral perfusion pressure
CPR	cardiopulmonary resuscitation
CRP	C-reactive protein

CRT	capillary refill time
CSF	cerebrospinal fluid
CSW	cerebral salt wasting
CT	computerised tomography
CVA	cerebrovascular accident
CVC	central venous catheter
CVP	central venous pressure
CVVH	continuous venovenous haemofiltration
CVVHD	continuous venovenous haemodialysis
CVVHDF	continuous venovenous haemodiafiltration
CXR	chest X-ray
2, 3-DPG	2, 3-diphosphoglyeric acid
DAI	diffuse axonal injury
DEAFF	detection of early antigen fluorescent foci
DI	diabetes insipidus
DIC	disseminated intravascular coagulation
DKA	diabetic ketoacidosis
DO_2	oxygen delivery
DO_2I	oxygen delivery index
DSA	digital subtraction angiography
DVT	deep vein thrombosis
ECG	electrocardiogram
ECMO	extracorporeal membrane exygenation
EDH	extradural haematoma
EDV	end diastolic volume
EEG	electroencephalogram
EF	ejection fraction
EFM	electronic foetal monitoring
EMG	electromyography
ERCP	endoscopic retrograde cholecystic pancreatogram
ESR	erythrocyte sedimentation rate
ESV	end systolic volume
ET(T)	endotracheal (tube)
$ETCO_2$	end-tidal carbon dioxide monitoring
FDPs	fibrin degradation products
FEV_1	forced expired volume in 1 second
FFP	fresh frozen plasma
FHR	foetal heart rate
F_IO_2	fractionated inspired oxygen concentration

FRC	functional residual capacity
FVC	forced vital capacity
g	gram
GBS	Guillain-Barre syndrome
GCS	Glasgow Coma Score
GFR	glomerular filtration rate
GHB	gamma hyroxybutyrate
GHRH	growth hormone-releasing hormone
GI	gastrointestinal
GIK	glucose-insulin-potassium
GM-CSF	granulocyte-macrophage colony-stimulating factor
GTN	glyceryl trinitrate
HADS	Hospital Anxiety and Depression Scale
HAI	hospital acquired infection
Hb	haemoglobin
HbA	adult haemaglobin
HbCO	carboxyhaemaglobin
HbS	sickle cell haemaglobin
HELLP	haemolysis, elevated liver enzymes and low platelets
HEPA	high efficiency particulate air
HHS	hyperosmolar, hyperglycaemic states
HIT	heparin-included thrombocytopenia
HIV	human immunodeficiency virus
HME	heat moisture exchange
HOCM	hypertrophic obstructive cardiomyopathy
HPA	hypothalamic-pituitary-adrenal
HR	heart rate
HRS	hepatorenal syndrome
HUS	haemolytic uraemic syndrome
I:E	inspiratory:expiratory
IAH	intra-abdominal hypertension
IAP	intra-abdominal pressure
ICH	intracerebral haematoma
ICP	intracranial pressure
ICS	intensive care society
ICU	intensive care unit
IDDM	insulin-dependent diabetes mellitus
IE	infective endocarditis
IGF	insulin–like growth factor

IHD	intermittent haemodialysis
im	intramuscular
IMV	intermittent mandatory ventilation
INR	international normalized ratio
IPPV	intermittent positive pressure ventilation
ITP	idiopathic thrombocytopenic purpura
IU	international unit
iv	intravenous
IVC	inferior vena cava
IVIg	intravenous immunoglobulin
JVP	jugular venous pressure
KCL	potassium chloride
Kg	kilogram
KPa	kilopascal
KPTT	kaolin partial thromboplastin time
L	litre
LAP	left atrial pressure
LBBB	left bundle branch block
LDH	lactic dehydrogenase
LFT	liver function test
LiCl	lithium chloride
LiDCO™	lithium dilution cardiac output
LMA	laryngeal mask airway
LMWH	low molecular-weight heparin
LOS	length of stay
LV	left ventricle
LVED	left ventricular end diastolic
LVEDV	left ventricular end diastolic volume
LVF	left ventricular failure
μg	microgram
μmol	micromole
MABP	mean arterial blood preassure
MAOI	monoamine oxidase inhibitor
MAP	mean arterial pressure
MARS	molecular adsorption recycling system
MC&S	microscopy, culture and sensitivity
mcg	microgram
MDMA	methylenedioxymethamfetamine
MET	medical emergency team

MetHb	methaemoglobin
MEWS	modified early warning score
MG	myasthenia gravis
mg	milligram
MI	myocardial infarction
MODS	multiple organ dysfunction syndrome
mOsmol	milliosmole
MPAP	mean pulmonary artery pressure
MRSA	methicillin-resistant *Staphylococcus aureus*
MV	minute volume
MW	molecular weight
NAC	*n*-acetylcysteine
ng	nanogram
NG	nasogastric
NICE	National Institute for Health and Clinical Excellence
NIDDM	non-insulin-dependent diabetes mellitus
NiPPY	non-invasive positive pressure ventilator
NIV	non-invasive ventilation
NMBA	neuromuscular blocking agents
NO	nitric oxide
NSAIDs	non-steroidal anti-inflammatory drugs
NSTEMI	non-ST elevation myocardial infarction
NYHA	New York Heart Association
O_2ER	oxygen extraction ratio
od	once daily
P_ACO_2	partial pressure of alveolar carbon dioxide
PA	pulmonary artery
P_aCO_2	partial pressure of arterial carbon dioxide
P_AO_2	partial pressure of alveolar oxygen
P_aO_2	partial pressure of arterial oxygen
PAOP	pulmonary artery occlusion pressure
PAWP	pulmonary artery wedge pressure
PCA	patient-controlled analgesia
PCI	percutaneous intervention
pCO_2	partial pressure of carbon dioxide
PCP	*Pneumocystis carinii* pneumonia
PCR	polymerase chain reaction
PCV	packed cell volume
PCWP	pulmonary capillary wedge pressure

PD	peritoneal dialysis
PE	pulmonary embolus
PEA	pulseless electrical activity
PEEP	positive end expiratory pressure
PEG	percutaneous endoscopic gastrostomy
PEJ	percutaneous jejunostomy tube
PERT	patient emergency response team
PiCCO	pulse contour cardiac output monitor
PImax	maximum inspiratory pressure
po	to be taken orally
pO_2	partial pressure O_2
PPI	proton pump inhibitor
ppm	parts per million
PR	per rectum
PRN	pro re nata – as required
PS	pressure support
PSTD	post-traumatic stress disorder
PSV	pressure support ventilation
PT	prothrombin time
PVC	polyvinyl chloride
PVR	pulmonary vascular resistance
PX	plasma exchange
QALY	quality-adjusted life year
Qs/Qt	shunt fraction
QT	Q-T interval
RA	right atrium
RAA	renin-angiotensin-aldosterone (pathway)
RASS	Richmond Agitation Sedation Scale
RBBB	right bundle branch block
RBC	red blood cell
RCT	randomized controlled trial
REM	rapid eye movement
ROC	receiver operating characteristic
ROM	range of movement
RQ	respiratory quotient
RR	relative risk
RR	respiratory rate
RRT	renal replacement therapy
RSBI	rapid shallow breathing index
rTPA	recombinant tissue plasminogen activator

RV	right ventricle
SA	sinoatrial
SAH	subarachnoid haemorrhage
SALT	speech and language therapist
S_aO_2	arterial oxygen saturation
SAPS	simplified acute physiology score
SARS	severe acute respiratory syndrome
SBAR	situation, background, assessment, recommendation
SBE	subacute bacterial endocarditis
SBP	systolic blood pressure
SBT	spontaneous breathing trials
SCUF	slow continuous ultrafiltration
SD	standard deviation
SDD	selective decontamination of the Digestive tract
SDH	subdural haematoma
SE	status epilepticus
SIADH	syndrome of inappropriate secretion of antidiuretic hormone
SIMV	synchronized intermittent mandatory ventilation
SIP	sickness impact profile
SIRS	systemic inflammatory response syndrome
S_iO_2	mixed venous oxygen saturation
$S_{jv}O_2$	jugular venous bulb oxygen saturation
SLE	systemic lupus erythematosus
SLT	speech and language therapist
SOFA	Sequential Organ Failure Assessment
S_pO_2	pulse oximeter oxygen saturation
STEMI	ST elevation myocardial infarction
SV	stroke volume
SVC	superior vena cava
S_vO_2	mixed venous oxygen saturation
SVR	systemic vascular resistance
SVT	supraventricular tachycardia
TB	tuberculosis
TBG	thyroxine-binding globulin
TBI	traumatic brain injury
TCD	transcranial Doppler
TED	thrombo-embolism deterrent
TENS	transcutaneous electrical nerve stimulation
TIPSS	transjugular intrahepatic portal systemic shunt
TISS	therapeutic intervention scoring system

TMA	thrombotic microangiopathy
TMP	transmembrane pressure
TNF	tumour necrosis factor
tPA	tissue plasminogen activator
TPN	total parenteral nutrition
TRALI	transfusion-related acute lung injury
TRH	thyrotrophin-releasing hormone
tSAH	traumatic subarachnoid haemorrhage
TSH	thyroid-stimulating hormone
TT	thrombin time
TTP	thrombotic thrombocytopenic purpura
TURP	trans urethral prostatectomy
TXA_2	thromboxane A_2
UA	unstable angina
U&E	urea and electrolytes
UPS	uninterrupted power supply
UTI	urinary tract infection
V	ventilation
V/Q	ventilation/perfusion
VAP	ventilator-associated pneumonia
VC	vital capacity
VC-IRV	volume controlled inverse ratio ventilation
V_D	dead space
VEs	ventricular premature contractions (ectopics)
VF	ventricular fibrillation
VMA	vanillylmandelic acid
VO_2I	oxygen consumption index
VSD	ventricular septal defect
V_T	tidal volume
VT	ventricular tachycardia
vWF	von Willebrand factor
VZE	varicella zoster encephalitis
WBC	white blood cell
WBPTT	whole blood partial thromboplastin time
WCC	white cell count
WFNS	World Federation of Neurological Surgeons
WG	Wegener's granulomatosis
WPW	Wolff–Parkinson–White (syndrome)
WTE	whole time equivalent

Chapter 1

The critical care continuum

Why hospital-wide critical care?

Knowledge, interventions, and skills once considered only necessary in intensive care are now an important component for effective patient care throughout the acute hospital. The right interventions made at the right time can impact strongly on disease progression and the development of organ failure. This contrasts sharply with outcomes following cardiac arrest that have seen little improvement, despite major investments in training and equipment, and management protocols.

Inpatients in acute hospitals are increasingly elderly, often have co-morbidities, and are undergoing increasingly complex surgery or other procedures. They are therefore at increased risk of deterioration and organ failure. This is compounded by reductions in the working hours of medical staff, which impacts on both continuity of care, and the ability to provide a suitably skilled and knowledgeable response to any decline in the patient's condition. Methods of ensuring these patients receive the care they need vary between hospitals. However, in recent years, there has been a shift in many countries towards:
- Sharing critical care skills.
- Improving early management of peri-arrest situations.
- Involving critical care earlier in ward patient management.
- Facilitating admission and discharge from critical care units.

As an example of proactive management, improved outcomes in sepsis can be achieved with early diagnosis and prompt, goal-directed treatment. However, this needs to occur in emergency departments and wards, rather than waiting to access a critical care bed. As sepsis is the leading cause of mortality and morbidity in the critical care patient, this makes good sense for both the patient and the use of limited hospital resources.

Causes of sub-optimal care in acutely ill ward patients have been identified and include:
- Failure of organization.
- Lack of knowledge.
- Failure to appreciate clinical urgency.
- Lack of experience.
- Lack of supervision.
- Failure to seek advice.

Improvement of skills in ward-based staff and changes in hierarchical culture are essential to protect patients. In essence, critical care must encompass patients according to their clinical need, rather than their location within the hospital. This is best achieved using an outreach service.

Further information

McGloin H, Adam S, Singer M. (1999) Unexpected deaths and referrals to intensive care of patients on general wards. Are some cases potentially avoidable? *J Roy Coll Physic*, **33**, 255.

McQuillan P, Pilkington S, Allan A, et al. (1998) Confidential inquiry into quality of care before admission to intensive care. *BMJ*, **316**, 1853–7.

Rivers E, Nguyen B, Havstad S, et al. (2001) Early goal-directed therapy in the treatment of severe sepsis and septic shock. *N Engl J Med*, **345**, 1368–77.

Models of critical care outreach

There are many variants of critical care outreach, from the individual attempting to improve skills and knowledge through education, to the full emergency team offering 24h per day, 7 days per week support to ward staff.

Critical care outreach

Critical care outreach teams focus on both emergency calls and follow-up, as well as providing post-ICU discharge support. Education is aimed at ward staff, and covers a range of acute skills and specific techniques, such as tracheostomy care, as well as recognition of acute deterioration and appropriate responses.

Medical emergency teams

Medical emergency teams focus predominantly on pre-critical care emergency calls from ward staff, and include education focused on recognition and response in acute emergencies.

Patients are categorized according to their needs in terms of support rather than their location within the hospital

Levels of care

- **Level 0:** patients whose needs can be met through normal ward care in an acute hospital.
- **Level 1:** patients at risk of deteriorating, or recently re-located from higher levels of care. Needs can be met on the ward with advice and support from the critical care team.
- **Level 2:** patients requiring more detailed observation or intervention. Includes single organ support/post-operative care/step-down care from level 3.
- **Level 3:** patients in multi-organ failure.

Aims of critical care outreach

- To facilitate appropriate admission to the critical care unit. This may consist of either:
  - identifying patients for whom critical care would not be suitable and ensuring this is clearly discussed between ward teams, patient, and relatives;
  - identifying and promptly treating any deterioration, such that critical care admission no longer becomes necessary;
  - transferring sick patients in an appropriate and timely manner with treatment already being commenced beforehand.
- To enable discharges from critical care by supporting ongoing care and recovery on the wards, thereby preventing new deterioration and the need for re-admission to critical care.
- To share critical care skills with staff in the wards and community, enhancing their knowledge and skills.

Up to 27% of patients die following discharge from critical care units to the ward. Some of these deaths are expected as part of end of life decisions; a significant number are not. There is a correlation between the discharge TISS (Therapeutic Intervention Scoring System) and mortality following discharge (Table 1.1). The highest number of deaths after discharge occurs in patients admitted with respiratory problems. For details of TISS scoring see 📖 p. 36.

Table 1.1 Correlation between the discharge TISS and mortality following discharge

TISS on day of ICU discharge	Post-discharge mortality
<10	3.7%
>20	21.4%

Further information

Smith L, Orts CM, O'Neil I. (1999) TISS and mortality after discharge from intensive care. *Intens Care Med*, **25**, 1061–5.

Intervening pre-critical care admission

The right interventions carried out at the right time can improve the patient's chance of survival. Hospital mortality rates in patients with sub-optimal care pre-ICU admission were 65% compared with 42% in those with appropriate management. The mortality rate increases in cardiac arrest to 82% overall and to 94% in those patients with a non-shockable rhythm. In septic patients, the transition to multiple organ failure has been labelled the 'golden hours', i.e. there is a possibility of reversal of organ dysfunction if appropriate action is taken.

Methods of improving responses to acute deterioration

- **Education and skills training for emergency situations:** these include specific courses aimed at developing recognition and management of the sick patient, comprising clinical skills workshops, scenario management, team building, and communication skills.
- **Sharing of critical care nursing skills:** teaching and providing hands on simulated practice in the following areas – tracheostomy care in the acute patient, caring for the unconscious patient, CVP measurement and management, oxygen therapy and respiratory support, chest drain management, etc.
- **Track and trigger systems:** these include call criteria and early warning scores for recognition of the sick patient. They must include protocols for responding to the trigger.
- **Emergency response teams:** known variously as medical or patient emergency response teams. They are usually drawn from critical care staff and are multi-disciplinary in nature. The aim is to provide skilled critical care capability to prevent pre-arrest situations from deteriorating to a full cardiorespiratory arrest. They should be available around the clock.

The outcomes for successful responses to acute deterioration should be monitored. These include:
- Cardiac arrest calls:
  - number of calls per 1000 hospital admissions;
  - outcomes from cardiac arrest;
  - number of inappropriate cardiac arrest calls.
- Unexpected admissions to critical care, and number of averted admissions to critical care.
- Length of stay, morbidity, and mortality associated with critical care admissions after acute deterioration.
- Severity scores (e.g. APACHE, SAPS) associated with critical care admissions.
- Number of hospital-wide unexpected deaths.
- Number of appropriate facilitated 'Do not attempt resuscitation' decisions associated with acute deterioration.

Intervening post-critical care discharge

Preventing re-admission

Re-admission to critical care is associated with a five–fold increase in mortality. Patients at high risk of re-admission should be carefully assessed by senior nursing or medical staff to ensure they are fit for discharge.

Factors associated with decreased risk of re-admission

- Discharge delayed by 48h.
- TISS <10 at discharge.
- Presence of critical care outreach services.
- Increased bed capacity in critical care.
- Decreased critical care occupancy.

Common interventions post-ICU discharge

The vast majority of interventions in these patients involve respiratory care such as nebulizers, suctioning, repositioning, physiotherapy and appropriate monitoring. Specific circumstances requiring intervention include a new septic episode, acute desaturation and dyspnoea, difficult fluid management, and oliguria.

Smoothing the transition from critical care to the ward

Relocation to the ward can be stressful for both patient and family, although the impact on individual patients can vary from highly traumatic to generally positive. Reassurance of the patient and their relatives is essential, especially as they will need to cope with fewer staff and a less monitored environment. The ward staff may also need reassurance and education regarding the special circumstances of the patient.

Interventions to improve the transition from critical care to the ward

- Pre-transfer preparation and teaching from critical care nursing staff.
- Written information as a leaflet or booklet for patients and families on the recovery period and what to expect in the ward.
- Accentuation to the patient of the positive association of transfer with becoming less sick.
- Comprehensive handover of information between critical care and ward staff.
- Discharge planning and assessment of patients' level of need.
- Critical care outreach follow-up post-discharge.

Emergency recognition and response

All healthcare professionals need to be able to identify acute patient deterioration and to know what should be done in response.

A structured framework for assessing the acutely sick patient will help to ensure that the problems most likely to result in death are identified and managed first.

The Airway, Breathing, Circulation (ABC) approach identifies the most serious problems, such as hypoxaemia and hypotension in the first moments of assessment, and are used as the basis of all types of emergency response training.

Recognition of the acutely unwell patient

Between 60 and 80% of patients exhibit clinical signs of deterioration in the 6–8h immediately prior to cardiac arrest. Studies also show it takes an average of 21min for the nurse to alert the doctor to this decline.

Physiological markers in ward patients of acute deterioration likely to precede cardiac arrest or admission to critical care

- Respiratory rate >36breaths/min
- Reduced GCS (Glasgow Coma Score) by 2 points or more
- Systolic blood pressure <90mmHg
- Heart rate >140bpm
- Airway at risk.

Call criteria based on such clinical signs have been developed to alert ward staff to summon the critical care outreach team and ensure that the patient receives a timely response. More complex scoring systems, such as the Modified Early Warning Score (Table 1.2), have also been developed to assist ward staff.

Patient Emergency Response Team call criteria:- University College London Hospital NHS Trust

Call the outreach nurse if:
- Respiratory rate <8 or >25breaths/min.
- Oxygen saturation <90% on ≥ 35% inspired oxygen.
- Heart rate <50 or >125bpm.
- Systolic BP <90 or >200mmHg (or has dropped >40mmHg from baseline).
- Sustained alteration in conscious level.
- Your patient looks unwell or you are worried about their clinical state.

Consider calling the outreach nurse and/or alert the patient's own doctor, plus increase monitoring frequency if:
- Urine output is <30ml/h for 2 consecutive hours.
- Hypoglycaemia continues in spite of glucose support.

Table 1.2 Modified early warning score. Trigger level is a score >4 for surgical patients

	3	2	1	0	1	2	3
Respiratory rate		<8		9–14	15–20	21–29	>30
Heart rate		<40	40–50	51–100	101–110	111–129	>130
Blood Pressure	<45%	<30%	<15%	Normal	>15%	>30%	>45% for patient
Conscious level	Responds to voice	Responds to pain	Unresponsive	Alert			
Temperature		<35.0		35–38.4		>38.4	
Urine		<0.5 ml/kg/h	<1 ml/kg/h		>3 ml/kg/h		

Further information

Gao H, McDonnell A, Harrison DA. (2007) Systematic review and evaluation of physiological track and trigger warning systems for identifying at-risk patients on the ward. *Intens Care Med*, **33**, 667–79.

Priestley G, Watson W, Rashidian A. et al (2004) Introducing Critical Care Outreach: a ward-randomised trial of phased introduction in a general hospital. *Intens Care Med*, **30**, 1398–404.

Assessment of the acutely unwell patient

- Use of a structured assessment in an acute situation helps to maintain focus on the right priorities and ensures important information is not missed.
- The ABCDE assessment structure is the most common format.
- Information should be gained by looking at, listening to, and, where appropriate, feeling the patient, as well as measuring variables, such as respiratory rate, heart rate, and blood pressure.

ABCDE assessment structure

- **A:** airway.
- **B:** breathing.
- **C:** circulation.
- **D:** disability or dysfunction.
- **E:** exposure or everything else.

Airway assessment

Indicators of airway compromise

- **Look:** increased respiratory effort, sweating, unable to lie down, drooling (unable to swallow own saliva), bleeding from mouth or tracheostomy site.
- **Listen:**
  - *talking in full sentences?* – probably not compromised;
  - *partial obstruction* – stridor, snoring, wheezing, gurgling, hoarse, unable to speak;
  - *complete obstruction* – no sounds, but frantic effort to breathe, seen as paradoxical chest and abdominal movements.
- **Feel:** any movement of expired air from mouth or nose, sweaty, clammy.

Breathing assessment

Indicators of respiratory compromise

- **Look:** using accessory muscles, stabilizing shoulder girdle by bracing arms, unable to lie flat.
- **Listen:**
  - talking, but only short sentences or single words between breaths;
  - chest auscultation with stethoscope: listen for air entry bilaterally and in all lobes, any added sounds.
- **Feel:**
  - for tracheal deviation, surgical emphysema, areas of tenderness over chest wall;
  - percussion changes in resonance, such as increased resonance with pneumothorax, dull sounds with fluid.
- **Measure:** respiratory rate (normal 12–20 breaths/min), oxygen saturation (normal >95% on air).

Circulatory assessment

Indicators of circulatory compromise

- **Look:** pallor, cyanosis (peripheral or central), sweating, increased jugular venous pressure.

- **Listen:** patient confusion, disorientation or drowsiness, complaints of chest pain, assess heart sounds.
- **Feel:** pulse (rate, rhythm, volume), peripheral temperature, capillary refill time (normal <3s), clammy skin, or warm and dilated.
- **Measure:** blood pressure, central venous pressure (CVP; if available), urine output, central temperature.

Disability assessment
- Indicators of decreased conscious level, e.g. AVPU score, GCS (Table 1.3), ACDU score. Measure blood glucose.

Exposure
- **Look:** view the whole patient to determine any specific areas of bleeding, bruising, swelling, inflammation, infection, pain.
- **Feel:** calves for any evidence of DVT, areas of swelling for associated pain.

Descriptors of consciousness

AVPU score
- **A:** alert.
- **V:** responds to voice.
- **P:** responds to pain.
- **U:** unresponsive.

ACDU score
- **A:** alert.
- **C:** confused.
- **D:** drowsy.
- **U:** unresponsive.

Table 1.3 Glasgow Coma Score

Eye opening		Verbal response		Motor response	
Spontaneous	4	Orientated	5	Obeys commands	6
To speech	3	Confused	4	Localizes to pain	5
To pain	2	Inappropriate words	3	Flexes to pain	4
None	1	Incomprehensible sounds	2	Abnormal flexion	3
		None	1	Extension	2
				None	1

Best − 15, worst − 3.

Immediate responses

Hypoxaemia and hypotension are the most imminent causes of cardiac arrest and death. Any emergency response should always deal with these first.

Hypoxia

Definitions

- **Hypoxia:** inadequate availability of oxygen for cell (tissue) metabolism
- **Hypoxaemia:** oxygen level <8 kPa in the blood when breathing room air, or <11kPa when breathing >40% oxygen.

Hypoxia is difficult to determine. Biochemical markers, such as an increasing arterial base deficit or lactate level are sensitive, but not specific measures of the degree of tissue hypoxia. Oxygen delivery to tissues depends on a combination of the haemoglobin (Hb) level, the cardiac output, and the oxyhaemoglobin level (i.e. arterial oxygen saturation). Thus, hypoxaemia does not automatically mean hypoxia because compensatory mechanisms, such as an increase in cardiac output, can supervene (see 📖 Hypoxaemia and hypoxia, p. 175). Nevertheless, severe hypoxaemia should be avoided.

After ensuring the patient's airway is patent, high flow oxygen via a non-rebreathe reservoir system should be commenced if the patient is still breathing spontaneously. The target is to raise the SaO_2 to an acceptable level, e.g. 97–99%, or perhaps lower in the chronic bronchitic, e.g. 92–94%. If the patient is ventilated, the inspired oxygen concentration should be increased and the adequacy of ventilation assessed.

Hypotension

Whilst hypotension is often used as a measure of poor organ perfusion (blood flow), patients may be perfectly well despite a low BP. Conversely, hypoperfusion may exist with a normal or even high BP, as compensatory vasoconstriction can often maintain an adequate BP until blood flow is extremely compromised. Accompanying signs of hypoperfusion should be sought (see 📖 Manifestations of poor organ perfusion, p.13).

Definitions

Hypotension is difficult to define as it depends on an individual patient's pre-morbid condition. A general rule of thumb is:
- Systolic blood pressure <90mmHg or a sustained decrease >40mmHg from normal values
- Mean blood pressure <60mmHg.

Manifestations of poor organ perfusion

- **Kidneys:** oliguria.
- **Brain:** drowsiness, confusion, agitation, syncope.
- **Skin:** pallor, cold peripheral temperature, CRT >3s.
- **Metabolic acidosis and raised lactate levels.**
- **Compensatory tachycardia and tachypnoea.**

Vascular access is essential to manage hypotension. The initial response is usually to optimize the circulating (intravascular) volume with rapid fluid administration unless the patient is clearly intravascularly overloaded, Once adequate intravascular volume has been achieved, if the patient remains poorly perfused and/or severely hypotensive, other strategies such as inotropic drugs or vasopressors should be considered. At the same time, it is crucial to identify and treat the underlying cause, e.g. relief of a tension pneumothorax or pericardial tamponade, emergency surgery, or angiographic embolization of a bleeding vessel.

Initial emergency responses

- Ensure airway is clear.
- Give high flow oxygen.
- Achieve intravascular access and give fluids to optimize circulating volume.
- Identify and manage precipitating causes.

Secondary transfer of critically ill patients

Secondary transfer refers to transfers from or within a hospital setting. Critically ill patients are highly vulnerable during transfer and a high level of expertise is required. Transfers undertaken by an experienced and well-trained critical care team are less likely to result in critical incidents and deterioration in the patient's condition.

Inter-hospital

This includes transfers between critical care units for tertiary specialist care or when a lack of critical care beds requires the patient to be transferred elsewhere.

Requirements for transfer

- Personnel should be specifically trained and experienced in transfer of critically ill patients.
- Equipment should be designed for transport – light, reliable, with a battery life >4h.
- Monitoring should include ECG, BP, SpO_2, and $ETCO_2$ if the patient is intubated.
- Adequate supplies for the expected journey time, plus an extra 2 h of oxygen, drugs, and fluids. Equipment such as infusion pumps should be adequately charged beforehand or connected to the ambulance electrical supply.
- Emergency equipment should include a full range of resuscitation drugs, defibrillator, intubation drugs and equipment, and suction.
- The patient should be stable prior to commencement of the journey (if interventions such as intubation are likely to occur during travel these should be undertaken before commencement; see Table 1.4).

A record should be kept of the patient's condition throughout the transfer. Any adverse incidents should also be recorded.

Prior to commencement the patient's family should be informed of the destination details, approximate length of journey, and reasons for the transfer. It is not usual for the patient's family to be allowed to travel with the patient due to vehicle insurance restrictions.

The receiving hospital should be informed of departure and estimated time of arrival. If the hospital is unknown to transferring staff, directions to the critical care unit should be requested.

Intra-hospital

Transfers take place within the hospital setting either as part of the admission process to critical care from the A&E/ward or to enable surgery, specialist procedures or imaging. A similar level of preparation to inter-hospital transfers is required for intra-hospital transfers, although these are commonly of a shorter duration. However, they also expose patients to a more risky environment than that of critical care itself and should never be treated lightly.

Table 1.4 Preparing the critically ill patient for safe transfer

Potential problem	Prior to transfer
Airway management and O_2 requirements	ABG/CXR if necessary
	Intubate if potential to deteriorate
	Chest physio/suction/nebulizers
Cardiovascular support	Insert vascular access (ideally triple lumen CVC) and arterial line (if not already in place)
	Correct electrolyte or pH abnormalities
	Set up drug infusions with back-up syringe and pump for inotropes/vasopressors
	Ensure adequate colloid and crystalloid available
	Insert urinary catheter
	If bleeding, carry cross-matched blood if available or O neg/Gp specific if not
	If necessary, insert nasogastric tube
Patient anxiety	Introduce self and team, briefly discuss reasons for transfer, destination, journey time, and location of critical care unit
Pain control and sedation	Assess level of pain and need for increased analgesia or sedation during journey. Ensure infusions and bolus drugs are available for journey
Pressure damage	Assess pressure areas and if possible avoid further pressure damage to vulnerable areas using pillows/pressure relieving devices
Wounds or fractures	Ensure fractures are stabilized prior to movement of patient. Check wound dressings are patent and unlikely to leak
Equipment or battery failure	Ensure batteries are charged and check function of all equipment prior to moving

The critical care environment

Who benefits from critical care?

Predicting which patient will benefit from critical care is extremely difficult, especially as medical advances extend the boundaries ever further. There is now a broader view of the type of patients likely to benefit from critical care and, in some cases, from earlier admission. Age was often used as a limiting factor until a number of studies showed that outcomes in specific disease states were often similar in matched older and younger age groups.

The single most important factor to consider is whether the patient has the potential for recovery and is not at the end-stage of a terminal disease. Even this is open to debate as many patients in the terminal phase of an illness may gain considerably from palliative symptom control and pain relief in an environment where opiate use is well-managed. However, critical care is a limited resource (constituting only 3.5% of acute hospital beds in the UK). Therefore, admission and discharge guidelines are essential to ensure appropriate use of available beds.

Defining critical care

Critical care offers the patient close observation and specialized treatment unavailable in general ward areas. In particular, organ support for patients with potential or established organ dysfunction is safely delivered in the critical care environment.

Negative aspects of critical care

Critical care can be both physically distressing and potentially hazardous for the patient. It is emotionally and psychologically traumatic for the patient and his/her family. It is a very expensive, labour-intensive resource, with costs per intensive care bed day averaging £1700 in the UK at the time of writing.

In spite of this, patients and their families are keen to access critical care; 90% of patients questioned following a period in critical care would wish to be re-admitted if necessary.

Components of critical care
- Close observation.
- Continuous monitoring of respiratory and cardiovascular function.
- Respiratory support.
- Cardiovascular support.
- Renal support.
- Neurological support.
- Intensive drug regimens.
- Adequate nutrition.
- Prevention of complications associated with critical illness.
- Rehabilitation.
- Psychological support.

Admission guidelines

Admission of critically ill patients should be guided by evaluation of clinical priority and predicted benefit. This should support decisions on individual patient need and allow triage (or transfer) where bed availability is limited.

An identified clinical lead should have responsibility for making these decisions. This is usually the consultant in charge of the critical care unit, although it could also be an experienced senior nurse.

Factors to be considered when evaluating a patient for admission are:
• The potential for reversal of the illness.
• The presence of significant co-morbidity.
• The existence of a stated or written preference against critical care by the patient.

Prioritizing admissions when beds are limited

Where more patients require a critical care bed than there are beds available, a system of prioritization must be used by the identified clinical lead (Table 2.1).

Table 2.1 Priorities for admission to critical care

Priority 1	Critically ill patient, unstable, in need of intensive treatment/monitoring that cannot be provided outside unit
Priority 2	Intensive monitoring is needed and immediate intervention may be necessary. No therapeutic limits are stipulated
Priority 3	The patient is critically ill, but has a reduced likelihood of recovery due to the underlying disease or nature of the acute illness
Priority 4	The patient is either too ill or too well for critical care intervention.
	The patient has made a stated or written decision against admission to critical care

Examples of types of terminal irreversible illness are:
• Unresponsive metastatic cancer.
• Severe irreversible brain damage or persistent vegetative state.
• End-stage cardiac failure where transplant is not an option.

Local policies are based on the above premises, but will also include detail of admission process, individual responsibilities for the lead clinician, the nurse in charge of the unit and bed managers.

Discharge guidelines

Discharge of a patient from critical care is usually dictated by the lead clinician (critical care consultant) and should be considered in the following circumstances:

- The patient is stable and no longer requires active organ support.
- The patient is no longer benefiting from the treatment available and is unlikely to die in the next few hours.
- The patient and/or family wish for transfer to palliative care facilities.
- A persistent vegetative state is confirmed.

Most discharges occur in the first circumstance, and every reasonable care should be taken to ensure discharge occurs at the optimum time and with the optimum outcome for the patient. In the last 3 circumstances, it is inappropriate to continue to care for the patient in the critical care environment; the objective in these situations is to ensure that the patient and family are comfortable and supported during their transfer to other care.

Factors increasing the likelihood of unexpected negative outcomes from discharge

- Discharge after 22.00 hours [relative risk (RR) – 1.7 × normal] or at weekends.
- Premature discharge dictated by need for the bed, rather than patient readiness.
- Poor communication and team working within the critical care unit.
- Poor communication and team working between unit and ward.
- Lack of critical care outreach/follow-up by critical care staff.
- Lack of a step-down facility.
- Initial illness severity (RR – 2.3 × normal).

Managing demand

Demand for critical care beds has increased and it is rare for units to be less than 90% occupied. Although this level of occupancy does not provide sufficient bed availability for all peaks of activity, it is possible to improve patient throughput by several workflow initiatives:

- Regular ward rounds throughout the day to identify and manage patients ready for discharge.
- Flexible use of high dependency and intensive care beds so that they can interchangeably take either level 2 or level 3 patients (see 📖 Models of critical care outreach, p. 3).
- Robust management of post-operative, overnight-stay patients to ensure ward bed availability the following morning.

Organization: design of units

Location within the hospital

Critical care units should be placed close to the source of patients:
- Emergency department.
- Operating theatres.
- Wards.

Other high dependency areas, and interventional radiology and endoscopy suites are also likely sources.

Ideally, critical care units should also be close to the services their patients need:
- Operating theatres.
- Specialist investigation suites.
- Imaging.

There should be close communication with:
- Pathology, for transfer of specimens.
- Transfusion, for blood and blood products.
- Pharmacy, for drugs, nutrition, and fluids.

Unit design

Few critical care units have been designed completely from scratch, and so many are a compromise between the ideal and the possible. However, there is no reason why the important principles of unit design cannot be adhered to.

Size

The suggested optimal number of beds in a critical care unit is 8 or multiples thereof, based on the assumption that this is the number that can be successfully managed by one intensivist and his/her team. Units of less than 8 beds are likely to be more costly to run per bed as there will be fixed costs, such as medical staff, senior nursing staff, and resources.

Arrangement of beds

Most units have a combination of open-plan bays and single cubicles. The recommended ratio currently is 2 cubicles per 10 beds. The rising incidence of multi-resistant organisms is increasing the need for cubicles. The ideal ratio is therefore uncertain, and depends on multiple factors including staffing ratios and case mix.

Arrangement of bed areas

Bed areas must offer unobstructed passage all round the bed and the minimum space requirements for open plan areas is 25 m^2 and 30 m^2 for cubicles.

Air conditioning will allow excellent environmental temperature control. In single cubicles it should support positive and negative pressure air flow control, which can be switched according to patient need for source or protective isolation.

All bed areas should have:
- Direct access to hand-washing facilities without having to cross through another bed area.
- Access to natural daylight and, ideally, an outside view from the windows.
- Electric or manual bed with the ability to raise head/feet, tilt to Trendelenberg (or reverse), adjust height, and with protective bed rails and rigid base/CPR flattening to allow cardiac compressions in emergency.
- Type of mattress according to the patient's risk of pressure damage.
- Provision for manual or computerized charting.
- Safe wall or pendant bracketing for monitoring facilities, suction, and oxygen delivery.
- Adequate electrical access (a minimum of 24 power sockets), half of these should have uninterrupted power supply (UPS).
- Adequate piped gas and vacuum outlets (4 oxygen, 2 air, 2 vacuum).
- Access to bedside emergency equipment, e.g. manual ventilation bags.
- Access to a wipe-clean surface for preparation of drugs, infusions, oral, and eye care, etc.
- Minimal storage space for drugs, infusions, dressings, and disposables.
- Minimal storage space for patient possessions and hygiene requirements.

Important additional facilities
- Emergency equipment (defibrillator, pacer, intubation equipment, drugs, etc.).
- Designated dirty utility area.
- Staff room.
- Visitors' room and interview/quiet room.
- Storage for equipment, drugs, fluids, disposables, linen.
- Reception area, staff base, and office space.

Organization: safety in critical care

Critical care carries potential risks associated with the type of patients and the work carried out. Risks apply to both patients and staff.

Increased risks in critical care

- Increased abundance of electrical equipment used in close proximity to combustible gases and fluids.
- Ubiquitous use of oxygen, which is highly combustible.
- Extra-corporeal blood circuits (haemofiltration) and high numbers of invasive tubes, cannulae, and procedures, exposing staff and patients to infection risk.

Essential safety precautions

- Electrical equipment should be checked before use by medical physics technicians, and regularly maintained thereafter. Any faults should be reported immediately and use discontinued until the fault has been checked and repaired.
- Precautions for oxygen use should be rigorously adhered to. No naked flames, antistatic flooring and footwear, increased atmospheric humidity, care during cardioversion/defibrillation.
- Back-up equipment for use in the event of power, medical gas, or technical failure of ventilators should be available at the bedside. Where possible equipment with battery back-up, such as syringe pumps, should be kept on charge, and used for emergencies or transfers.

Essential back-up equipment at the bedside

- Manual ventilation bag/mask/catheter mount.
- Oxygen cylinder (in safety stand).
- Torch.
- Battery syringe pumps.

Safety visors should be used in addition to gloves and aprons at the bedside when there is a risk of body-fluid splashing or contamination. Local infection control procedures should be rigorously followed (see 📖 Preventing complications: hospital acquired infection, p. 80).

Fire safety

- Evacuation equipment should be kept at every bedside and staff trained in their use.
- All staff should attend fire training on a yearly basis, which should cover alarms, control procedures, such as fire doors and shutters, exit strategies, moving patients, and prioritizing responses.

Organization: staffing

There are five main groups of staff associated with critical care. Their number, seniority, and level of skill will reflect the unit activity and focus.

Essential staff in critical care include:
- Nurses (the largest group).
- Medical staff.
- Allied health professionals, such as physiotherapists, pharmacists, dietitians, medical technicians, and speech and language therapists.
- Administrative staff.
- Cleaning and portering staff.

Nursing, senior medical staff, and administrative staff are usually permanently based in critical care. Allied health professionals are either rotated to cover critical care, attend for ward rounds, etc., or may be permanently based in larger units.

Nursing staff

Critically ill patients require considerable amounts of nursing skill, expertise, and time if they are to avoid secondary complications and recover from their illness.

The level of knowledge and skill required to work as a nurse in critical care is high; most will undertake a post-registration qualification in critical care.

Nursing workload and patient outcome

Although several studies have shown an association between patient outcome and the ratio of trained nurses to patients in critical care, these have all been observational, without risk adjustment for illness severity. Impact on morbidity, e.g. infectious complications, length of weaning, and length of stay has also been demonstrated and may be more representative of the effect of levels of nurse staffing.

There is a minimum number of nurses below which the patient's recovery is put at risk, but it remains difficult to determine this due to the number of confounding factors involved.

At present, the gold standard (in the UK) is considered to be a 1:1 nurse:patient ratio for level 3 patients, with additional back-up from senior nursing staff.

Although most critical care units are ≥ 95% occupied, there are variations in this occupancy level. Employment of nursing staff cannot vary in quite the same way. It is usual to calculate nursing establishment on average occupancy.

Calculating nursing establishment

- If average occupancy is 90% in a 10-bed unit, then the number of nurses employed should be enough to cover 9 beds.
- Using the 5.6 nurses per bed formula, **50.4 nurses** are needed to cover bedside nursing.
- A nurse in charge per shift and a support nurse will require another 11.2 nurses to cover.
- The total number employed would need to be **61.6** WTE nurses.
- WTE = whole time equivalent and constitutes 1 nurse's full time working hours.
- Any part-time nurses are expressed as a fraction of this depending on how many hours they work. Thus, a nurse working 22.5h per week will be working 0.6 WTE (22.5/37.5h).

Nursing roles in critical care

Registered nurses (UK model)
- Novice/nurse in training.
- Experienced nurse (usually with post-registration critical care course).
- Team leader/clinical facilitator/clinical expert.
- Sister/charge nurse.
- Nurse manager/senior nurse lead.
- Nurse consultant.

Non-registered nurses
These require supervision at all times and cannot take responsibility for the patient.
- Nursing students.
- Health care or nursing assistants.

Medical staff
Several studies have shown an association between a full-time intensivist leading the critical care team and improved patient outcome. Better outcomes are also associated with 'closed' units, i.e. primary patient management is by the critical care team, rather than the patient's admitting team. It is recommended that critical care units should have dedicated intensive care specialists leading medical management around the clock.

Medical leadership should encompass:
- Dealing with clinical issues for each patient.
- Management of admission and discharge of patients.
- Education and supervision of junior medical staff.
- Audit/evidence-based practice.
- Resource management (such as staffing, equipment, drug prescribing, etc.).

Competency-based training programmes (e.g. CoBATrICE) have recently been introduced and are likely to be the future of medical assessment and training.

The number of junior medical staff required by a critical care unit is difficult to establish, but depends on unit size, case mix, and external factors, such as legislative working time directives and mandatory training requirements.

Allied health professionals (AHPs)
These groups form an essential part of the team, but require fewer staffing numbers and generally do not provide a 24h service.

Allied health professionals in critical care

- **Dietician:** advice on nutritional needs, feeding methods, special requirements.
- **Occupational therapist:** rehabilitation in long-term critical illness and specific injuries.
- **Pharmacist:** advice on specialist prescribing, dispensing and resource management, drug interactions and dosing, financial aspects of prescribing practices, education.
- **Physiotherapist:** secretion clearance and chest management, maintenance of musculoskeletal function, mobilization, weaning, and rehabilitation.
- **Speech and language therapist:** assistance with/assessment of communication, assessment of swallow function, and risk of aspiration.

Further information

Numata Y, Schulzer M, Van der Wal R, Globerman J, Semeniuk P, Balka E, Fitzgerald JM. (2006) Nurse staffing levels and hospital mortality in critical care settings: literature review and metaanalysis. *J Adv Nurs*, **55**, 435–48.

Organization: team working

Collaborative working is another organizational feature that has particular patient benefit in critical care. It can be described as critical care health-care professionals working positively together, sharing responsibility for solving problems, and making and acting on decisions to deliver the best possible outcome for the patient. The essential focus of this is the multi-professional ward round, although the approach should be the same whenever patient management is being discussed. Historically, the team co-ordinator and lead for decisions is the intensive care consultant, but this may not always be appropriate, particularly in the long-term weaning/rehabilitation patient.

A single multi-professional patient record is essential to support a collaborative approach. This can be facilitated by computerized documentation, but paper records should also be integrated to prevent loss of valuable information.

Standards that support effective critical care team working identified by Manley & Hardy (2006) are:
• Patient-centred care.
• Staff empowerment, support, and development.
• Evidence-based approaches, monitoring, and evaluation.
• Early warning and outreach systems in place.
• Developing effective teams and a culture of shared governance.
• Leadership and culture.
• Flexible service planning.
• Effective communication systems.
• Effective resource use.

Features of effective team working are
• Common goals and values.
• Mutual respect.
• Clarity of roles and job purpose.
• Willingness to address and resolve causes of conflict.
• A range of qualities, skills, and knowledge.
• Commitment to the team.
• Shared achievement of success and responsibility for failure.

Further information

Manley K, Hardy S. (2006) *Improving services to patients through ongoing development of critical care teams.* Department of Health. Available at: http://www.dh.gov.uk/en/Publicationsandstatistics/Publications/PublicationsPolicyAndGuidance/DH_4134609

Stress and burnout in critical care

Critical care is a fast-paced, high technology, and relatively high mortality environment, meeting complex patient needs, which demands enormous concentration, skill, and personal effectiveness. This can make it a high stress area for many staff who may find it difficult to cope.

The main stressors identified by nursing staff are:
- Shortage of staff.
- Issues concerning patients' families.
- Unnecessary prolongation of life.
- Apathetic or incompetent nursing staff.
- Critically unstable patients.
- Inexperienced medical staff.
- Fear of making an error.
- Poor or inadequate communication.
- Slow response of medical staff to emergencies.

When staff are unable to cope or use maladaptive coping mechanisms over a prolonged period of time, symptoms of burnout are evident.

Adaptive or direct coping mechanisms employed include:
- Active problem solving.
- Seeking support from other team members or peers.
- Use of clinical supervision.
- Confrontation of the issue.

Maladaptive or palliative coping mechanisms include:
- Avoidance/detachment.
- Crying.
- Humour.
- Emotional distance.
- Increased alcohol intake or other substance abuse.

Methods of decreasing staff stress which can be employed by critical care units include:
- Providing adequate training for staff.
- Improving communication between individuals and groups of staff.
- Optimizing staffing and supporting staff during times of increased workload.
- Developing an open atmosphere.
- Involving staff in decisions about unit management, e.g. staff rotas, changes to policies, etc.

Burnout

Defined as a syndrome of negative self-concepts, accompanied by loss of concern or caring for patients and their families

Performance: ensuring quality of care

Major iatrogenic adverse events (adverse incidents associated with treatment) occur in at least 1% of the 12 million admissions to UK acute hospitals – approximately 120,000 incidents/year. Adverse incidents in critical care are associated with increased costs (just under £2700/incident) and increased length of stay (0.77 days). Quality and safety initiatives could potentially prevent many of these potentially devastating incidents from occurring. Quality can be examined using three main components of healthcare delivery:

- Structure, e.g. setting, organization, equipment.
- Process, e.g. techniques, staffing, protocols.
- Outcome, e.g. mortality, critical incident rates, infection rates.

Traditionally, most emphasis has been on outcome though processes and structures are probably equally important. This is the premise behind the development of clinical governance for acute healthcare organizations.

Quality initiatives can also be based on reviewing best practice seen and evidenced in some healthcare areas, and transferring it to other organizations.

Clinical governance

Clinical governance is the framework through which healthcare organizations are responsible for continuously improving the quality of their services and safeguarding the standard of care through management of risk and development of clinical excellence.

In order to deliver clinical governance the organization must have:

- Clear lines of accountability and responsibility for the overall quality of clinical care.
- A comprehensive programme of quality improvement systems such as clinical audit, staff development programmes, evidence-based practice, and clinical standards/guidelines.
- Programmes for education and training.
- Clear policies and processes for identifying and managing risk.
- Integrated procedures aimed at all professions to identify and manage poor performance.
- Systems to ensure patient and other user groups' views are sought and responded to.

In critical care this is seen as:

- An identified leader responsible for the critical care area and to whom other professionals answer for their actions. This may be a clinical director or clinical lead for medical staff, and a senior nurse or manager for nursing staff.
- Ongoing audit programmes, regular personal development review with line managers, evidence-based guidelines, and protocols.
- Continuing professional development and education for all staff.
- Critical or adverse incident reporting and review.

- Competency-based assessments and regular (usually yearly) review of performance.
- A formal complaints process, as well as informal comments systems and satisfaction surveys.

Further information

Kaushal R, Bates D, Calvin F. (2007) Costs of adverse events in intensive care units. *Crit Care Med*; **35**, 2479–83.

Clinical audit

Audit has been defined as the systematic and public examination of factors that affect the delivery of good quality care. Both quantitative and qualitative methods of data collection are required.

Ensuring effective clinical audit

- A programme of regular audit meetings, where data can be presented to a multi-professional forum.
- Participation in the collection of a common dataset so that comparison between critical care units can be made.
- Systems in place to ensure recommendations based on audit findings are incorporated into unit practice (also known as loop closure).
- Systems in place to allow dissemination of information to all staff from audit findings.
- An audit lead within the critical care unit to ensure that all the above takes place.

Benchmarking

Nursing benchmarking refers to the comparison of audited processes of care against an agreed optimum standard, based on published evidence and expert opinion (see Fig. 2.1).

Benchmarking allows comparison of nursing care delivery between critical care units through these agreed standards.

Standards of care

A standard is a professionally agreed level of performance appropriate to the population addressed. It must be both desirable and achievable.

Traditional components of standards of care have been based on:
- Structure of care delivery (staffing numbers, facilities, environment, etc.).
- Process of care delivery (methods of care delivery, attitudes to care, collaboration between groups of carers, etc.).
- Outcome of care delivery (discharge home from hospital, rates of infection, temporary or permanent levels of dysfunction, etc).

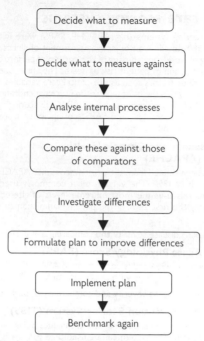

Fig. 2.1 The benchmarking process

Critical care scoring systems

Critical care scoring systems (e.g. APACHE, SAPS) were initially developed in the 1980s to allow an objective assessment of illness severity, an understanding of workload, a means of comparison of performance and, in some cases, prediction of patient risk of death. They have been criticized for failing to include factors such as pre-critical care variables, and organizational variables within the unit, such as the nurse:patient ratio. However, they continue to be commonly used, with APACHE scoring systems predominating in the US and UK, and SAPS scoring systems predominating across most of mainland Europe.

Acute Physiology and Chronic Health Evaluation (APACHE)

APACHE has been refined from the original score into APACHE II in 1985 and APACHE III in 1990. The version most commonly used in the UK is APACHE II. This uses the most extreme levels of altered physiology recorded during the first 24 h of the patient's admission to critical care (Table 2.2).

Used for indexing disease severity and comparing unit performance.

Simplified Acute Physiology Score (SAPS)

SAPS was devised in 1984 and is very similar to APACHE. It has also been refined, most recently in 2006 with publication of SAPS III (Table 2.3).

Used for indexing disease severity and comparing unit performance.

Therapeutic Intervention Scoring System (TISS)

TISS attaches a score to procedures and techniques being carried out on an individual patient. The system can be used on a daily basis to measure workload and, in some cases, to cost the patient's use of resources. It has also been used to estimate the likelihood of re-admission of patients about to be discharged from critical care.

Used for measuring workload, risk of re-admission to ICU, and costing.

Sequential Organ Failure Assessment (SOFA)

This is one of several systems designed to enable daily scoring of patient severity to take place [others include the Riyadh Intensive Care Programme (RIP) and the Multiple Organ Dysfunction Score]. SOFA incorporates a combination of biochemical and physiological markers with organ support interventions in order to reflect the level of critical illness and the degree of organ support required:

- PaO_2:FiO_2 ratio (with degree of ventilatory support).
- Creatinine or urine output.
- Bilirubin.
- Mean arterial pressure (with dosage of inotropes used).
- Platelet count.
- Glasgow Coma Score.

Table 2.2 Acute Physiology and Chronic Health Evaluation II Score

Variable	+4	+3	+2	+1	0	+1	+2	+3	+4
Temperature (rectal) (°C)	≥41	39–40.9		38.2–38.9	36–38.4	34–35.9	32–33.9	30–31.9	≤29.9
Mean BP (mmHg)	≥160	130–159	110–129		70–109		50–69		≤49
Heart rate (bpm)	≥180	140–179	110–139		70–109		55–69	40–54	≤39
Respiration rate (per min)	≥50	35–49		25–34	12–24	10–11	6–9		≤5
If FiO2 ≥0.5: A–aDO2 (mmHg)	≥500	350–499	200–349		<200				
If FiO2 <0.5: PO2 (mmHg)					>70	61–70		55–60	≤55
Arterial pH	≥7.7	7.6–7.69		7.5–7.59	7.33–7.49		7.25–7.32	7.15–7.24	≤7.15
Serum Na (mmol/l)	≥180	160–179	155–159	150–154	130–149		120–129	111–119	≤110
Serum K (mmol/l)	≥7	6–6.9		5.5–5.9	3.5–5.4	3–3.4	2.5–2.9		<2.5
Serum creatinine (μmol/l), double if acute renal failure	≥300	171–299	121–170		50–120		<50		
Haematocrit (%)	≥60		50–59.9	46–49.9	30–45.9		20–29.9		<20
Leucocytes (per mm³)	≥40		20–39.9	15–19.9	3–14.9		1–2.9		<1

Neurological = Glasgow Coma Score.

Age points:

Years	≤44	45–54	55–64	65–74	≤75
Points	0	2	3	5	6

Chronic health points: 2 points for elective post-operative admission or 5 points if emergency operation or non-operative admission, if patient has either cirrhosis, heart failure (NYHA Grade 4), respiratory failure, dialysis-dependent renal disease, or is immunocompromised.

Table 2.3 Simplified Acute Physiology Score

Age	<40 (0 points); 40–59 (7); 60–69 (12); 70–74 (15); 75–79 (16); ≥80 (18)
Heart rate (bpm)	<40 (11); 40–69 (2); 70–119 (0); 120–159 (4); ≥160 (7)
Systolic BP (mmHg)	<70 (13); 70–99 (5); 100–199 (0); ≥200 (2)
Body temp	
(°C)	<39 (0); ≥39 (3)
PaO$_2$/F1O$_2$ (kPa) (only if ventilated or CPAP)	<13.3 (11); 13.3–26.5 (9); ≥26.6 (6)
Urine output (l/day)	<0.5 (11); 0.5–0.999 (4); ≥1(0)
Serum urea (mmol/l)	<10 (0); 10–29.9 (6); ≥30 (10)
White blood count/mm^3	<1(12); 1–19.9 (0); ≥20 (3)
Serum potassium (mmol/l)	<3 (3); 3–4.9 (0); ≥ 5 (3)
Serum sodium (mmol/l)	<125 (5); 125–144 (0); ≥ 145 (1)
Serum bicarbonate (mmol/l)	<15 (6); 15–19 (3); ≥20 (0)
Serum bilirubin (µmol/l)	(<68.4 (0); 68.4–102.5 (4); ≥ 102.6 (9)
Glasgow Coma Score	<6 (26); 6–8 (13); 9–10 (7); 11–13 (5); 14–15(0)
Chronic disease, type of admission	Metastatic cancer (9); haematological malignancy (10), AIDS (17)

Scheduled surgical (0); medical (6); unscheduled surgical (8).

Infection and the critical care environment

Hospital acquired infection (HAI) is a huge problem with approximately 9% of hospital patients contracting HAI each year. The cost to the UK health service is estimated at more than £1 billion per year and it is thought to cause up to 5000 deaths/year. Critically ill patients are highly vulnerable to infection and the rate of HAI rises to 25% in these patients. Their immune systems are weakened by the stress of critical illness and many of the features of their care, e.g. cannulae, tubes, and drains, provide portals of entry for invading organisms.

Unit layout and design

- Units must have sufficient single rooms to allow appropriate isolation of patients either (a) at increased risk of infection (neutropenic, immunocompromised) or (b) who are colonized, and thus able to transmit resistant or highly infectious organisms to other patients (droplet spread/multi-resistant organisms, e.g. MRSA).
- All single rooms should be under negative pressure air flow (or be able to switch from positive to negative pressure) with HEPA (high efficiency particulate air) filters and closed doors, as well as a minimum of 6 air changes per hour.
- Hand-washing basins must be placed at every bed space or at a minimum of 1 hand basin to 2 beds.
- Distinct sluice areas should be in close proximity to allow disposal of body fluids, etc.
- Bed areas must be a minimum of 25m^2 for open plan and 30 m^2 for cubicles.

Factors affecting nosocomial infection rates in intensive care

- Architecture (open bays versus single rooms).
- Environment (cleaning and ergonomics).
- Hand hygiene.
- Universal precautions.
- Staffing levels.
- Patient population.
- Antibiotic prescribing practice.
- Invasive monitoring and procedures.
- Essential nursing care methods.

Hand washing and disinfection

Poor hand hygiene is the most important and persistent source of cross-infection in patients. Opportunities (indications) for hand hygiene occur between 5 and 80 times/h for each member of staff caring for a critically ill patient. Hand-washing is time-consuming (requiring approx 2min in total) and in spite of the use of gel-based alcohol products to supplement hand washing, staff compliance can be poor at between 15 and 50%.

Reasons for poor compliance are complex and there are many other factors that impact:

Negative factors impacting on hand hygiene compliance

- Increased workload and bed occupancy.
- Increased patient acuity and other priorities of care.
- Poor staffing levels.
- Poor availability of hand washing facilities (hand basins, soap dispensers, towels).
- Lack of availability of alcohol-based hand rubs.
- Poor training and policing of hand hygiene.
- Lack of senior role models and emphasis on hand hygiene.

Infection control measures

Each unit must develop policies that cover standard precautions, cleaning schedules, antibiotic prescribing practice, evidence-based preventive measures for specific risks, such as ventilator associated pneumonia. Standard precautions should apply to all patients (see Table 2.4).

Table 2.4 Standard infection control precautions

Hand hygiene	After contact with body fluids, after removing gloves, between patient contacts
Gloves	For anticipated contact with body fluids, mucous membranes, non-intact skin
Masks/eye protection/face shield	To protect mucous membranes during procedures likely to splash or spray body fluids
Gowns/aprons	To protect clothing/skin during procedures likely to splash or spray body fluids
Sharp object handling	No recapping of needles, use of puncture resistant sharps containers
Patient care equipment handling	Discard of single use items, appropriate cleaning of re-usable items, avoidance of contamination from used equipment

Further information

Pittet D, Hugonnet S, Harbarth S, et al. (2000) Effectiveness of a hospital-wide programme to improve compliance with hand hygiene. *Lancet*, **356**, 1307–12.

The patient in the critical care environment

Stress: the physiological response

Although almost all patients experience stress in the critical care environment, their ability to deal with it will alter according to their physical and psychological make-up. Whatever the stressor, whether physical or psychological, the patient will experience the same physiological processes of response. This has been termed the general adaptation syndrome.

Definition of stress

Stress occurs when the demands made of an individual (either physically or psychologically) exceed the personal, physical, and social resources the individual is able to mobilize in order to cope.

Definition of a stressor

A stimulus (physical or psychological) that is perceived as threatening by the individual.

Physiological response to stress

The response to a perceived physical stressor, such as the organ dysfunction associated with critical illness, involves three major activation streams (see Table 3.1).
- The hypothalamic-pituitary-adrenal (HPA) axis.
- The autonomic nervous system response.
- The somatotropic axis.

The hypothalamus releases growth hormone-releasing hormone (GHRH). Growth hormone acts on insulin–like growth factor (IGF-1), which stimulates cell-division and growth.

Response to a psychological stressor is mediated through the limbic system (a rim of cortical tissue, the hippocampus, the amygdala, and the hypothalamus). These structures are associated with emotions and memory. The HPA and autonomic response are then as for a physical stress.

The physiological effects of stress enhance the body's capability to resist a stressor in the acute situation.

They are detrimental in the chronic situation leading to muscle wasting, fatigue, vulnerability to infection, poor tissue healing, and ongoing fluid retention/displacement.

Table 3.1 Physiological effects of stress

Physiological pathway	Physiological effect
HPA	Increased tissue utilization of glucose
	Protein and fat catabolism and mobilization
	Gluconeogenesis
	Adrenaline-linked anti-inflammatory effect
	Increased extracellular fluid volume through sodium and water re-absorption
	General CNS effect increases rate of learning
	Inhibition of granulation tissue
Autonomic nervous system	Increased heart rate and blood pressure
	Increased oxygen consumption and metabolic rate
	Redistribution of blood flow from non-essential to essential
	Increased glycogen breakdown and tissue glucose uptake
	Increased gut motility, constriction of GI, and bladder sphincters
Somatotrophic system	Increased growth hormone release and enhancement of immune function

Stressors in critical care

The major perceived stressors for patients in critical care are:
• Fear and anxiety.
• Pain.
• Dyspnoea.
• Sleep deprivation.

These perceptions are representative of only half of patients as up to 48% of patients claim to have no memory of their experience in critical care and are unable to report stressors.

Up to a quarter of patients show evidence of anxiety whilst in critical care. These stressors are over and above the ongoing stress of critical illness itself and increase the pre-existing physiological stress response.

The inability to communicate is recognized as being a compounding factor in many of the perceived stressors, particularly for intubated or tracheotomized patients.

Elements likely to increase patient stress are:
• Loss of autonomy and control (powerlessness).
• Lack of information.
• Lack of contact with loved ones.
• Increased meaningless environmental noise and light.
• Social isolation.

The critical care nurse is responsible for ameliorating the effects of these additional stressors where possible. Being alert to the presence of the stressors and having an awareness of their impact as well as utilizing potential interventions, such as informing the patient, and reassuring and using therapeutic touch, are essential.

High meaningless noise levels at the bedside can cause disorientation and sleep deprivation. Patients have mentioned particular contributors to this include:
• Radios played at high volume.
• Nurses who speak unnecessarily loudly when talking to patients.
• Staff chatter that does not include the patient.

Further information

Thomas L. (2003) Clinical management of stressors perceived by patients on mechanical ventilation. *AACN Clin Iss*, **14**, 73–81.

Anxiety and fear

This is one of the most common non-physical stressors, but only half of the patients who show signs of anxiety and depression in critical care are identified and treated by the staff.

Anxiety

Anxiety is defined as a state of disequilibrium or tension caused by apprehension of a potential non-specific threat. It is a natural response to the knowledge of critical illness and potential closeness of death associated with admission to critical care.

Assessment of the level of anxiety depends almost wholly on subjective judgement as use of complex tools, such as the Hospital Anxiety and Depression Score (HADS) is commonly beyond critically ill patients.

Recent development of a facial expression scale for judging anxiety has yet to be validated fully, but may help to identify anxiety in the critically ill.

Interventions to reduce anxiety

Nursing interventions which may help are listed in Table 3.2.

Fear

Fear is defined as a state of distress and apprehension causing sympathetic arousal.

The physiological response invoked by fear reflects the levels of sympathetic stimulation, and is mediated by adrenaline (epinephrine) and noradrenaline (norepinephrine) release. Symptoms include:

- Increased heart rate and blood pressure.
- Dilated pupils.
- Dry mouth.
- Peripheral and splanchnic vasoconstriction.
- Sweating.

The patient's behavioural response can be affected by background, culture and social conditioning.

Table 3.2 Coping mechanisms for anxiety

Patient mechanisms	Nursing interventions to enhance
Denial	Encouragement to verbalize fears. Recognition of the need to deny
Rationalization	Give appropriately worded and timed information
Substituting positive thoughts for negative ones	Positive feedback for coping techniques
Retention of control of environment, timing of care, etc. (this is often via the nurse who must facilitate this)	Facilitation of patient retention of control
Additional nursing interventions	
Use of empathetic and therapeutic touch	Access to spiritual counselling as needed
Support unrestricted family visiting	Amelioration of environmental stressors, e.g. noise from alarms, etc.
Offer relaxation and/or meditation techniques	Appropriate background music, e.g. slow, flowing rhythms
Speak calmly and slowly using warm tones	If necessary, administration of anxiolytics, e.g. lorazepam
Ensure pain relief is adequate	Nursing presence, attentiveness, and reassurance
Biofeedback, e.g. patient view of heart rate on monitor	

Pain

Pain is a complex phenomenon involving social, cultural, emotional, psychological, and physiological components.

It is aggravated by anxiety and fear, and compounded in the critically ill by difficulty in communicating, and the limiting effect of analgesia on blood pressure or respiratory rate that may be life-threatening.

Relief of pain is important in order to:
- Improve patient comfort, and relieve stress and anxiety.
- Reduce the physiological stress response (see 📖 Stress: the physiological response, p. 42), which otherwise can lead to increased metabolic rate and oxygen requirements, as well as water/sodium retention.
- Reduce immobility and reluctance to breathe deeply, which increases risk of chest infections and DVTs.

Patient recollections show that their greatest worries in critical care were pain and the inability to lie comfortably. Pain was also the leading cause of sleeplessness.

Perception of pain
- Noxious stimuli are generated by the release of products from tissue damage, which bind to nerve receptors initiating impulse generation in the nociceptive fibres.
- Thalamic and forebrain level perception, i.e. there is conscious awareness of the pain, as well as spinal reflex causing rapid withdrawal to avoid the stimulus.
- Sensation of pain occurs at similar intensity of stimulus in different individuals, but reaction to the sensation is individually varied. Factors such as cultural background, previous experience of pain, mood, site, and pathology of injury are part of this variation.
- Endorphin release will modulate perception of pain and occurs in situations, such as fear, stress, restraint, elevated blood pressure, and hypoglycaemia.

Gate control theory
Pain stimuli transmitted by small-diameter nerve fibres can be inhibited by large-diameter nerve fibres carrying innocuous information. This is due to competition between the different signals from the affected area passing to the thalamus that modulates the pain sensation. This theory is used to explain the pain-relieving effects of rubbing, transcutaneous electrical nerve stimulation (TENS) and massage that preferentially stimulate large-diameter nerve fibres.

Assessing pain in critical care
Nurses in critical care frequently underestimate the patient's level of pain and in 40% of cases do not re-assess patient's pain levels after administering analgesia. In addition, patients report that analgesia does not always bring total relief. As a result, pain management is often less than optimal.

Assessment is strongly affected by:
- The patient's ability to communicate.
- Ventilatory status.

Use of a visual analogue (commonly a 1–10 linear scale) or pain chart is essential to allow patients to clearly express the level of pain they experience and to judge the effectiveness of interventions.

Pain levels must be re-evaluated after administration of analgesia.

Further reading

McKinley S, Coote K, Stein-Parbury J. (2003) Development and testing of a faces scale for the assessment of anxiety in critically ill patients. *J Adv Nurs* **41**, 73–9.
Puntillo K, Stannard D, Miaskowski C. (2002) Use of a pain assessment and intervention notation (P.A.I.N) tool in critical care nursing practice: nurses evaluations. *Heart Lung* **31**, 303–14.

Management of pain

Different management techniques will be appropriate depending on the level of pain.

Non-pharmacological methods of pain management

- **Repositioning of the patient to reduce discomfort:** joint stiffness and pressure-related pain, firm support for flaccid limbs to maintain neutral position, etc.
- **Massage:** foot massage and other techniques.
- **Relaxation techniques:** slow, deep-breathing, guided visual imagery.
- **Localized warmth:** relief of aches and muscular spasm.
- **Localized cooling:** particularly for burn pain.
- **Effective communication and provision of information** to relieve underlying fear/anxiety.
- **TENS:** more successful in reducing analgesic requirements than total alleviation.

Pharmacological methods of pain management

Opioids are the mainstay of analgesia in critical care, delivery of which is mostly managed by nurses. Delivery is usually intravenous and commonly by infusion to ensure consistent analgesia. Other methods of delivery include PCA (in the conscious patient), intramuscular, and oral routes. Dose depends on age, weight, haemodynamic status, renal and hepatic function, as well as clinical effect (Table 3.3).

Paracetamol or NSAIDs (non-steroidal anti-inflammatory drugs) can be used for less severe pain or in addition to opioids as a background to reduce requirements.

NSAIDs have a number of serious side effects including GI bleeding (due to increased likelihood of gastric ulceration), general bleeding (due to platelet inhibition), renal impairment, and sodium retention, and should be used with caution (see Table 3.4).

Patient-controlled analgesia

PCAs (patient-controlled analgesia) have the enormous advantage of allowing the patient to control their own pain management, rather than wait for the nurse. This reduces dose requirements by avoiding excessive levels of pain (the patient doesn't have to wait for the nurse to deliver the dose) and reduces the likelihood of overdose as a drowsy patient will not self-administer ongoing doses of pain relief.

Assessment of the number of demands for analgesia a patient makes against the number of delivered doses allows effectiveness of the regimen to be evaluated.

Table 3.3 Doses for opioid analgesia: intravenous route

Opiate	Type	Dose - bolus	Dose - infusion
Morphine	Natural opiate	0.1–0.2mg/kg	0.05–0.07mg/kg/h
Diamorphine	Semi-synthetic opiate	0.05–0.1mg/kg	0.03–0.06mg/kg/h
Fentanyl	Synthetic opiate	5–7.5µg/kg	5–20µg/kg/h
Alfentanil	Synthetic opiate	15–30µg/kg	20–120µg/kg/h
Remifentanil	Synthetic opiate	1µg/kg	0.05–2µg/kg/h
Pethidine	Synthetic opiate	0.5mg/kg	0.1–0.3mg/kg/h

Table 3.4 Effect and side-effects of opioids

	Use	Side effects	Notes
Morphine	A, S, Rd, V	$\downarrow$BP, nausea, H_2 release, Rd, $\downarrow$CNS, $\downarrow$gut motility, $\uparrow$muscular tone	Poor GI absorption, accumulation in renal failure
			Avoid in asthmatics
Diamorphine	A, S, Rd, V	$\downarrow$BP, nausea, H_2 release, Rd, $\downarrow$CNS, $\downarrow$gut motility, $\uparrow$muscular tone	Poor GI absorption, accumulation in renal failure
			Avoid in asthmatics
Fentanyl	A, Rd, V	$\downarrow$BP, nausea, Rd, $\downarrow$gut motility, $\uparrow$muscular tone	Muscular rigidity seen with high doses
Alfentanil	A, Rd, V	$\downarrow$BP, nausea, Rd, $\downarrow$gut motility, $\uparrow$muscular tone	Muscular rigidity seen with high doses
Remifentanil	A, Rd, V	$\downarrow$BP, nausea, Rd, $\downarrow$gut motility, $\uparrow$muscular tone	Ultra-short acting may cause re-bound pain if stopped suddenly
Pethidine	A, S, Rd,	$\downarrow$BP, nausea, Rd, $\downarrow$gut motility, $\uparrow$muscular tone, cardiac depression	Respiratory depression occurs in spite of maintained respiratory rate
			May cause seizures with accumulation

A = analgesia, Rd = respiratory depression, S = sedative, V = vasodilatation in heart failure.

Delirium

Delirium is defined as an acute change or fluctuation in the course of a patient's mental status, including inattention, disorganized thinking, or an altered level of consciousness. However, it is commonly under-diagnosed in critical care.

It has 4 essential elements:
• Disordered attention or arousal.
• Cognitive dysfunction.
• Acute development of signs and symptoms (hrs/days).
• Medical, rather than psychiatric cause.

Incidence rates in critical care have been reported as between 19 and 87% depending on study population and methods used to identify delirium.

Delirium in the critically ill is associated with increased lengths of stay and morbidity, such as unplanned extubation. There are a number of risk factors predisposing to delirium (Table 3.5).

Table 3.5 Risk factors pre-disposing to delirium

In ICU patients generally	In elderly ICU patients	In hospital patients
Benzodiazepine use	Raised urea-creatinine ratio	Malnutrition
Morphine	Prior history of depression, cognitive impairment or dementia	>3 drugs added during hospital stay
Epidural	Visual/hearing impairment	Urinary catheter
History of hypertension	Severe illness	Iatrogenic complications
History of smoking		Use of physical restraint
Raised bilirubin level		
Age >70 years		

There are 2 sub-types of delirium:
• **Hypoactive:** the patient is withdrawn, lethargic, and apathetic, occasionally completely unresponsive. This type is less commonly identified by ICU staff.
• **Hyperactive:** the patient exhibits extreme levels of agitation and emotional lability, they may refuse care, or exhibit other forms of disruptive behaviour, such as shouting, violence, self-removal of cannulae and catheters, and attempting to leave the ICU.

Management of delirium

Assessment and identification of delirium in the critically ill should be carried out using a validated tool, such as the CAM-ICU (confusion assessment method for the ICU).

- Early identification and correction of precipitating factors, such as metabolic abnormalities, infection, and renal impairment.
- Ensure alcohol, benzodiazepine, or opiate withdrawal are treated to alleviate withdrawal.
- Haloperidol can be used to treat symptoms: the recommended starting dose is 5mg (po) or 2.5–5mg slowly iv every 12h. Increasing up to a maximum of 20mg/day.

Further information

Ely EW, Margolin R, Francis J, et al. (2001) Evaluation of delirium in critically ill patients: validation of the confusion assessment method for the intensive care unit (CAM-ICU). *Crit Care Med*, **29**, 1370–9.

Sedation

In order to facilitate mechanical ventilation most patients require some form of sedation at least initially. The goals of sedation in the critically ill patient are:
- Alleviation of anxiety.
- Relief of discomfort.
- Promotion of sleep.
- Facilitation of procedures/treatment.
- Obtundation of detrimental physiological responses, e.g. increased oxygen requirements, increased intra-cranial pressure, etc.

Over-sedation can cause increased ventilator days and LOS, as well as other problems, such as hypotension, gastrointestinal stasis, etc.

Assessment of sedation level

Monitoring of sedation level using an assessment tool such as the UCL Hospitals Sedation Score (Table 3.7) or the Richmond Agitation Sedation Scale (RASS) is essential (Table 3.6). The target for most nurses should be a calm patient who is easily aroused and who maintains a diurnal rhythm that is normal for them. Specific circumstances may require deeper sedation. Examples of these include facilitation of 'difficult to tolerate' modes of ventilation like inverse ratio ventilation or hypoxaemia on maximal oxygen therapy.

The patient's sedation target should be reviewed on a daily basis. Some critical care units employ a daily sedation break in order to assess the patient's underlying levels of sedation.

Sedative drug doses should be adjusted and infusion rates titrated according to ongoing hourly monitoring to maintain the level of sedation at target.

Bispectral index monitoring (BIS™)

Bispectral index monitoring is an objective method of assessing awareness using a processed signal electroencephalogram (EEG). This is measured on a numeric scale of 1–100, where 0 is a flat line EEG and 100 is fully awake. Anaesthesia is achieved at BIS levels below 50. The sedation level suggested for patients in critical care is 60–80, although this has not been validated.

Table 3.6 The Richmond Agitation-Sedation Score (RASS)

Score	Term	Description
+4	Combative	Overtly combative, violent, danger to staff
+3	Very agitated	Pulls or removes tubes or catheters; aggressive
+2	Agitated	Frequent non-purposeful moves, fights ventilator
+1	Restless	Anxious, but moves. Not aggressive or vigorous
0	Alert and calm	
−1	Drowsy	Not fully alert, but sustained awakening; eye opening/eye contact to voice (>10s)
−2	Light sedation	Briefly awake with eye contact to voice (<10s)
−3	Moderate sedation	Movement or eye opening to voice, but no eye contact
−4	Deep sedation	No response to voice, but movement or eye opening to physical stimulation
−5	Unrousable	No response to voice or physical stimulation

Procedure for RASS assessment

Observe patient
- Patient is alert, restless or agitated   score +1 to +4

If not alert, state patient's name and ask to open eyes and look at speaker
- Patient awakens with sustained eye opening/contact   score −1
- Patient awakens with unsustained eye opening/contact   score −2
- Patient moves in response to voice, but no eye contact   score −3

If no response to verbal stimulation, physically stimulate patient by shaking shoulder/rubbing sternum
- Patient makes any response to physical stimulation   score −4
- Patient makes no response to any stimulation   score −5

Table 3.7 UCL Hospitals Sedation Score. Frequent objective assessment of patient behaviour is carried out and scored using the descriptors below

Behaviour	Score
Agitated and restless	+3
Awake and uncomfortable	+2
Aware, but calm	+1
Aroused by voice, but calm	0
Roused by movement	−1
Roused by painful or noxious stimuli	−2
Unrousable	−3
Natural sleep	A

Further information

Sessler CN, Gosnell MS, Grap MJ, et al. (2002) The Richmond agitation–sedation scale validity and reliability in adult intensive care unit patients. *Am J Resp Crit Care Med*, **166**, 1338–44.

Sedative drugs

The ideal sedative drug has rapid onset, does not accumulate, and is easily titratable with a short duration and no unwanted effects. Unfortunately, a drug with all these qualities is not yet available and current types of sedation all have some unwanted effects.

Types of sedative drugs

Benzodiazepines: e.g. diazepam, lorazepam, midazolam

Sedatives with anxiolytic and amnesiac effect

These are mainly used intravenously and in combination with analgesia:

- **Propofol:** developed as an anaesthetic agent, it is now used in lower doses for short-term sedative infusions (48–72h). It has vasodilator and negative inotropic properties so should be used with caution where hypovolaemia has not been fully corrected or cardiac function is poor.
- **Ketamine:** an anaesthetic agent that is also a powerful analgesic. It is associated with good airway maintenance, spontaneous respiration, bronchodilation, and cardiovascular stimulation. Drawbacks are hypertension and tachycardia, as well as hallucinations and psychotic episodes, which usually require concurrent benzodiazepines to invoke amnesia.
- **Inhalational agents:** e.g. isoflurane, desflurane, sevoflurane. Anaesthetic agents used for short-term sedation in critically ill patients. Cumulative effects may be a problem. The delivery system requires adapted ventilator circuits and as the gas is exhaled virtually unchanged, scavenging systems are essential.
- **Antipsychotics:** e.g. chlorpromazine, haloperidol. Caution is necessary as arrhythmias and extrapyramidal disorders are associated with their use.
- **α_2 Agonists:** e.g. dexmedetomidine, clonidine. Act as synergistic analgesics with opiates, but cause minimal respiratory depression and the patient is easily rousable. Drawbacks are hypotension and bradycardia. The patient will experience a dry mouth.

Table 3.8 Sedative drugs and doses

Drug	Bolus dose	Infusion	Adverse effects
Diazepam	0.05–0.15 mg/kg	Not recommended	Rd, ↓BP,
Lorazepam	1 mg PRN		
Midazolam	50 µg/kg	10–50 µg/kg/h	ATN, LA at ↑doses
Propofol	0.5–2 mg/kg	1–3 mg/kg/h	Rd, ↓BP
Dexmedetomidine		*0.2–0.7 µg/kg/h	↓BP
Ketamine	1–2 mg/kg added doses of 0.5 mg/kg	5–25 µg/kg/h	↑BP, ↑HR, hallucinations, psychosis

*Dexmedetomidine requires a loading dose: 1.0 µg/kg over 10 min.

Please note doses are a guide and may need to be altered widely according to individual patient circumstance.

Clonidine has also been used for sedation.

Rd = respiratory depression, BP = blood pressure, HR = heart rate, ATN = acute tubular necrosis, LA = lactic acidosis.

Communication

Normal communication is disrupted in the critically ill patient by sedative and opiate drugs, endotracheal tubes, ventilation, fluctuating consciousness, anxiety, and fear.

In spite of this, it is likely that patients hear and understand far more than their level of awareness would lead us to assume. It is essential that nurses communicate as much information to their patients as they can and that they remember that other conversations may be overheard by the patient.

Inability to talk is cited by critical care survivors as one of the key stressors, and the use of effective technological support and communication strategies is vital.

Insufficient communication can invoke frustration, isolation, anxiety, and fear in the patient, particularly when survival may not be possible.

Communication between the multidisciplinary team members is also vital so that communication barriers and strategies to deal with them are passed on.

Strategies to facilitate communication with the patient

- Assess the patient for potential barriers to communication,
  e.g. deafness, blindness, language barriers.
- Use eye contact and give the patient full attention during any communication.
- Identify and use appropriate communication aids (see 📖 p. 61).
- Develop simple agreed gestures or movements depending on the patient's ability to move (blinking, eye brow raising, nods, etc.), to denote simple responses.
- Orientate to time and place, and ensure the patient always knows who is speaking to them.
- Use touch as a means of communicating empathy and attention.
- Use closed questions for patients who can only nod or gesture.
- Use open questions for patients who can speak or communicate more fully in other ways, such as in written or electronic formats.
- Where language barriers exist, obtain translations of lists of common words, and involve translators and the family in enhancing communication.

Communication aids

- Pen/pencil and paper.
- Magic slates.
- Alphabet boards.
- Symbol boards/book.
- Lip-reading.
- Passy-Muir valve (one-way valve that, when attached to a fenestrated, cuff-down tracheostomy tube, allows the patient to speak).
- Electronic communication devices, such as light writer or laptop computer.
- Possum portascan (device that can be operated using the lips or other movement).

Further information

Happ M, Tuite P, Dobbin K. (2004) Communication ability, method and content among non-speaking, nonsurviving patients treated with mechanical ventilation in the intensive care unit. *Am J Crit Care* **13**, 210–20.

Patak L, Gawlinski A, Fung N, et al. (2006) Communication boards in critical care: patients' views. *Appl Nurs Res* **19**, 182–90.

Patient perceptions of critical care

The narratives of patients who have experienced critical care can give a good understanding of the effect of the environment on patients.

Although up to 60% of patients do not have any recollection of their stay in the critical care unit, those who do outline the following problems.

Discomfort due to the endotracheal tube

Oral tubes are uncomfortable, particularly during turning or movement of the patient. They cause a continuous gagging sensation and stimulation of salivary production.

Nasal tubes are thought to be less uncomfortable, although they can be traumatic to insert and discomfort is associated with this trauma.

Nursing interventions
- Support the tube during movement or turning.
- Use of commercial tube holders, rather than tape to secure the tube.
- Inspect the mouth, lips, ears, and back of head daily for evidence of pressure damage from tube holder.
- Regular 2–4h mouth care is vital.

Fear of disconnection from the ventilator

Patients can develop considerable psychological, as well as physical dependence on the ventilator. They describe a disconnection experience as terrifying and feel it goes on interminably. The level of fear may be associated with the degree of confidence in the staff.

Hearing ventilator alarms is also frightening as the patient cannot identify whether it comes from their own ventilator or other patients.

Nursing interventions
- Develop the patient's trust and confidence.
- Only disconnect after full explanation and rationale for the need for disconnection.
- Cancel ventilator alarms as quickly as possible, fix the problem, explain the reason for them, and any interventions needed to the patient.

The importance of touch

Patients describe the comfort of caring human touch and of hand-holding in particular. This is felt to be an important indicator of caring and is distinguished by patients from procedural touch (touch associated with a required intervention). Touch may be the only non-threatening sensation the patient is aware of when sedated and ventilated. The risks of cross-infection mean that many nursing interventions must be carried out using gloves, limiting the opportunity for non-procedural touch. However, comforting touch is possible without gloves providing that full hand hygiene measures are adhered to.

Nursing interventions
- Use touch during communication, and to support the patient during painful or difficult interventions.
- Encourage the patient's families to touch and hold them when it is appropriate to do so.

Other patient perceptions discussed elsewhere

- **Communication**: 📖 p. 60.
- **Pain**: 📖 p. 48.
- **Dreams and hallucination**: 📖 p. 542.
- **Sensory deprivation and temporal disorientation**: 📖 p. 64.
- **Staff noise/talking at the bedside**: 📖 p. 44.
- **Transition to the ward**: 📖 p. 20.

Further information

Rotondi A, Chelluri L, Sirio C, et al. (2002) Patients' recollections of stressful experiences while receiving prolonged mechanical ventilation in an intensive care unit. *Crit Care Med*, **30**, 746–52.

Sensory imbalance and temporal disorientation

Sensory imbalance occurs when the levels of stimulation are too great or too minimal to be meaningful or recognizable to the patient. Interpretation of stimuli is confounded by numerous other factors, such as drugs, hypoxia, and critical illness.

Five main types of sensory alteration in the critically ill have been identified:
• Reduction in the amount and variety of stimuli.
• Monotony of indistinct meaningless stimuli.
• Physical or social isolation.
• Confinement, immobilization, or restriction of movement.
• Increased sensory input

Pre-disposing factors in the critically ill

• Alcohol/drug addiction.
• Previous cerebral damage.
• Psychological illness.
• Chronic illness.
• Increasing age.
• Previous episodes of delirium.
• Previous psychological stressors.

Contributory environmental factors

Most contributory factors are open to modification by staff.

High noise levels

High noise levels are common within the critical care unit. Equipment alarms, buzzers, telephones, and staff and family conversation all contribute.

Decibel levels as high as 80dB with a constant level of 50dB have been recorded. Talking amongst staff contributed the highest recorded decibel level.

Unfamiliar/incomprehensible sounds

Patients are unable to interpret many of the sounds heard in critical care. These sounds are a meaningless background, which may result in the bizarre dreams or illusions that many patients suffer as their brain struggles to interpret what is happening.

High and/or constant levels of artificial light

Patients often report an inability to distinguish the passage of time. This is compounded by a lack of exposure to natural light, and the loss of an obvious difference in light levels between day and night.

Nursing interventions

Day–night phasing

- Long-term patients should have access to natural light and windows.
- Phase the patient's routine to reflect day and night.
- Ensure the patient is settled for the night, e.g. analgesia, comfortable positioning, reduced light, night sedation.
- Limit and cluster night-time interventions to protect sleep periods of a minimum of 90min.

Supporting sensory balance and orientation

- Reduce meaningless, unnecessary noise.
- Place large clocks and calendars in the patient's line of sight.
- Repeatedly re-orientate the patient to time, day, place, person, and events.
- Introduce the patient to staff or others entering their room or bed space.
- Formally greet and leave-take the patient when starting and finishing a shift.
- Involve the patient in conversation with visitors.
- Place familiar objects and photos in the patient's line of sight.
- Offer stimulation from music, radio, television, computers, newspapers (ascertaining the patient's likes and dislikes first).

Further information

Jones C, Griffiths R, Humphris G, et al. (2001) Memory, delusions, and the development of acute posttraumatic stress disorder-related symptoms after intensive care. *Crit Care Med,* **29**, 573–80.

Diurnal rhythm and sleep disturbance

The 24h diurnal cycle is resistant to change and long-term disruption to sleep can be fatal. In the critically ill patient, care, monitoring, and interventions must continue round the clock, and this makes patients vulnerable to diurnal rhythm and sleep disturbance. Restorative processes, including protein synthesis and mental restoration, are affected by sleep deprivation. Cortisol levels vary in a 24h cycle (see Fig. 3.2), which leaves the patient most vulnerable during the early hours of the morning.

Factors other than noise and interventions are involved in the sleep disturbance seen in the critically ill. Studies using polysomnography in critical care have shown that only 20% of patient arousals are due to environmental noise and only 10% are due to patient care activities, suggesting that other factors are involved in sleeplessness. Early work suggests that disturbances in melatonin secretion may be responsible in some cases and melatonin supplementation may be effective in this case.

Effects of sleep disturbance
- Physical exhaustion and fatigue.
- Irritability and anxiety.
- Disruption of immune function.
- Reduced endurance of respiratory muscle activity.
- Increased energy expenditure and negative nitrogen balance.
- Cognitive dysfunction.

Contributing factors to sleep disturbance
- Inadequate pain relief.
- Frequent nursing interventions.
- High levels of background noise.
- Inappropriate nursing routines (e.g. bed baths at 05.00 hours).
- Suppression of REM (rapid eye movement) and slow wave sleep by benzodiazepines and narcotics.

Nursing interventions to limit sleep disturbance
- Dim lights and reduce noise for the night period.
- Institute a unit-wide minimal noise and intervention time between 01.00 and 05.00 hours.
- Offer earplugs or noise-cancellation headsets and eye masks.
- Carry out only vital observations and interventions at night.
- Cluster interventions to allow a minimum of 90min protected sleep.
- Avoid procedures likely to stress the patient between 01.00 and 05.00 hours (lowest cortisol secretion level; see Fig. 3.2).

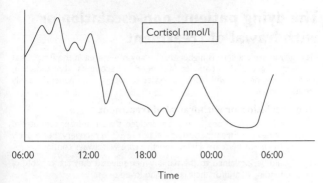

Fig. 3.2 Graph of cortisol levels over a 24-h period to show diurnal cycle.

Further information

Gabor J, Cooper A, Shelley A, et al. (2003) Contribution of the intensive care unit environment to sleep disruption in mechanically ventilated patients. *Am J Resp Crit Care Med*, **167**, 708–15.

The dying patient: non-escalation or withdrawal of treatment

Mortality in critical care is higher than in any other area in the hospital at between 15 and 25% of patients. Staff need to become familiar and comfortable with dealing with death in order to support the patient's family and loved ones.

Non-escalation or withdrawal of treatment

In certain futile situations it may be decided that it is inappropriate to continue or extend treatment that will not result in recovery, but merely prolong the point of death. Full supportive care will always continue.

This should be explained to the patient themselves if they are capable of comprehending it, and/or their family and loved ones.

The final decision should be taken by the critical care consultant, but prior discussion should take place between all those concerned with the patient's care, including nursing and medical staff, family and loved ones, other medical, nursing, and AHP teams involved, and spiritual advisors.

Communication of the decision to the patient's family and loved ones should be undertaken by the critical care consultant and should include:
• Reasons for the decision.
• Treatments that will continue.
• Treatments that will not continue.
• Alternative treatments that would be futile.
• Reassurance that full supportive care will continue.
• Reassurance that pain/discomfort will be relieved.

Once the decision has been taken, altered priorities will apply to the patient's care. Adequate pain relief, comfort, and psychological support are pre-eminent priorities. Decisions about requirements for personal hygiene needs, repositioning, and non-essential therapies should be judged on the situation, and require sensitivity and thought.

Breaking the news of impending death

• The critical care consultant or a senior doctor, accompanied by a nurse, should break this news to family and loved ones.
• The setting should be private, available for as long as needed, and away from the hubbub of the unit. Water and tissues should be available.
• After a preparatory statement, the news should be given in clear, short sentences without the use of euphemisms. Where there is likelihood of misperception, explanation should be given. Recognition of the family and loved one's distress should be included, and an opportunity given for recovery.
• Details may need to be repeated a number of times, with frequent invitations to ask questions and check clarification.
• Nursing staff should be available to interpret or clarify afterwards.

Priorities that dying patients rate most important

- Freedom from pain.
- Being at peace with God.
- Presence of their family.
- Being mentally aware.
- Knowing their treatment choices are being followed.
- Having their finances in order.
- Feeling life was meaningful.
- Able to resolve conflicts.
- Able to die at home.

Further information

Steinhauser K, Christakis N, Clipp E, et al. (2000) Factors considered important at the end of life by patients, family, physicians, and other care providers. *J Am Med Ass*, **284**, 2476–82.

The dying patient: supporting family and loved ones

Coping with the experience of death is stressful for all concerned, but the effect on family and loved ones is the greatest. When it becomes clear that the patient is dying, they will have their hopes of recovery extinguished and will have to face the reality of death. This may trigger a crisis point with a range of responses from grief, through denial, to anger. Dealing with this requires the nurse to be comfortable with his/her own feelings about grief and loss.

Family and loved ones of dying patients have identified the following issues:
- Uncertainty is the prevalent experience.
- There is a lack of information.
- There is conflicting or confusing information from different carers.
- They need privacy and opportunities to say goodbye.
- They feel a responsibility to protect the patient.

They identify the best methods of dealing with these issues as:
- Frequent effective communication with staff.
- Provision of concrete and objective information.
- Effective communication between staff to ensure information is congruent.
- Provision of opportunities to be with the patient and to have privacy.

Nursing interventions for support

Effective verbal communication
- Grief should be acknowledged.
- Open and honest communication.
- Frequent repetition of information.
- Effective listening to pick up cues for help or information.

Effective non-verbal communication
- Sitting with the family.
- Comforting touch (shoulders/forearms, but be aware of cultural sensitivities).
- Facial expression should reflect concern.
- Silence.

Encouraging participation by family and loved ones in the patient's care
- Mouth care.
- Hair brushing and washing.
- Reading to the patient.
- Re-positioning for comfort.
- Help with taking oral fluids.
- Massage.

Establishing routines to support family and loved ones
- Discussion of preferred level of privacy (the nurse can remain close by).
- Discussion of spiritual support.
- Organizing a room for the family and loved ones to stay close by.
- Determining whether they wish to be there at the time of death.

The ten most important needs of the family of critically ill, dying patients

- To be with the person.
- To be helpful to the dying person.
- To be informed of the dying person's condition.
- To understand what is being done to the patient and why.
- To be assured of the patient's comfort.
- To be comforted.
- To ventilate emotions.
- To be assured that their decisions were right.
- To find meaning in the dying of their loved one.
- To be fed, hydrated, and rested.

(Truog et al. 2001)

Further information

Bryce C, Lowenstein G, Arnold R, et al. (2004) Quality of death: assessing the importance placed on end-of-life treatment in the intensive-care unit. *Med Care*, **42**, 423–31

Steinhauser K, Christakis N, Clipp E, et al. (2000) Factors considered important at the end of life by patients, family, physicians, and other care providers. *J Am Med Ass*, **284**, 2476–82.

Truog R, Cist A, Bracket S, et al. (2001) Recommendations for end-of-life care in the intensive care unit: The Ethics Committee of the Society of Critical Care Medicine. *Crit Care Med*, **29**, 2332–48

Nursing skills to support critical care patients

The nursing effect

Although impossible to quantify and difficult to link to formal outcomes, there is little doubt that skilled nursing care can make a difference to patients in critical care.

Some data suggest that numbers of nurses alone can affect outcome with a nurse:patient ratio of greater than 1:2 (i.e. 1:3 or 1:4) being associated with increased mortality, infection rates, and possibly increased weaning time.

Other studies have shown that more experienced nurses are more likely to assist patients to wean from ventilation.

Patients refer to the effect of nursing care as being positive to their recovery and stress their feelings of relief when cared for by competent nurses. This is also echoed by families and loved ones, who feel the patient is safe when cared for by a nurse perceived as skilled or competent.

This effect can be negated by burnout and increased workload so that even the most competent and skilled nurse is unable to perform safely.

Priorities of care

The priorities are always to keep the patient safe, and should reflect the situation and the level of threat imposed to the patient. In an emergency, supporting airway, breathing, and circulation are critical. Where there is no direct threat to life, then other issues, such as psychological support, routine drugs, and lower impact care, such as enteral nutrition, can assume a higher priority.

Top priorities of care
- Airway.
- Breathing (patient/ventilator).
- Circulation.

Good critical care prevents life-threatening events by:
- Close observation/monitoring.
- Skilled interpretation and analysis.
- Early identification of problems.
- Effective intervention.

Checking emergency equipment

Nurses taking responsibility for a patient must check their emergency equipment to ensure it is not only available, but functional.

The bedside emergency equipment should be checked, as well as the unit cardiac arrest trolley and emergency equipment.

Bedside emergency equipment checks

Airway

- **Suction:** check suction builds to set pressure when tubing is occluded. Set pressure should not be higher than 30 KPa to reduce risk of trauma.
- **Suction catheter:** yankauer sucker, and closed or open catheters of an appropriate size (see 🕮 Suctioning, p. 210).
- **Closed suction catheter:** check connections, patency of transparent sleeve, and test with a small amount of normal saline flushed through the irrigation port.
- **Oropharyngeal airway:** of appropriate size (commonly size 2 for women, 3 for men).
- **Tracheostomy tube:** replacement tubes, the same size and 1 size smaller.
- **Tracheal dilator.**

Breathing

- Self-inflating resuscitation bag with reservoir – tested for leaks by screwing pressure relief valve closed and applying pressure on the bag.
- Check connection is to oxygen supply.
- Catheter mount and mask as appropriate.
- Emergency oxygen supply (in case of central supply failure).

Circulation

- Re-zero arterial (and other) pressure monitoring, ensure waveform is optimal, and transducers at the correct height. (see 🕮 Central venous pressure, p. 104 for details).
- All nurses should be competent to recognize life-threatening rhythm changes and respond accordingly.
- All nurses should be competent to perform cardiac compressions.
- Ensure patient has patent intravenous access and fluid available should it be required.
- Re-calculate drug infusions and check against prescription.

Prevention of immobility complications

The potential complications of restricted mobility are well-documented. Critically ill patients can remain immobile due to a combination of factors, including physiological instability, weakness, sedation, traction, multiple invasive devices, etc.

Ideally, these patients should be repositioned frequently with early mobilization as soon as their condition permits.

Complications of restricted mobility

- **Chest infection:** due to decreased sputum clearance, impaired functional residual capacity (FRC), and reduced cough.
- **Muscle atrophy due to disuse:** occurs rapidly with lack of use and requires long periods to rebuild.
- **Joint stiffness and contractures:** stronger flexor muscles increase flexion commonly plantar, shoulder hand, and hip flexors.
- **Demineralization and loss of long bone density:** loss of weight-bearing pressure decreases osteoblastic activity within 1–2 days.
- **Pressure sores:** high risk due to immobility plus altered tissue perfusion, reduced sensory function, malnutrition, and chronic disease factors.
- **DVT and peripheral oedema:** venous stasis and increased coagulability due to loss of muscle pumps.
- **Urinary tract infection:** urinary stasis in the supine position due to dependent bladder portion filling, increased infection risk with urinary catheter.
- **Nephrolithiasis:** increased urinary calcium excretion due to disuse bone density loss.
- **Decreased gut motility and constipation:** partly due to muscle atrophy compounded by sedation and loss of enteral stimuli if not enterally fed.
- **Peripheral nerve injury:** ulnar nerve is at particular risk from pronation and elbow flexion when the patient is supine.

Interventions to reduce risk of complications

Regular repositioning

- Use right and left lateral, as well as supine, but maintain 30–45° head up.
- Correct alignment and positioning of limbs to prevent nerve damage and contractures.
- Early mobilization to chair.
- Use hoists and stretchers for highly dependent patients.
- Passive limb movements.
- Maintain normal range of movement (ROM) and stretch flexors.
- Maintain muscle strength and joint mobility.
- Active isotonic limb and ROM exercises at regular intervals.
- Spread the pressure load.
- Use special support mattresses and surfaces, and check dependent points over bony structures (high risk areas) each shift.
- Active chest physiotherapy.
- Use humidification, deep breathing, suction, and repositioning, plus specific physiotherapy techniques, such as vibration and hyperinflation.
- Bowel management.
- Commence enteral feeding as soon as possible.
- Observe and document bowel function, intervening as necessary (see ⬚ Gastrointestinal dysfunction: diarrhoea, p. 360; ⬚ Constipation, p. 362).
- Scrupulous infection control (see ⬚ Preventing complications: hospital acquired infection, p. 80).
- DVT prophylaxis.
- Use prophylactic anticoagulation (unless contraindicated) and thrombo-embolism deterrent (TED) stockings, and intermittent pneumatic compression devices.

Preventing complications: hospital acquired infection

Critically ill patients have a 10–15% incidence of hospital-acquired (noso-comial) infections. There are three main reasons for this:

- Many infections have a greatly increased risk associated with invasive devices, such as central venous catheters (9.2-fold increase in infec-tion if site is reddened), urinary catheters (3.2-fold increase) and endotracheal tubes (21-fold increase). This is due to the breaching of skin integrity and the facilitation of colonization by bypassing normal defence mechanisms.
- Increased requirement for antibiotics amongst the critically ill creates resistant strains of organisms, which can be transmitted rapidly from patient to patient.
- Compromised immune function related to sepsis or other disease processes.

Other factors that may be involved are possible genetic predisposition, the presence of nasogastric tubes for enteral nutrition increasing tracheal reflux/aspiration risk and supine body positioning. Levels of nurse staffing that are less than 1:1 can also increase cross-infection.

Hand washing/alcohol gel disinfection

The single most important factor in preventing transmission of infection.
- Before any patient contact.
- After any patient contact.
- Prior to preparation of drugs, iv fluids, procedures, dressings, etc.
- Before leaving the bedside.

Limiting infection in critical care (general)

- Strict adherence to local infection control policies.
- Local infection control standards and protocols for staff.
- Local antimicrobial use policy.
- Hand washing/alcohol rub between patient contacts.
- Aprons and gloves for patient contact.
- Maintenance of 30–45° semi-recumbent patient position.
- Maintenance of staffing ratios appropriate to patient workload.
- Strict aseptic technique for any invasive line dressing/procedure.
- Minimize use of invasive devices or remove as soon as possible.
- Minimal manipulation of IV lines, catheters, dressings.
- Regular feedback to staff of infection rates.
- Avoidance of antacid ulcer prophylaxis in combination with H_2 blockers.
- Avoidance of endotracheal intubation wherever possible.

Limiting ventilator-associated pneumonia infection

- Use of HME humidifiers (with bacterial filters).
- Disposable ventilator circuits, changed at 48h intervals if no HME.
- Closed suction systems, changed at 48-h intervals or as needed.
- Disposable or in-line nebulizers.
- Semi-recumbent patient position (30–45° head up).
- Regular left/right lateral position change alternating with semi-recumbent.

(For full details see 📖 Pneumonia, p. 230)

Limiting intravascular device infection

- Aseptic technique for insertion.
- Use of 2% chlorhexidine gluconate in alcohol for skin preparation/site cleaning.
- Central venous catheters replaced according to clinical indicators, e.g. reddening, swelling, pus at site, or signs of infection, e.g. temp. ↑WCC.
- Immediate removal of device if infection suspected.
- Aseptic technique for any manipulation of connection, dressing of site, etc.

Limiting urinary tract infection

- Avoid bladder catheterization if at all possible.
- Early removal of urinary catheter.
- Aseptic catheter insertion.
- Closed circuit drainage system with minimal manipulation.
- Anchoring of catheter to prevent urethral drag.

Oral hygiene

The lining of the mouth and oropharynx consists of squamous epithelial cells, which are highly vulnerable to the effects of poor blood flow, malnutrition, and drug toxicity. In addition, the loss of normal cleansing mechanisms, such as salivary flow, and frequently the presence of an endotracheal tube increase the risk of infection and damage.

Saliva has a strong protective antimicrobial effect, but intubated patients have greatly reduced or absent salivary flow. This is associated with increased oral colonization and increased risk of mucositis.

Research has been mainly inconclusive in supporting firm recommendations regarding best practice in oral hygiene. However, the use of 0.1%–0.2% chlorhexidine mouth rinse or spray has been shown to be effective in reducing oral colonization by gram-negative bacteria and subsequent respiratory infections in cardiac surgical patients.

The use of a formal assessment tool may be beneficial in identifying patient's oral hygiene requirements.

The best oral hygiene tool is a small, soft toothbrush used with neutral pH solution or water in a circular motion, or with short horizontal strokes. This allows removal of plaque and should be used with a flexible suction device when rinsing the mouth following cleaning.

The minimum frequency of care is twice daily and more frequent care should be instigated according to assessment of the patient's need using a mouth assessment tool (Table 4.1).

Table 4.1 Assessment and intervention for oral problems

	Normal	Abnormal	Intervention
Mucosa	Pink, moist, intact, smooth	Reddening, ulceration, other lesions	Hydration, use of neutral mouthwash solution, pain-relieving anaesthetic gels for ulcers
Tongue	Pink, moist, intact, papillae present	Coated, absence of papillae, smooth shiny appearance, debris, lesions, crusted, cracks, blackened	Hydration, frequent, neutral mouthwashes, use of a debriding agent (e.g. sodium bicarbonate) for blackened areas
Lips	Clean, intact, pink	Dry skin, cracks, reddened, encrusted, ulcerated, bleeding	Hydration, protection using petroleum jelly or lubricant jelly
Saliva	Watery, white, or clear	Thick, viscous, absent, blood-stained	Hydration, use of artificial salivas
Gingiva	Pink, moist, firm	Receding, overgrown, oedematous, reddened, bleeding	Teeth brushing 2–3 times daily with small soft brush
			Chlorhexidine 0.1–0.2% mouthwash
Teeth	White, firm in sockets, no debris, no decay	Discoloured, decayed, debris, wobbly	Teeth brushing 2–3 times daily with small soft brush
			Dental assessment

Further information

Berry A, Davidson P, Masters J, Rolls K. (2007) Systematic literature review of oral hygiene practices for intensive care patients receiving mechanical ventilation. *Am J Crit Care*. **16**, 552–63.

Dennesen P, Van der Ven A, Vlasveld M, et al. (2003) Inadequate salivary flow and poor oral mucosal status in intubated intensive care unit patients. *Crit Care Med*, **31**, 781–6.

Eye care

Normal eyes are protected from dehydration by the tear film. This is continuously replenished by the lacrimal gland at a rate of approximately 1–2µl/min. These are spread over the surface of the eye by the blink reflex.

This protective mechanism can be disrupted in critically ill patients due to a reduced ability to blink, dehydration affecting tear production, incomplete lid closure, drug side effects, and occasionally orbital oedema.

The patient is also at risk of eye infections due to the decreased immune function and increased likelihood of cross-infection.

Increased intra-thoracic pressure related to IPPV will increase the risk of orbital oedema.

The two eye care problems associated with the critically ill are dry eyes and exposure keratopathy.

Dry eyes are due to a combination of the above factors and exposure keratopathy is due to incomplete lid closure in the unconscious patient. Drying occurs as a result of exposure to air with the onset of epithelial erosion and ultimately corneal ulceration as a result.

Infection is a particular risk in both cases, and should be identified and managed early (see Table 4.2).

Table 4.2 Assessment and management of the eyes

	Normal	Abnormal	Intervention
Eyelid closure	Upper eyelid completely covers the eye	Eyelids do not fully meet, or cornea are swollen and extruded	Close eyelids with hydropolymer dressing, Lacri-Lube® ointment or moisture seal chamber
Hydration status	No fluid restriction, no signs of dehydration, corneal surface is moist.	Other features of dehydration or restricted fluid intake, plus dry corneal surface	Use sterile water for cleansing the eye, apply artificial tears (hydroxyethylcellulose) or hypromellose
Corneal surface	Moist, clear, white	Purulent, coated, or crusting exudate, clouding, oedematous, haemorrhage	Swab for culture, clean as above, apply appropriate topical antibiotic as per culture result
Orbital oedema	Cornea and orbital area are not swollen or extruded	Corneal and orbital area are swollen, reddened, or extruding	Maintain a head-up position to reduce pressure, ensure tapes securing ET or trach tube are not too tight

Communication: the patient

Normal communication processes are disrupted in the critically ill patient by sedation, opiates, endotracheal and tracheal tubes, and fluctuating consciousness. This is complicated by pain, fear, and anxiety.

Communicating with the critically ill patient

- Communication requires patience, motivation, the ability to see the patient as an individual, perseverance, a willingness to try new methods and experience.
- Many patients are able to hear, understand, and respond emotionally to what is said to them, even when they are not thought to be aware by critical care staff.

Most communication in critical care is procedural or task-related, although there is also often acknowledgement of discomfort or distress. Patients can feel isolated, alienated, and fearful. This should be recognized in any communication with empathy, information-giving, and acknowledgement of these concerns.

Critical care survivors have given accounts of their experiences, which are a valuable source of information about what is important.

Time, day, and situation orientation is an important baseline, as well as a clear introduction of self and others.

Communicating effectively with critically ill patients

- Ensure the patient can see and hear you by positioning yourself in their line of sight, making eye contact, and speaking clearly.
- Use touch to signal that he/she has your attention and empathy.
- Use positive feedback – smiling, nodding attentively, focusing full attention on the patient's face.
- Orientate the patient to time, day, place, and your own identity.
- Assess the patient's ability to respond – speech, signs, mouthing, nodding and facial gestures, writing, etc.
- Enhance the response using communication devices such as word or symbol boards/computers.
- Use appropriate levels of questioning:
  - open questions for patients who can speak/communicate fully;
  - closed questions for gestures and nodding communication.
- Where possible agree appropriate gestures for communication, and ensure these are documented or handed over.
- Where language difficulties exist obtain phonetic translations of simple words, such as pain, or use symbol boards (available from speech and language therapists).
- Involve the patient's family in planning and executing the right method of communication.

Communication assistance devices for intubated patients

- Passy-Muir valve.
- Possum portascan.
- Pen/pencil and paper.
- Alphabet or symbol boards.
- Laptop computer.
- Magic writers/slate.
- Electronic communicator (e.g. light writer).

Nursing skills to enhance communication

- Lip reading.
- Knowledge of other languages.
- Use of mime, gesture, and facial expression.
- Eye contact.
- Touch.

Communication: the family and loved ones

The term 'family' refers to all those providing the patient's intimate support structure at home.

When a family member is critically ill, family inter-relationships experience considerable stress. This is compounded by the loss of normal family rituals and day-to-day routines, as well as the loss of routine interaction and normal communication. The situation can often highlight tensions between family members and become a trigger for overt disagreement.

Family needs when a loved one is in critical care have been extensively studied.

Five common factors identified are the need for:
• Support.
• Comfort.
• Information.
• Proximity.
• Assurance.

Families require a positive, supportive relationship with the staff, with a common record of any contacts, so that the whole multi-professional team are aware of what has been communicated.

The main response identified by families that is required from staff is the offering and updating of information about the patient, their prognosis and diagnosis, and support. However, families also need psychological and spiritual support as well.

Strategies for staff to manage large families include:
• Asking the family to appoint one spokesperson, information receiver, transmitter.
• Limiting concurrent visiting numbers and organizing relays of attendance at the bedside. Ensuring visitors are aware of rest periods.
• Specifying a daily update time.
• Encouraging mutual support within the family.

Meeting family needs in critical care

Information
- Anticipate and supply information needs.
- Supplement information with printed booklets and explanations.
- Ensure information is not conflicting.

Communication and explanation
- Communication should be open and honest.
- Distressing communications should be delivered in a private environment.
- Ensure explanations are delivered in appropriate language.
- A common record of all communication between the family and the multi-professional team should be maintained.

Involvement in care
- Support family time, both at the bedside and away from it.
- Involve families in non-technical patient care as appropriate.
- Involve families in patient diaries, in personalizing the environment, and stimulating the patient when they are more awake.
- When English is a second language, be highly active in involving families in reassuring the patient.

Support of the family
- Access to the patient should be tailored to meet both the patient's best interests and the family's needs.
- The staff should monitor the family carefully for stressors, and offer advice, support, and links to alternative support mechanisms as necessary.
- Assign consistent nurses to maintain continuity.
- Use volunteers and pastoral carers, as well as ancillary staff to give added support.

Further information

De Jong MJ, Beatty DS. (2000) Family perceptions of support interventions in the intensive care unit. *Dimens Crit Care Nurs*, **10**, 244–51.

Leske J. (1991) Internal psychometric properties of the critical care family needs inventory. *Heart Lung*, **20**, 236–44

Communication: the team

Collaborative working is essential within the critical care unit. It is one of the few organizational features clearly shown to have benefit for patient outcome and staff satisfaction.

The process requires mutual respect between professionals and recognition that all team members' contributions are necessary to give the patient the best outcome.

Teams should have a recognized team leader, which in critical care tends to be the medical consultant or their deputy. However, there are often several different team groupings such as:
• **Unit clinical team:** team leader = medical consultant.
• **Unit nursing team:** team leader = sister or charge nurse.
• **Bedside team:** team leader = nurse at bedside.
• **Unit management team:** general manager or clinical director.

Effective team working requires a key decision-making point, such as the traditional ward round, during which the patient's case can be discussed and a plan of care decided on. The key to effective and safe teams, however, is the opportunity for all team members to raise concerns and question decisions.

Handover between nurses and other professions should take place at the bedside so that the patient's current situation can be assessed. Use of a handover structure, such as the nursing care plan or SBAR (situation, background, assessment, recommendation) will ensure essential information is handed over.

Markers of effective teamwork
• Team members monitor each other's performance and step in to help out—trust is implicit in this.
• Giving and receiving feedback is the norm for all team members and is seen as part of their role.
• Team members understand each other's role.
• Communication is made real, i.e. senders check that messages are received as they intended.
• Teams should ensure that they are able to hear the voices of those staff with the most experience of what can go or has gone wrong in patient care, whether or not they are of lower rank than their colleagues.

Methods of improving team effectiveness
• Enhancing multidisciplinary decision-making to allow a broad spectrum of knowledge of the patient's condition. This could also include listening to the patient.
• Rewarding teams as a whole.
• Encouraging innovative solutions to problems.

Cardiovascular monitoring

Electrocardiogram

Basic principles

- Electrodes are placed on the chest wall to detect electrical activity initiated by the heart. Activity moving towards an electrode will produce an upward (positive) deflection, and away from the electrode produces a downward (negative) deflection. The baseline (isoelectric line) is where the positive and negative deflections begin and end.
- The electrodes are connected by a cable to the monitor, which displays a continuous waveform reflecting each phase of the heart's electrical activity.
- These impulses are amplified so that their height is increased 1000-fold.
- The waveform on the monitor can be adjusted so that optimal size, brightness, and position are seen. A choice of leads is possible, but lead II is usually selected. This is because the direction of electrical current passing through the ventricles is directed towards lead II, resulting in a large, positive waveform that can easily be interpreted.

Placement of electrodes

Usually three electrodes are used, but some equipment may require 4–5. Attach the electrodes by peeling off the backing paper and pressing firmly to the skin. The skin must be clean and dry, and chest hair may need to be shaved to facilitate contact. The electrodes can remain *in situ* for several days, but should be re-sited regularly to avoid soreness. Skin irritation can occur due to the adhesive used on the electrode or the conducting gel.

Adjusting the monitor

The displayed waveform must be clear and distinct. The amplitude of the R wave is particularly important as the heart rate is calculated by recognizing and counting this wave. If the height of the wave cannot be increased sufficiently to record an accurate heart rate, change the position of the electrodes or the lead displayed to obtain a greater electrical potential.

High and low alarm limits should be set according to the patient's condition. False heart rate readings will occur if the R and T waves are the same height, there is electrical interference from other devices at the bedside, or there is shivering, muscle tremors, or movement by the patient.

A wandering baseline can occur due to movement of the chest wall during respiration – alter the electrode position to the lowest ribs and the apex of the chest.

Timing of the ECG

ECG paper is made up of small and large squares. Each small square measures 1mm and each large square 5mm. The paper is run at a speed of 25mm/s. Thus, each small square represents 0.04s and each large square 0.2s. This allows the time of conduction and the heart rate to be calculated.

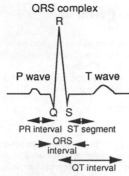

Fig. 5.1 The QRS complex. Reproduced with permission from *Critical Care Nursing*, Adam and Osborne (2005), Oxford University Press.

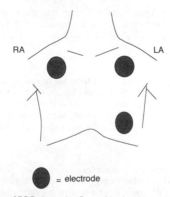

Fig. 5.2 Placement of ECG electrodes. Reproduced with permission from *Critical Care Nursing*, Adam and Osborne (2005), Oxford University Press.

Analysis of the rhythm strip
- Determine the rate.
- Determine the regularity of the rhythm.
- Identify the P wave and its shape.
- Identify the QRS complex.
- Determine the relationship between P waves and QRS complexes.
- Calculate the P–R interval.
- Examine the shape and calculate the width of the QRS complex.
- Calculate the Q–T interval.

Further information
Adam SK, Osborne S. (2005) *Critical Care Nursing*. Oxford: Oxford University Press.

Arrhythmias: general

Classified as:
- **Disorders of impulse formation:** dysfunction of the pacemaker rate of the sinoatrial node allows escape rhythms from other pacemakers within the heart (e.g. the AV node).
- **Disorders of impulse conduction:** conduction is either slowed, blocked or uses an alternative pathway.

Causes of arrhythmias
- Cardiac disease.
- Myocardial ischaemia.
- Autonomic control affected by central neurological damage.
- Electrolyte and acid-base balance disturbance.
- Endocrine influences, particularly thyroid hormone.
- Effects of drugs.

Monitoring the Q–T interval

The normal value depends on the heart rate. As heart rate increases the Q–T interval shortens and as it decreases the interval lengthens. The formula for correcting the Q–T interval to a heart rate of 60 bpm (QTc) is:

$$QTc = QT/\sqrt{(R\text{-}R)}$$

where QT is the interval measured from the beginning of the QRS to the end of the T wave, and $\sqrt{(R\text{-}R)}$ is the square root of the time between two successive R waves. The QTc is prolonged if >0.44 s. This is associated with hypokalaemia, hypocalcaemia, hypomagnesaemia, and tricyclic drugs. It can lead to torsades de pointes, a very rapid and potentially life-threatening rhythm.

Axis

The sum of the ventricular electrical forces during depolarization. The normal axis of the heart lies between $-30°$ and $+90°$ (i.e. towards the left as the left ventricular mass is greater than the right). Left axis deviation is when the axis lies outside $-30°$. Right axis deviation is when the axis is greater than $+90°$ (Fig. 5.4).

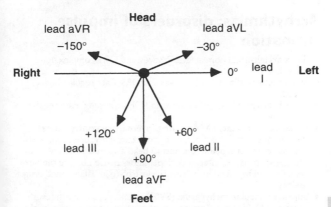

Fig. 5.3 Orientation of the limb leads. Reproduced with permission from *Critical Care Nursing*, Adam and Osborne (2005), Oxford University Press.

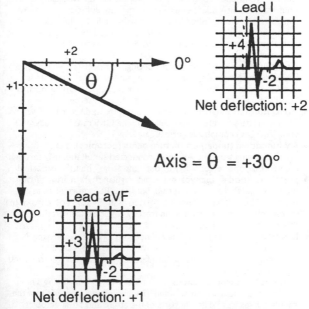

Fig. 5.4 Calculation of the axis. Reproduced with permission from *Critical Care Nursing*, Adam and Osborne (2005), Oxford University Press.

Further information

Adam SK, Osborne S. (2005) *Critical Care Nursing*. Oxford: Oxford University Press.

Arrhythmias: disorders of impulse formation

- **Sinus arrhythmia:** normal rate, P waves, and QRS complex. Rate irregular.
- **Sinus tachycardia**: normal P waves and QRS. Rate regular, but >100bpm.
- **Sinus bradycardia**: normal P wave and QRS complex. Rate regular, but <60bpm.
- **Atrial ectopic beats (APCs – atrial premature contractions)**: stimulus arising from part of the atrium occurs early, producing a ventricular contraction before the normal beat. This may be followed by a longer than normal interval ('compensatory pause') before the next beat. Caused by infection, ischaemia, electrolyte imbalance, and drug toxicity.
- **Supraventricular tachycardia (SVT)**: a rapid, regular rhythm with a rate of 140–250bpm. P waves may be abnormal or obscured by the rapid rate QRS complex. There may difficulty in distinguishing SVT with aberrant ventricular conduction from ventricular tachycardia. Carotid sinus massage or iv adenosine can slow the rate sufficiently to make a diagnosis. It is distinguished from sinus tachycardia by the lack of a P wave, and its sudden onset and cessation. Caused by heart disease and arrhythmogenic conditions, such as Wolff–Parkinson–White (WPW) syndrome.
- **Atrial flutter**: an atrial rhythm producing 'sawtooth' or 'picket fence' P waves. The atrial rate is 250–300bpm, but the ventricular rate is variable depending on the degree of AV nodal block. QRS is normal. Usually caused by ischaemic or rheumatic heart disease.
- **Atrial fibrillation (AF)**: an irregular rate with no discernible P waves. Atria fibrillate at a rate of 400–600bpm. The QRS rate is usually >100 bpm. The QRS complex is normal.
- **AV junctional (nodal) premature beats (ectopics)**: a premature stimulus arising from the AV node, conducted simultaneously through the ventricle and retrogradely through the atria. The QRS is normal.
- **Junctional (nodal) tachycardia**: rapid, regular rhythm arising from the AV node. P waves are inverted, but the QRS is normal. Rate can rise to 140bpm. If paroxymal, it is treated as an SVT. A non-paroxysmal rhythm may be caused by digoxin toxicity, myocardial infarction, rheumatic fever, and myocarditis.
- **Junctional nodal rhythm:** The AV node acts as the pacemaker. No discernible P waves, but QRS is normal, rhythm is regular, and rate is 40–70bpm. Caused by myocardial infarction, increased vagal tone, and digoxin toxicity.
- **Sick sinus syndrome**: various rhythm disturbances, including sinus bradycardia, sinoatrial arrest, wandering pacemaker (the origin of the impulse arises from different parts of the atria), and atrial ectopics. May be accompanied by episodes of atrial flutter, atrial fibrillation, and SVT. Caused by intrinsic disease of the SA node and conducting system

producing palpitations and episodes of fainting (Stokes–Adams attacks). Can be associated with infarction of the atria, rheumatic heart disease, and pericarditis.

- **Ventricular premature contractions (ectopics) (VEs)**: impulse stimulus arises in the ventricles. No P wave is seen prior to a premature, widened QRS complex, which is often bizarrely shaped and increased in amplitude. An inverted P wave may be seen after the beat due to retrograde conduction. A compensatory pause may follow the beat. Bigeminy is when an ectopic beat alternates with a normal beat. Trigeminy occurs when an ectopic beat follows every second normal beat. Multifocal ectopics appear as different shaped QRS complexes and arise from different areas within the ventricle. VEs can occur at any age at any time. Common in myocardial irritability (hypoxia, hypokalaemia, digoxin toxicity). They are associated with heart disease in the over 40s if frequent, occur in runs and multifocal.

- **Ventricular tachycardia (VT)**: a ventricular ectopic focus stimulates a series of rapid and regular beats. No P waves are present, and the QRS is bizarrely shaped and widened. Rate is between 100 and 200 bpm. It often occurs following myocardial infarction or from digoxin toxicity. The fast rate and the loss of co-ordinated atrial contractions cause a severe drop in cardiac output, which may require CPR.

- **Ventricular fibrillation (VF)**: rapid, chaotic, and ineffectual contractions of the ventricle accompanied by complete loss of cardiac output. If CPR is not instituted, the patient will die. VF is associated with ischaemic heart disease, metabolic disturbances, and following electrocution and drug toxicity (e.g. digoxin, tricyclic antidepressants).

- **Torsades de pointes**: a specific type of fast ventricular rate transitional between VT and VF. The QRS complex is widened, but the axis alternates between positive and negative. It is associated with a prolonged QT interval (>0.44s). Precipitating conditions include low serum K^+, Mg^{2+}, and Ca^{2+}, or anti-arrhythmic agents, such as disopyramide. Prolonged Q–T with torsades de pointes can occur with tricyclic antidepressants, phenothiazines (e.g. haloperidol) and insecticide poisoning. The rhythm must be recognized correctly, as conventional treatment for VT may cause the condition to worsen.

Arryhthmias: disorders of impulse conduction

First degree heart block

Caused by a delay in conduction at the AV node. The P–R interval exceeds 0.2s. It occurs in normal or diseased hearts, and may be a precursor to second or third degree block.

Second degree heart block

There are two types:
• **Mobitz type I (Wenkebach):** a delay at the AV node (seen as a lengthening P–R interval) gradually increases through a series of beats until conduction of the impulse does not occur. The whole process is then repeated. The QRS complex is normal. Usually associated with acute reversible conditions and is relatively benign.
• **Mobitz type II:** a varying ratio of P waves to QRS complexes are conducted through the AV node (e.g. two P:1 QRS or three P:1 QRS). The P–R interval remains constant. Indicates more severe impairment of the AV node and is associated with myocardial infarction. It may precede complete heart block.

Third degree (complete) heart block

• There is a complete block of conduction between the atria and ventricles at the AV node, with no relationship between P waves and QRS complexes. The atrial rate thus continues at a normal or slightly faster rate, but the ventricular rate is slower. If the QRS originates in the AV node the rate will be 50–60bpm and the QRS will be normal. If it originates more distally, the rate will be 30–40bpm, and the QRS will be widened and enlarged. Common causes are myocardial infarction, post- cardiac surgery, and idiopathic degeneration of the conducting system.

Wolff–Parkinson–White syndrome (WPW)

Bouts of paroxysmal tachyarrhythmia characterized by a widened QRS and shortened P–R interval. In the non-tachyarrhythmic state the QRS complex has a notch called a delta wave. This indicates early ventricular stimulation via the accessory conduction pathway, which bypasses the AV node. The P–R interval is shortened due to rapid conduction through the accessory pathway, which unlike the AV node, does not slow conduction. It is due to strands of myocardial tissue – the bundle of Kent – acting as a bridge of conducting tissue across the non-conducting AV ring. This accessory pathway is capable of supporting arrhythmias, such as AF and paroxysmal SVT.

Table 5.1 Arrhythmias caused by metabolic changes

Metabolic change	Disorder
Hyperkalaemia	Tall (tented) T waves
	±Wide QRS complexes
	±Absent P waves
Hypokalaemia	Flattened T waves
	U waves (waves seen after T wave)
Hypercalcaemia	Short QT interval
Hypocalcaemia	Prolonged QT interval
Hypothermia	J wave (small wave appearing immediately after QRS complex)
	Bradycardia
Digoxin effect	ST depression
	Inverted T wave ('reverse tick'); not a sign of toxicity
	Any arrhythmia may occur with toxicity

Reproduced with permission from *Critical Care Nursing*, Adam and Osborne (2005), Oxford University Press.

Further information

Adam SK, Osborne S. (2005) *Critical Care Nursing*. Oxford: Oxford University Press.

The 12-lead electrocardiogram

This can assist clinical diagnosis and can also be serially monitored, depending on the patient's condition. It records flow of current in several planes to obtain a more comprehensive view of the heart. One electrode is placed on each limb and six on the chest wall. The right leg electrode acts as an earth and is not an electrical lead. Electrodes should be placed over positions of least muscle mass to avoid interference from skeletal muscle (i.e. inside of wrist and inner aspect of ankle). Use the same position for each serial ECG.

The electrodes

The complete 12-lead ECG consists of:

- Three limb leads I, II, and III. These form a hypothetical triangle with the heart at its centre.
- Three augmented (modified) limb leads termed aVL (augmented view left), aVR (augmented view right) and aVF (augmented view foot or left leg).
- Six chest leads: V1, V2, V3, V4, V5, and V6.

Positions of the chest leads

- **V1:** fourth intercostal space to the right of the sternum.
- **V2:** fourth intercostal space to the left of the sternum.
- **V3:** midway between V2 and V4.
- **V4:** fifth intercostal space, mid-clavicular line.
- **V5:** anterior axillary line at same level as V4.
- **V6:** mid-axillary line at same level as V4.

All 12 leads show different electrocardiographic patterns due to the different positions of the electrodes. The direction of deflection depends on the view of the heart in that particular lead. Some waves may change polarity due to disease.

The ECG should be analysed for rate, rhythm, axis, P wave, QRS complex, QT interval, S–T segment, and T wave to enable diagnosis of:

- Abnormal rhythms and conduction.
- Changes secondary to ischaemic heart disease.
- Changes secondary to pericardial disease.
- Changes secondary to metabolic and other diseases.
- Ventricular hypertrophy.

Analysis of the 12-lead electrocardiogram

Changes secondary to ischaemic heart disease

- Changes in the anteroseptal area are indicated by leads V1–4.
- Changes in the anterolateral area are indicated by leads I, aVL, V5, and V6.
- Changes in the inferior area are indicated by leads II, III, and aVF.
- Changes in the posterior area are indicated by a mirror image (i.e. upside down changes) in leads V1 and V2.

Changes secondary to pericardial disease

Concave ST segment elevation and tachycardia is seen in pericarditis. Low voltage (and, occasionally, alternating QRS complexes) is seen with large pericardial effusions.

Changes due to ventricular and atrial hypertrophy

Large QRS complexes are suggestive of hypertrophy though this is not applicable in young adults. Left ventricular hypertrophy is present when the sum of the R wave in V5 or V6 plus the S wave in V1 >35 mm. In right ventricular hypertrophy a 'dominant' R wave is seen in lead V1 with a normal width QRS. A 'strain pattern' is seen when ST depression and T wave inversion co-exist in the appropriate leads, and is suggestive of ischaemia in the hypertrophied ventricle.

Changes due to other diseases

Changes due to pulmonary embolism and acute right heart strain may include:

- Sinus tachycardia.
- Right axis deviation and peaked P waves in Leads V1 and V2 suggestive of right ventricular strain.
- 'S1-Q3–T3', i.e. a deep S wave in lead 1, and a pathological Q wave and inverted T wave in lead III.
- Partial right bundle branch block, i.e. an M-shaped, non-widened (width <0.12s) QRS complex.
- Atrial fibrillation.

Blood pressure

Non-invasive

Automated, but intermittent techniques. These include oscillometry (arterial pulsations sensed as a function of cuff pressure), detection of arterial turbulence under the cuff, ultrasonic detection of arterial wall motion under the cuff, and detection of blood flow distal to the cuff. Direct intra-arterial pressure can be expected to be 5–20mmHg greater than by indirect measurement. To ensure accuracy:

- Use cuff bladder width that is 40–50% of upper arm circumference.
- The bladder length should encircle 80% of the upper arm.
- Ensure cuff is at the level of the heart to maintain a true zero level.

Invasive (direct) arterial monitoring

Radial, and to a lesser extent, femoral and dorsalis pedis arteries are most commonly used. The radial artery is preferred as it has a good collateral circulation, is near to the skin surface, and the cannula site can be easiliy observed. The femoral approach is often used in shocked patients as the femoral pulse can be easier to palpate. The dorsalis pedis artery is small, often difficult to cannulate, makes mobilization difficult, and may not produce a good waveform.

Safety

- Regular assessment of skin colour, temperature, and pulses distal to the cannula. Contact a doctor promptly if change is noted.
- The site must be easily observed.
- It should not be located in an area prone to contamination/soiling or where a wound exists.
- It should not be inserted in a limb that has a vascular prosthesis.
- Alarm limits must be set on the monitor (particularly a lower limit).
- Arterial lines must be clearly labelled to avoid accidental injection.
- Luer lock connections must be used and firmly connected.

Complications

- Infection.
- Local haematomas, pain.
- Exsanguination due to disconnection.
- Thrombus formation or embolization, leading to distal necrosis.
- Accidental intra-arterial injection of drugs.
- Air embolus (from within flush system).
- Arteriovenous fistula, aneurysm.

Removing the cannula

Pressure must be applied for as long as necessary to achieve haemostasis. Check frequently for haemorrhage when the external pressure is removed. Assess the peripheral circulation as thrombosis can occur after removal.

Setting up the transduced pressure monitoring system

This system can continuously display pressures (e.g. arterial, CVP, pulmonary artery). A transducer (small, usually fluid-filled device) in the circuit measures and transmits the pressure to the monitor. Tubing from the patient cannula is connected to one side of the transducer and a giving set connected to a bag of 0.9% saline attached to the other side. Before patient connection, the system should be pre-primed using this solution, expelling all air. The solution is kept under continuous pressure (approximately 300mmHg for arterial lines, less for central venous lines) to prevent back-flow of blood from the circulation). Adjacent to the transducer, a flushing device ensures continuous (3ml/h) ± intermittent delivery of fluid (often containing a small amount of heparin) through the cannula, to keep it patent. The monitor displays the waveform trace and a digital pressure reading. To ensure accuracy:

- The transducer must always be level with the zero reference point (usually the right atrium).
- The system must be calibrated to atmospheric pressure ('zeroed') pre-use, intermittently during use (e.g. at each change of nursing shift), and if the tubing is disconnected. To calibrate, turn the 3-way tap at the cannula or transducer 'off' to the patient and 'open' to air. Press the zero button on the monitor. When zero is displayed turn the 3-way tap back 'on' to the patient.
- Only dedicated manometer tubing should be used in the system.
- Excessively long tubing or air bubbles in the tubing or transducer may cause dampened, trace, and inaccurate readings.

The arterial waveform

- *Anacrotic notch:* this is due to a pre-systolic rise in pressure occurring before opening of the aortic valve. It is seen only with central aortic pressure monitoring or in some pathological conditions.
- *Peak systolic pressure:* the maximum left ventricular systolic pressure generated by the outflow of blood from the ventricle into the arterial circulation.
- *Dicrotic notch:* reflects aortic valve closure caused by a rise in intra-aortic pressure. It marks the end of systole and the onset of diastole. It is elevated in patients with decreased cardiac output and increased peripheral vascular resistance.

Pulse pressure

The difference between systolic (SBP) and diastolic (DBP) pressures.

Mean arterial pressure (MAP)

The average pressure in the arterial system during one complete cycle of systole and diastole. Measured automically or calculated by:

$$MAP = DBP + (SBP - DBP)/3$$

Central venous pressure

Measured by a catheter inserted into internal jugular or subclavian veins, or via a long femoral or brachial line. The tip of the catheter should lie within one of the larger veins leading to the heart and must be within the thoracic cavity. CVP is right atrial pressure, which in turn, is equal to right ventricular end diastolic (filling) pressure. Post-insertion, a transduced pressure monitoring system is attached. The catheter tip position should be checked by X-ray before the catheter is used.

Types of catheter
- Single, double, triple, or quadruple lumens.
- Sheaths for pacing wire or PA catheter insertion.
- Tunnelled for long-term use.
- Large bore, double lumen for renal replacement therapy.
- Long catheters for insertion into brachial or axillary veins.

Uses
- Haemodynamic monitoring.
- Multiple infusions.
- Use of drugs that cause peripheral phlebitis or tissue necrosis if tissue extravasation occurs (e.g. TPN, catecholamines, amiodarone).
- Renal replacement therapy, plasmapheresis, exchange transfusion.
- Access for pacing wires.
- Rapid volume infusion.
- Emergency access when peripheral circulation is 'shut down'.

Potential problems during insertion
- Arrhythmias (usually from guidewire 'tickling' tricuspid valve).
- Pneumo/haemo/chylothorax.
- Haematoma caused by trauma to the vein or surrounding tissue.
- Catheter in incorrect position.
- Air embolus, venous thrombosis.

Measuring central venous pressure
'Zero' the pressure transducer by opening the 3-way tap to air at the level of the right atrium (mid-axillary line). Ensure a correct waveform is seen on the monitor. Record the reading.

The central venous pressure waveform
The monitor display should show small undulations reflecting pressure changes within the right atrium. Excessive undulations are seen in tricuspid regurgitation or if the tip is in the right ventricle. Normal values are 3–10mmHg. Any increase in intrathoracic pressure (from mechanical ventilation or PEEP) will increase the CVP (Fig. 5.5).

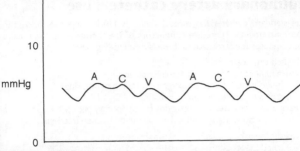

Fig. 5.5 The right atrial pressure waveform. Reproduced with permission from *Critical Care Nursing*, Adam and Osborne (2005), Oxford University Press.

- The A wave reflects right atrial contraction while the descent afterwards represents atrial relaxation. It is elevated in right ventricular failure and tricuspid stenosis.
- The C wave represents tricuspid valve closure.
- The V wave represents the pressure generated to the right atrium by the contracting right ventricle. A large 'V' wave is associated with tricuspid regurgitation.

Conditions affecting the central venous pressure

Increased in:
- Right ventricular failure.
- Pericardial tamponade.
- Fluid overload.
- Pulmonary hypertension.
- Tricuspid regurgitation.
- Pulmonary stenosis.
- Peripheral vasoconstriction.
- Superior vena cava obstruction.

Decreased in:
- Hypovolaemia (n.b. may initially rise due to compensatory constriction).
- Peripheral vasodilation (includes sepsis, drugs, regional analgesia, sympathetic dysfunction).

Removal of the central venous pressure

If their condition allows, the patient should lie flat or head tipped down, while the catheter is removed in order to minimize the risk of air embolism. Turn off or transfer any infusions. Slowly withdraw the catheter, ideally during expiration in the spontaneously breathing patient to avoid air embolism. Cover site with a sterile, occlusive dressing.

Further information

Adam SK, Osborne S. (2005) *Critical Care Nursing*. Oxford: Oxford University Press.

Pulmonary artery catheter: use

The standard catheter has three lumens, is 110cm long, and marked in 10cm increments. There are connectors to the thermister at the tip and the computer for cardiac output measurement (Fig. 5.6).

Modified catheters enable:
- Extra lumens for drug/fluid administration.
- Continuous mixed venous oxygen saturation monitoring.
- Continuous cardiac output monitoring.
- Pacing wire or external electrodes for temporary pacing.
- Measurement of right ventricular volume or ejection fraction.

Uses
- Pressure monitoring.
- Flow monitoring and calculation of oxygen delivery.
- Derived variables such as SVR, PVR, VO_2.
- Mixed venous oxygen saturation (i.e. blood draining from the upper and lower body is well mixed).
- Temporary pacing.
- Right ventricular ejection fraction and end diastolic volume.

The catheter

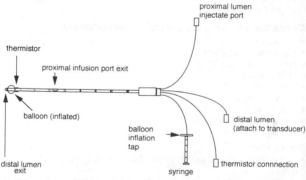

Fig. 5.6 The standard pulmonary artery catheter. Reproduced with permission from *Critical Care Nursing*, Adam and Osborne (2005), Oxford University Press.

- The proximal lumen: opens 30 cm from the tip and should lie in the right atrium. Used to monitor RA pressure and drug/fluid infusions.
- The distal lumen: runs the entire length of the catheter, opening at the tip, which lies in the pulmonary artery. Connects to the transducer to continually monitor PA pressure. Blood ('mixed venous') can be withdrawn from this lumen.
- The thermister connection: connected to the monitor to enable core temperature to be monitored.
- The thermister lies 4cm from the tip of the catheter and senses blood temperature. Connected to two insulated wires running the length of a lumen and ends at the thermister connection.

- Balloon inflation lumen is used to inflate/deflate the balloon to record pulmonary artery wedge pressure. A 1.5ml syringe is attached at this point and a tap allows the lumen to be turned off when not in use.

Measuring the wedge pressure

- Inflate balloon slowly until a flattened waveform appears on the monitor.
- Stop inflating as soon as this is seen – over-inflation may cause rupture of the pulmonary branch artery.
- Freeze the monitor screen and deflate the balloon rapidly (do not leave inflated for more than 15s).
- Move the cursor on the monitor to the correct position on the waveform (see Fig. 5.7).
- Unfreeze the screen to restore the continuous pulmonary artery waveform.

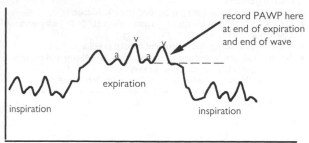

(a) In a spontaneously breathing patient

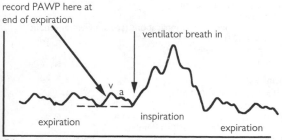

(b) In a mechanically ventilated patient

Fig. 5.7 Where to measure the wedge pressure. Reproduced with permission from *Critical Care Nursing*, Adam and Osborne (2005), Oxford University Press.

Further information

Adam SK, Osborne S. (2005) *Oxford Handbook of Critical Care Nursing*. Oxford: Oxford University Press.

Pulmonary artery catheter: insertion and removal

Insertion

Common insertion sites are the internal jugular, subclavian, and femoral veins:

- Before insertion, flush all lumens of the catheter (connect and use the transducer system for this).
- Check balloon integrity by inflating with 1.5ml of air.
- Connect distal lumen of the catheter to the transducer.
- Insert introducer sheath using a Seldinger technique. The catheter passed through a self-sealing valve into the blood vessel.
- Observe monitor continuously, while advancing the catheter with the balloon deflated.
- Inflate balloon when the tip is beyond the introducer.
- The catheter tip should enter the right atrium at 10–15 (using internal jugular approach).
- Advance into the right ventricle and record pressures.
- Advance catheter into the pulmonary artery (40–45cm) and continue advancing until a 'wedged' trace is seen.
- Deflate balloon and continually monitor waveform thereafter to ensure catheter tip does not migrate forward and 'wedge', causing a pulmonary infarct if allowed to persist.

Complications

- Pulmonary artery rupture/perforation.
- Rupture of the right atrium.
- Air embolism.
- Ventricular arrhythmias.
- Pulmonary artery infarction.
- Valvular damage.
- Central venous insertion complications (see ▢ Central venous pressure, p. 104).
- Knotting of the catheter.
- Infection.

Normal values

- Stroke volume (SV) 70–100ml.
- Cardiac output (CO) 4–6l/min.
- Right ventricular pressure 20–25/0–5mmHg.
- Pulmonary pressure 20–25/10–15mmHg.
- Pulmonary artery wedge pressure (PAWP) 6–12mmHg.
- Mixed venous oxygen saturation 70–75%.

Removal

The catheter can be removed leaving the introducer *in situ*:

- Transfer all infusions to the side arm of the introducer or other cannulae.
- Disconnect cardiac output monitoring cables.
- Emergency defibrillation equipment should be available.

- Explain the procedure to the patient.
- Lay the patient supine to reduce risk of air embolism.
- Ensure the balloon is deflated and a PA trace is seen on the monitor.
- Unclip the sleeve adapter from the introducer sheath.
- Remove the dressing and cut sutures.
- While observing the ECG, gently withdraw the catheter.
- Ventricular arrhythmias can occur as the tip passes through the ventricle, if this occurs continue withdrawing the catheter as these will often terminate once it is removed.

Cardiac output: thermodilution

A technique utilizing the pulmonary artery catheter (or peripheral catheters) to measure cardiac output. A bolus (5 or 10ml) of cooled 5% glucose is injected through the proximal lumen of the catheter into the right atrium. The temperature change is detected by a thermister at the catheter tip. Cardiac output can be calculated by modification of the Hamilton-Stewart equation (incorporating the injectate volume, temperature, and specific heat of the injectate) from a temperature change curve generated by the computer as the bolus is injected.

Technique

• Set the computer constant for the volume and temperature of the injectate bolus used (10ml of ice-cold glucose provides the most accurate measure).
• Press 'start' button on computer.
• Inject smoothly over 2–3s.
• A temperature change curve will be generated on the monitor.
• Repeat at least twice more.
• Average three measurements that fall within 10% of each other. Reject values from curves that are irregular.

Potential errors

• Erroneous readings in septal defects, tricuspid regurgitation, leakage of injectate.
• Operator variability.

Disadvantages

• Non-continuous.
• Repeated measurements may result in considerable volumes of fluid being injected. Injectate volumes must be recorded in the fluid balance chart.

'Continuous' thermodilution cardiac output

Modified pulmonary artery catheters release frequent pulses of heat upstream at varying short time intervals. These are detected at the downstream thermister sited near the catheter tip. The data are computed into cardiac output values. Calibration can be performed against a bolus thermodilution measurement (see above). Values displayed are not 'continuous' as such, but represent an average of 2–7min data. Averaging takes longer during rapidly changing circulatory conditions, such as rapid haemorrhage. As with the bolus technique, similar errors are introduced in patients with tricuspid regurgitation and septal defects.

Table 5.2 Summary of problems associated with measuring cardiac output (CO)

Problem	Potential cause	Action
Difficulty injecting solution through proximal lumen	Proximal lumen occluded or kinked	Inform medical staff
	Catheter tip against wall of vessel	Unkink or replace catheter
		Reposition catheter
Blood temperature not displayed	Faulty thermistor. Fibrin growth on thermistor	Replace catheter
Injectate temperature not displayed	Faulty injectate temperature probe	Replace probe
Wide discrepancies in serial CO recordings	Inaccurate amounts of injectate drawn up	Ensure exact injectate volume is drawn up
	Poor technique (uneven injection)	Inject evenly and within 4s
	Arrhythmias (atrial fibrillation, ventricular ectopics)	Observe ECG, avoid injection during arrhythmias
	Valvular disease (tricuspid insufficiency) causing turbulent flow	Use alternative method for obtaining CO
	Patient movement during recordings	Limit patient movement during measurements
	Malfunction of CO computer	Replace computer
Inappropriately high values for CO	Incorrect injectate volume (usually too low or leaking connection)	Check correct volume to be used (5 or 10ml)
	Injectate temperature too low	Check temperature of injectate
	Incorrect computer constant	Check computer constant
	Poor injection technique	Inject evenly within 4s

Continued

Table 5.2 Summary of problems associated with measuring cardiac output (CO)—Cont'd

Problem	Potential cause	Action
Inappropriately low values for CO	Incorrect injectate volume (usually too much)	Ensure correct injectate volume
	Injectate temperature too high	Check temperature of injectate
		Do not hold barrel of syringe while injecting
	Start button pressed after beginning of injection	Press start button at the same time or just before beginning the injection
	Incorrect computer constant	Check computer constant
	Delivery of injectate longer than 4s	Ensure injection is within 4s
	Concomitant infusions at high flow rates (>150m/h) through distal lumen	If possible, turn off concomitant infusions during measurements

Reproduced with permission from *Critical Care Nursing*, Adam and Osborne (2005), Oxford University Press.

Cardiac output: peripheral dilution techniques

Dye dilution

Involves injection of a dye/chemical into the bloodstream (usually via a central venous line) and measuring the subsequent dilution after a designated time. Indocyanine green was traditionally used. Its dilution can be measured by a downstream densitometer or by repeated sampling of arterial blood. A time–concentration curve is constructed with a rapid upstroke and exponential decay. Plotting the dye decay curve semi-logarithmically and extrapolating values to the origin produces the cardiac output.

Lithium dilution

This uses the dye dilution method but the 'dye' used is lithium chloride (LiCl). Lithium chloride is injected as a bolus via the central venous catheter and an arterial plasma concentration curve is measured by a disposable sensor, housing a lithium-selective electrode. The voltage across the lithium-selective membrane is related by the Nernst equation to plasma $Li+$. A correction is applied for plasma sodium concentration.

Cardiac output is calculated by:

$$CO = (LiCl \ dose \times 60)/[area \times (1 - PCV)] \ l/min$$

where LiCl dose is in mmol, area is the integral primary curve, and PCV is packed cell volume. The haematocrit thus needs to be known.

The dose of lithium used is 1/300th of the therapeutic dose and should not cause adverse effects.

Cautions

- Measurements should be limited to 12/day.
- It should not be used in patients on lithium therapy.
- It cannot be used on patients being given non-depolarizing neuromuscular blocking agents as they interfere with the sensor.
- Similar issues to thermodilution apply with regard to erroneous measures (fluid leakage via loose connectors, tricuspid regurgitation, etc.).

Peripheral thermodilution

This uses the same principle as central thermodilution, but in this situation, a bolus of 5% glucose is injected via a central vein and temperature change is assessed in an artery. This usually requires a femoral artery catheter as doubts exist over the accuracy of measuring at more peripheral arterial sites, such as the radial artery.

Similar issues to central thermodilution techniques apply with regard to erroneous measures (fluid leakage, tricuspid regurgitation, etc.).

Cardiac output: Doppler ultrasound

Doppler ultrasound

An ultrasound beam is reflected by red blood cells, causing a frequency shift proportional to the blood flow velocity. The actual velocity can be calculated from the Doppler equation, which requires the cosine of the vector between the direction of the ultrasound beam and that of blood flow. For suprasternal and oesophageal approaches the vector is assumed to be 0° and 45°, respectively. Spectral analysis of the Doppler frequency shifts produces time-velocity waveforms, the area of which represents the 'stroke distance', i.e. the distance travelled by a column of blood with each left ventricular systole (see Fig. 5.8). The product of stroke distance and aortic cross-sectional area (measured by echocardiogram or assumed from nomograms) is stroke volume. It is quick, safe, and easy to perform, and can be measured suprasternally (intermittent readings) or via the oesophagus (continuous readings).

Cautions and relative contraindications for use

- During surgery when the aorta is cross-clamped.
- When an intra-aortic balloon is *in situ* (causes local turbulence).
- With aortic co-arctation.
- Patients who have oesophageal pathology.
- Recent surgery to the mouth/oesophagus/stomach.
- Severe bleeding disorders.
- Under epidural or spinal anaesthesia as the ratio of upper:lower blood flow will be altered from the normal 30:70 split.

Insertion of the oesophageal probe

- Explain procedure, ensure adequate sedation.
- Position patient appropriately.
- Apply lubricating gel to probe.
- Connect probe to monitor.
- Gently insert probe orally into the oesophagus until the patient's teeth are midway between the external depth markers (35–40cm from tip in normal height adult).
- Confirm position by achieving a correct descending aortic waveform trace – this should be sharp and well-defined on the monitor, and with the highest frequency signal audible through the loudspeaker.
- Secure to the endotracheal tube or catheter mount to prevent movement (avoid pressure from probe on lips).

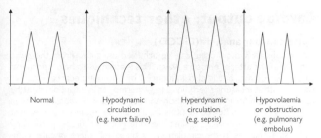

Fig. 5.8 Normal blood velocity profile of oesophageal Doppler. Reproduced with permission from *Critical Care Nursing*, Adam and Osborne (2005), Oxford University Press.

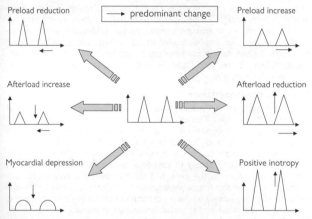

Fig. 5.9 Waveform responses to clinical interventions. Reproduced with permission from *Critical Care Nursing*, Adam and Osborne (2005), Oxford University Press.

Further information

Adam SK, Osborne S. (2005) *Critical Care Nursing*. Oxford: Oxford University Press.

Cardiac output: other techniques

Pulse contour analysis (PiCCO)

Continuous flow monitoring can be achieved using data from the pulse contour of the arterial pressure wave. This is assumed to be proportional to stroke volume, but is also influenced by aortic impedance. Another cardiac output measuring technique (e.g. thermo- or dye dilution) must be used in tandem for initial calibration and regular recalibration. It can then be used as a method of continuous cardiac output monitoring. Frequent re-calibration is necessary against the reference technique, particularly with rapid changes in the circulation, as these will affect vascular compliance and impedance. The arterial line must be non-obstructed with a good waveform.

Pressure waveform analysis

This new technique also measures cardiac output from the arterial pressure waveform using a proprietary formula, but it differs from the pulse contour techniques in that no cardiac output calibration is needed to another device. The arterial line must be non-obstructed with a good waveform. Its accuracy in cardiac output measurement needs to be validated in intensive care populations where arterial compliance and impedance can change rapidly.

Thoracic bio-impedance

Impedance changes originate in the thoracic aorta when blood is ejected from the left ventricle. This effect is used to determine stroke volume from formulae utilizing the electrical field size of the thorax, baseline thoracic impedance, and fluctuation related to systole and ventricular ejection time. A correction factor for sex, height, and weight is also introduced. The technique simply utilizes four pairs of electrodes placed in proscribed positions on the neck and thorax; these are connected to a dedicated monitor that measures thoracic impedance to a low amplitude, high (70KHz) frequency 2.5mA current applied across the electrodes. It is a quick, safe technique and reasonably accurate in normal, spontaneously breathing subjects. However, there can be significant discrepancies in critically ill patients, especially those with arrhythmias, tachycardias, intrathoracic fluid shifts, anatomical deformities, and aortic regurgitation, and if there is any metal within the thorax.

Respiratory monitoring

Pulse oximetry

This refers to continuous, non-invasive measurement of oxygen saturation in arterial blood (SpO_2). A probe is placed over a digit, earlobe, cheek, or the bridge of the nose. It emits light at two specific wavelengths – red and infrared. Light passes through the tissue and is sensed by a photodetector at the base of the probe. Most of the emitted light is absorbed by skin (including pigment), bone, connective tissue, and venous vessels (baseline measurement). This amount is constant so the only relevant fluctuations are caused by increases in blood flow during systole. The peaks and troughs of the pulsatile and baseline absorption for each wavelength are detected and the ratios of each compared. This provides the ratio of oxyhaemoglobin to total haemoglobin, i.e. the saturation. Pulse oximetry does not measure the oxygen content of the blood as this depends on how much haemoglobin is present. An anaemic patient may still have an oxygen saturation of 100%.

Accuracy

The accuracy is within 2% when measuring above 70% arterial O_2 saturation.

Certain conditions may make the readings inaccurate:
- The presence of dysfunctional haemoglobin, e.g. in smoke inhalation (raised carboxyhaemoglobin), drugs producing methaemoglobinaemia, and administration of certain dyes and pigments (such as methylene blue).
- Low peripheral perfusion.
- High levels of ambient light (sunlight, phototherapy, or surgical lamps).
- Strong-coloured nail varnish.
- Restrictive tape at probe site.
- Probe distal to blood pressure cuffs, iv infusions, arterial cannulae.

Care

- Attach securely.
- Ensure a clearly pulsatile waveform or bar is seen on the monitor.
- Set alarm limits.
- Change probe site regularly to avoid pressure necrosis. Older probes emitted more heat and could cause local burns.
- Check abnormal readings by blood gas analysis.

Capnography

Capnography is the measurement of carbon dioxide (CO_2) in each breath of the respiratory cycle. The capnograph continuously displays a waveform of CO_2 and displays the CO_2 value at end-exhalation – the end-tidal CO_2 ($ETCO_2$).

Capnography is used to assess the adequacy of ventilation, to detect oesophageal intubation (no/very little CO_2 is detected), to indicate disconnection from the ventilator, and to diagnose circulatory problems, such as pulmonary embolus (sudden fall in $ETCO_2$).

Method

Gas in the ventilator circuit can be sampled either by a sidestream or mainstream analyser. With sidestream analysis gas is drawn through narrow impermeable tubing connected near the patient end of the circuit to the capnograph. With mainstream analysis, the sample chamber is positioned within the patient's gas stream near the patient end of the circuit.

Most analysers work using infrared absorption spectroscopy, whereby gases of molecules containing at least two dissimilar atoms absorb infrared radiation. The amount of infrared radiation absorbed by CO_2 at a wavelength of 4.3mm is measured by a photodetector. By Beer–Lambert's law this is proportional to the number of CO_2 molecules in the chamber, i.e. the partial pressure of CO_2. Other techniques for measuring CO_2 include photo-acoustic spectrometry, Raman scattering, and mass spectrometry.

End-tidal carbon dioxide ($ETCO_2$)

The $ETCO_2$ approximates to $PaCO_2$ if there is cardiorespiratory stability and normothermia. It is not so reliable in patients with respiratory failure, as V–Q mismatch or significant air trapping (e.g. asthma) widens the gradient between arterial and $ETCO_2$ values.

A large difference between end-tidal and arterial pCO_2 may represent an increased dead space to tidal volume ratio, poor pulmonary perfusion, or intra-pulmonary shunting. A progressive rise in end-tidal pCO_2 may represent hypoventilation, airway obstruction, or increased CO_2 production due to an increase in metabolic rate.

The capnogram

There are four phases (see Fig. 6.1). If significant amounts of CO_2 are recorded in Phase 1 this implies rebreathing of exhaled gas. The commonest cause is failure of the expiratory valve to open during manual ventilation or an inadequate amount of fresh gas into the rebreathing bag. The slope of Phase 3 depends on the rate of alveolar gas exchange. A steep slope can indicate a V–Q mismatch. Alveoli that are poorly ventilated, but well perfused will discharge late in the respiratory cycle. A steep slope is seen in patients with significant auto-PEEP.

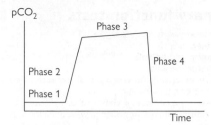

Fig. 6.1 The normal capnogram. Reproduced with permission from *Critical Care Nursing*, Singer and Webb (2005), Oxford University Press.

Phase 1

During the early part of the exhaled breath anatomical dead space and sampling device dead space gas are sampled. There is negligible CO_2 in phase 1.

Phase 2

As alveolar gas begins to be sampled there is a rapid rise in CO_2 concentration.

Phase 3

This is known as the alveolar plateau and represents the CO_2 concentration in mixed expired alveolar gas. There is normally a slight increase in pCO_2 during phase 3 as alveolar gas exchange continues during expiration. Airway obstruction or a high rate of CO_2 production will increase the slope. $ETCO_2$ will be less than the pCO_2 of ideal alveolar gas since the sampled exhaled gas is mixed with alveolar dead space gas.

Phase 4

As inspiration begins there is a rapid fall in sample pCO_2.

Further information

Singer M and Webb AR. (2005) *Critical Care Nursing*, 2nd edn. Oxford: Oxford University.

Pulmonary function tests

- **Arterial blood gases:** PaO_2, SaO_2, $PaCO_2$.
- **Pulse oximetry:** SpO_2.
- **Capnography:** end-tidal pCO_2.
- **Wright meter:** peak flow.
- **Spirometry, electronic flowmetry:** peak expiratory flow rate, FEV_1, FVC, vital capacity, tidal volume.
- **Pressure–volume curve:** lung/chest wall compliance.
- **Pneumotachograph, manometry:** flow–volume loop, pressure–volume loop.

Lung volumes

- **Tidal volume (V_T):** volume of air that will move in or out of the lungs in a normal breath. Normal range 5–9ml/kg.
- **Minute volume (MV):** volume of air that will move in and out of the lung in 1min. Normal range $5–9/kg \times 12 = 5–6l$ ($V_T \times$ respiratory rate).
- **Vital capacity (VC):** maximum volume of gas exhaled after a maximum inspiration. Normal range 3000–4800ml.
- **Anatomical dead space:** volume of gas filling conducting airways (nose to lower airways but not bronchioles). Normal value 2ml/kg.
- **Functional residual capacity (FRC):** volume of air remaining in the lungs after normal exhalation. Normal range 1800–2400 ml.

Compliance

Compliance equals the change in pressure during a linear increase of 1l in volume above FRC. It is decreased by:

- Pulmonary congestion.
- Pulmonary vascular constriction.
- Increased surface tension.
- Pulmonary fibrosis, infiltration, or atelectasis.
- Pleural fibrosis.

Increased by:

- Pulmonary oligaemia.
- Decreased pulmonary smooth muscle tone.
- Augmented surfactant release.
- Destruction of lung tissue (e.g. emphysema).

Ventilation/perfusion match

The relationship between pulmonary capillary perfusion (Q) and alveolar ventilation (V).

These equations allow estimation of ventilation/perfusion mismatch:

- **V/Q = 1:** ventilation and perfusion are well-matched.
- **V/Q > 1:** increased dead space (where alveoli are poorly perfused, but well ventilated).
- **V/Q < 1:** increased venous admixture or shunt (where alveoli are perfused, but poorly ventilated).

Blood gas analysis

The blood gas analyser

A sample of blood (arterial, venous, or capillary) is injected into or aspirated by the machine for measurement of gas tensions and acid-base status. The machine contains three electrodes that measure pH, pO_2, and pCO_2. Bicarbonate values are calculated by the Henderson–Hasselbach equation. Actual base excess (deficit), standard base excess (deficit), standard bicarbonate values, and oxygen saturation are also derived. Blood gas values can be given as 'pHstat' or 'alphastat'. The former corrects for body temperature, which is entered into the machine. A CO-oximeter, which uses at least five wavelengths of light, which may be incorporated into the device, can also calculate total and foetal Hb, carboxyHb, metHb, and sulph-Hb (Table 6.1).

Taking the sample

- Use a 1 or 2ml syringe that may be pre-heparinized, or requires addition of heparin 1000 IU/ml solution to just fill the hub. Too much heparin may give an excessively acidic reading.
- After taking the sample (0.5ml is adequate), expel any air bubbles, mix well, and insert into the blood gas analyser without delay.

Table 6.1 Normal values of arterial blood gases.

Property	Value
pH	7.35–7.45
PO_2	4.6–6.0kPa
PO_2	10.0–13.3kPa
HCO_3	22–26mmol/l
Base excess	−2 to +2
O_2 saturation	>95%

Reproduced with permission from *Critical Care Nursing*, Adam and Osborne (2005), Oxford University Press.

Table 6.2 Alterations in different types of acidosis and alkalosis.

	pH	pCO_2	HCO_3
Acute respiratory acidosis	pH low	pCO_2 high	HCO_3 normal
Acute respiratory alkalosis	pH high	pCO_2 low	HCO_3 normal
Acute metabolic acidosis	pH low	pCO_2 normal or low	HCO_3 low
Acute metabolic alkalosis	pH high	pCO_2 normal	HCO_3 high

There may also be mixed or combined acidosis or alkalosis due to a combination of causes. Reproduced with permission from *Critical Care Nursing*, Adam and Osborne (2005), Oxford University Press.

Acid-base disturbances

- *Respiratory acidosis*: excess production and/or inadequate excretion of CO_2. Causes include:
  - obstructive lung disease;
  - over-sedation/other causes of respiratory depression;
  - neuromuscular disorders;
  - hypoventilation during mechanical ventilation;
  - pain, chest wall deformities, respiratory muscle fatigue.
- *Respiratory alkalosis*: reduction in pCO_2 due to hyperventilation. Causes include:
  - hypoxia;
  - anxiety states;
  - pulmonary embolus;
  - pregnancy;
  - hyperventilation during mechanical ventilation;
  - brain injury;
  - high salicylate levels;
  - fever;
  - asthma;
  - severe anaemia.
- *Metabolic acidosis*: excess acid/loss of base. Causes include:
  - uraemia;
  - acid ingestion (e.g. aspirin, ethylene glycol);
  - acid from abnormal metabolism (e.g. ketoacidosis);
  - hyperchloraemia (from excess n-saline/colloid administration);
  - lactic acidosis (exercise, shock, hypoxia, liver failure, trauma);
  - loss of alkali (diarrhoea, bowel fistula, renal tubular necrosis).
- *Metabolic alkalosis*: excess alkali or loss of acid. Causes include:
  - excess bicarbonate or buffer infusions;
  - loss of acid from large gastric aspirates or vomiting;
  - renal disorders;
  - hypokalaemia;
  - drugs (e.g. diuretics, ingestion of alkali).

Further information

Adam SK, Osborne S. (2005) *Critical Care Nursing*. Oxford: Oxford University Press.

Neurological monitoring

Neurological assessment

Observation

Clinical observation is the most sensitive measure of neurological function (Table 7.1).

Impaired consciousness is an expression of dysfunction of the brain as a whole and changes in conscious level provide the best indication of complications following brain injury.

Table 7.1 Clinical observation

Observation	Appearance	Possible causes
Conscious level	Reduced	• Neurological deterioration • Drug therapy • Uraemia • Metabolic causes • Hypoperfusion states
Behaviour	Restless, agitated, aggressive, confused	• Hypoxaemia • Sepsis • Neurological deterioration • Metabolic causes • Pain, discomfort • Need to open bowels • Full bladder or stomach • Haemorrhage • Reaction to the environment & illness • Drug therapy
Expression	Grimacing, worried	• Pain, discomfort, fear, anxiety

Neurological assessment

Includes:
• Assessment of conscious level.
• Limb assessment.
• Pupil size and reaction to light.
• Vital signs.

Assessment of conscious level

The Glasgow Coma Score defines conscious level in terms of 3 modes of behaviour: eye opening, verbal, and motor response. Each category assesses responses to different stimuli. An increasing stimulus required to elicit a response indicates a falling level of cerebral functioning. Each response is given a score ranging from 3 to 15.

Table 7.2 The Glasgow Coma Score

Eye opening	Score	Verbal response	Score	Motor response	Score
Spontaneous	4	Orientated	5	Obeys commands	6
To speech	3	Confused	4	Localizes to pain	5
To pain	2	Inappropriate words	3	Flexes to pain	4
None	1	Incomprehensible sounds	2	Abnormal flexion	3
		None	1	Extension	2
				Bone	1

Limb assessment
A difference in responsiveness in one limb indicates focal brain damage or nerve injury. Hemiparesis or hemiplegia usually affects the limbs on the opposite side to the lesion. However, it may also affect the limbs on the same side as the lesion due to pressure on the contralateral hemisphere.

Pupillary response
This depends upon intact optic and oculomotor nerves. A dilating pupil indicates an expanding lesion on the same side. The presence or absence of the light reflex is the single most important sign distinguishing structural from metabolic coma.
- Pupils should be assessed for size, shape, equality, and reaction to light.
- Muscle relaxants do not affect pupil reaction. In the paralysed, ventilated patient, this is an important but late clinical sign of raised ICP.
- Damage to the cervical cord or brachial plexus can cause inequality of the pupil due to Horner's syndrome (pupillary constriction, sunken eye, ipsilateral loss of sweating due to interruption of the sympathetic supply to the pupil).

Temperature
Temperature regulation may be disrupted due to damage to the hypothalamus. Hyperthermia may exacerbate cerebral ischaemia.

Electrocardiogram changes associated with neurological dysfunction
- Bradycardia: in the later stages of raised ICP or with associated cervical injury.
- Tachycardia: in terminal stages of raised ICP.
- Arrhythmias: in posterior fossa lesions or where there is blood in the CSF. Also peaked P waves, heightened T waves, prolonged QT interval, S–T elevation/depression can occur.

Blood pressure

The brain is usually protected from changes in BP by autoregulation, but this may be impaired following cerebral insult allowing further damage to occur.

• Hypertension (+ bradycardia) is associated with a rising ICP (+ widening pulse pressure).
• Hypotension (+ bradycardia) is associated with cervical injury.
• Hypotension (+ tachycardia) may indicate extracranial haemorrhage.
• Hypotension alone is rarely attributable to cerebral injury except in children.

Respiration

A rise in ICP will decrease respiratory rate. Respiratory support is often required.

Intracranial pressure (ICP) monitoring

ICP is the CSF pressure within the lateral ventricles. Normal adult ICP is <10mmHg. ICP 20–25mmHg is usually treated in head injury. There may be sustained rises in ICP to 50–100mmHg lasting 5–10min. These may increase in frequency as the baseline ICP rises. This is associated with a 60% mortality. Cerebral perfusion pressure (CPP) is the difference between mean BP and mean ICP. Treatment aimed at reducing ICP may also reduce mean BP. CPP should be maintained >50–60mmHg.

Uses of intracranial pressure monitoring

- To confirm the diagnosis of raised intracranial pressure.
- To monitor treatment.
- To allow measurement of CPP and estimation of cerebral blood flow.
- In cases of severe head injury, particularly if mechanically ventilated, GCS <8 and/or abnormal CT scan.
- Post-neurosurgery.

Types of intracranial pressure monitoring

ICP can be measured using a subdural, intraparenchymal, or intraventricular catheter. The catheter is inserted via a burr hole, and is either connected to a pressure transducer or can admit a fibre optic pressure monitoring device. Calibration and patency testing must be performed regularly.

Subdural monitoring

The dura is opened and a hollow bolt inserted into the skull. It is easier to insert than ventricular monitors, but tends to under estimate ICP.

Intraventricular monitoring

The catheter is inserted into the lateral ventricle. CSF may be drained via the catheter to reduce ICP.

Complications

- Infection (particularly after 5 days).
- Haemorrhage.

Jugular venous bulb oximetry

Jugular venous bulb saturation can be measured by placing a sampling catheter in the internal jugular vein, directed upwards, so that the tip rests in the jugular vein bulb at the base of the brain. Blood samples taken at this point measure the mixed venous oxygen saturation (SjO_2) of blood leaving the brain.

$SjvO_2$ management

Normal values are 50–75% in the absence of anaemia. $SjvO_2$ falls when there is an imbalance between oxygen delivery and consumption.

When SaO_2 values are normal, values of $SjvO_2$ of:
- <50% imply a fall in cerebral blood flow (CBF) or a rise in oxygen consumption.
- >85% imply hyperaemia with a rise in CBF, shunting of blood away from the neurons or impending cell/brain death. It is usually associated with increased cerebral lactate production.

Troubleshooting

Erroneous readings can occur:
- If the catheter is sited too low in the jugular bulb (due to mixing of intracerebral and extracerebral venous blood).
- If the light intensity reading is too high (the catheter may be abutting against a vessel wall).
- If the light intensity reading is too low (the catheter may not be patent or have a small clot over the tip).

Electrocardiogram, Bispectral Index, cerebral function monitor, and transcranial Doppler monitoring

Electroencephalogram (EEG)

Currents generated by the combined synaptic activity of neurons in the cerebral cortex give rise to electrical activity that can be recorded directly from the scalp using surface or needle electrodes.

Uses

- To monitor cerebral ischaemia intra-operatively.
- To confirm the diagnosis of epilepsy.
- To monitor seizure activity in patients with status epilepticus under the effects of muscle relaxants.
- To predict the outcome of coma.
- As an ancillary tool for the confirmation of brain death.

Bispectral index monitor (BIS)

This uses a processed EEG parameter to provide a direct means of measuring the effects of anaesthetic and sedative agents on the brain. A sensor on the forehead captures the EEG signals, which are translated into a single number ranging from 100 (wide awake) to 0 (absence of brain electrical activity). Usual levels during anaesthesia are 30–40 and during sedation 50–70. It may be useful for titrating sedation in patients receiving muscle relaxant infusions and patients with status epilepticus, where subclinical seizures can be detected and therapy titrated against the BIS value.

Cerebral function monitor (CFM)

A device for monitoring background neurological activity using 2–3 needle electrodes to obtain an EEG signal. The signal is filtered and the output displayed on a chart. This output is a representation of the overall endo-cortical activity of the brain. A high reading indicates a high level of activity, and a low reading low activity.

Drugs such as anticonvulsants and sedatives may transiently suppress the CFM record, and administration must be recorded on the chart.

Periods of increasingly prolonged electrical silence (burst suppression) may provide an early warning of cerebral ischaemia. Seizure activity may also be detected in patients, despite apparently adequate clinical control or where muscle relaxants have been used.

Transcranial Doppler (TCD) ultrasound

A non-invasive method of assessing the intracranial circulation by measuring the velocity of blood flow in the middle, anterior, or posterior cerebral arteries, the ophthalmic artery or internal carotid. Vascular spasm leads to an increase in flow velocity Doppler waveform analysis and can give information about the state of blood flow (acceleration and pulsatile index). TCD can be used in patients with intracranial hypertension where cerebral perfusion pressure cannot be maintained by standard therapy.

Electroencephalogram, Bispectral Index, cerebral function monitor, and transcranial Doppler monitoring

Electroencephalogram (EEG)

Uses

Bispectral Index (BIS)

Cerebral function monitor (CFM)

Transcranial Doppler (TCD) ultrasound

Laboratory monitoring

Electrolytes (Na^+, K^+, Cl^-, HCO_3^-)

Electrolytes are measured from plasma or urine samples by direct-reading ion-specific electrodes.

Causes of hypernatraemia: H_2O and Cl^- usually retained
- Excessive intake of NaCl.
- Fluid loss without water replacement.
- Diabetes insipidus.
- Osmotic diuresis.
- Primary or secondary hyperaldosteronism.
- Chronic renal failure.

Causes of hyponatraemia: H_2O and Cl^- usually in deficit
- Excessive sweating.
- Burns.
- Loss via gut (e.g. diarrhoea, fistulae).
- Small bowel obstruction.
- Diabetes mellitus (causing an osmotic diuresis).
- Excessive diuretic therapy.
- Inappropriate ADH secretion syndrome (e.g. due to malignancy, neurological disorders, metabolic disorders, drugs).
- Post-TURP syndrome.

Causes of hyperkalaemia
- Acute/chronic renal failure – inadequate renal excretion.
- Potassium sparing drugs given in the presence of renal dysfunction (e.g. amiloride, spironolactone).
- Metabolic acidosis (e.g. diabetic ketoacidosis).
- Addison's disease.
- Sodium depletion.
- Severe tissue damage, e.g. rhabdomyolysis.
- Anorexia.
- Massive blood transfusion.
- Lithium toxicity.

Causes of hypokalaemia
- Prolonged vomiting.
- Severe diarrhoea/intestinal fistulae.
- Laxative or liquorice abuse.
- Thiazide and loop diuretics.
- Renal tubular failure.
- Steroid therapy.
- Hyperaldosteronism, Cushing's syndrome.
- Metabolic alkalosis.
- Ureterosigmoid anastomosis.
- Low potassium intake.

Chloride and bicarbonate

Levels vary with acid-base balance. In the kidney, Cl^- re-absorption is increased when HCO_3^- re-absorption is decreased and *vice versa*. Plasma chloride tends to vary inversely with plasma bicarbonate, keeping the total anion concentration normal. Hypochloraemia can be found in salt water drowning, but otherwise is rarely seen. Hyperchloraemia may be seen when large volumes of n-saline or saline-containing fluids, such as albumin or artificial colloids are given.

Normal plasma ranges

- Sodium: 135–145mmol/l.
- Potassium: 3.5–5.3mmol/l.
- Chloride: 95–115mmol/l.
- Bicarbonate: 23–28mmol/l.

Anion gap

The difference between serum anions (e.g. phosphate, protein, bicarbonate, sulphates, chloride) and cations (e.g. calcium, magnesium, potassium, sodium). The gap exists because more anions than cations are routinely unmeasured (normal range 8–16mmol/l).

Excess anions in the blood are buffered by bicarbonate, as well as Hb and albumin.

In metabolic acidosis with an elevated anion gap, extra unmeasured anions are added to the blood.

In metabolic acidosis with a normal anion gap, there is no gain of unmeasured anions because serum chloride replaces depleted bicarbonate. Hyperchloraemia develops as a result.

Calculated anion gap = plasma $[Na^+] + [K^+] - [HCO_3\text{-}] - [Cl^-]$

Causes of metabolic acidosis with an increased anion gap
- Ingestion of acid (e.g. aspirin, ethylene glycol, methanol).
- Renal failure.
- Ketoacidosis (diabetes mellitus, starvation, alcohol).
- Hyperlactataemia (e.g. exercise, shock, hypoxia, liver failure, trauma).

Causes of metabolic acidosis with a normal anion gap
- Failure to excrete acid (e.g. renal tubular disease, Addison's disease).
- Loss of base (e.g. diarrhoea, proximal renal tubular acidosis, acetazolamide, ureterosigmoidostomy).

Urea and creatinine

Measured in blood, urine, and occasionally other fluids, such as abdominal drain fluid. These are commonly used as markers of renal function, although estimated glomerular filtration rate (GFR) is now also available.

Urea

A product of the urea cycle resulting from ammonia breakdown, it depends upon adequate liver function for its synthesis and adequate renal function for its excretion. Low levels are seen in cirrhosis and high levels in renal failure. Uraemia is a clinical syndrome including lethargy, drowsiness, confusion, pruritus, and pericarditis, resulting from high plasma levels of urea and other waste products, such as ammonia. Urea levels can be high without decreased GFR with increased catabolism, dehydration, and increased protein intake

The ratio of urine urea to plasma urea may be useful in distinguishing oliguria of renal or pre-renal origins. Higher ratios (>10:1) are seen in pre-renal conditions (e.g. hypovolaemia), whereas low levels (<4:1) occur with direct renal causes.

Creatinine

A product of creatinine breakdown, it is predominantly derived from skeletal muscle and is renally excreted.

Causes of low levels
- Malnutrition and chronic wasting diseases.
- Extremes of age.
- Alcoholism.

Causes of high levels
- Rhabdomyolysis (muscle breakdown).
- Renal failure.

The usual ratio for plasma urea (mmol/l) to creatinine (μmol/l) is approximately 1:10. A lower ratio in a critically ill patient suggests rhabdomyolysis, whereas higher ratios are seen in cirrhosis, malnutrition, liver failure, and hypovolaemia. The ratio also may help distinguish between oliguria of renal or pre-renal origins. Higher ratios (>40) are seen in pre-renal conditions and low levels (<20) with direct renal causes.

Creatinine clearance

This is a measure of glomerular filtration. Once filtered by the kidney, only small amounts of creatinine are re-absorbed. Normal values are >100ml/min.

To measure creatinine clearance, urine is collected over 24h. A sample for plasma creatinine is taken once during this period.

Substituting the results in the following equation, where Cr = creatinine:

$$[\text{plasma Cr}] \times \text{Cr clearance} = \text{urine Cr} \times \text{urine flow rate}$$

It can be unreliable if not all the urine is collected, if renal function is unstable, or the patient is very obese or oedematous.

Urea and creatinine

Normal plasma range

- Urea: 2.5–6.5mmol/l.
- Creatinine: 70–120μmol/l (depends on lean body mass).

Calcium and magnesium

Calcium

About 40% of plasma calcium is bound to albumin, although this can vary. Traditionally, calcium levels have been corrected to plasma albumin levels, but this is now considered irrelevant, particularly at the low albumin levels seen in the critically ill. Measuring the ionized fraction is now considered more important, since this fraction is responsible for the extracellular actions of calcium. Changes in ionized fraction causes the symptoms related to high and low calcium levels.

Causes of hypercalcaemia
- Hyperparathyroidism.
- Sarcoidosis.
- Malignancy (e.g. myeloma, bone metastases).
- Prolonged immobility.

Causes of hypocalcaemia
- Severe pancreatitis.
- Chronic renal failure.
- Hypoparathyroidism.
- Osteomalacia.
- Over-hydration.
- Hypomagnesaemia.
- Rhabdomyolysis.

Magnesium

Plasma levels poorly reflect intracellular or whole body stores, 65% of which is in bone and 35% in cells. The ionized fraction is approximately 50% of the total level. Supranormal plasma levels are often targeted when administered for treatment of ventricular and supraventricular arrhythmias, eclampsia, seizures, asthma, and after myocardial infarction.

Causes of hypermagnesaemia
- Renal failure.
- Excessive administration of magnesium.

Causes of hypomagnesaemia
- Severe diarrhoea.
- Diabetic ketoacidosis.
- Alcohol abuse.
- Accompanying hypocalcaemia and hypokalaemia.
- Diuretic therapy.

Calcium and magnesium

Normal plasma values
Calcium: 2.2–2.6mmol/l.
Ionized calcium: 1.05–1.2mmol/l.
Magnesium: 0.7–1.0mmol/l.

Full blood count

Haemoglobin

A low haemoglobin (anaemia) may be due to reduced cell mass (resulting from decreased production or shortened survival), or to haemodilution by excess fluid where anaemia is seen despite a normal total circulating red cell and Hb mass. Following major blood loss there may be no apparent anaemia as total blood volume is reduced. When the circulating volume is repleted with non-blood fluids, the anaemia becomes apparent.

A raised Hb (polycythaemia) can be primary (polycythaemia vera) or secondary (chronic hypoxaemia, inappropriate erythropoietin, over-transfusion, contracted circulating volume).

White blood cells

A raised and lowered white cell count is common in critical illness.

Neutrophils
- Barrier nursing is usually instituted if the patient is neutropenic (< 0.5 × 10^9/l).
- **Decreased in:** sepsis (especially in elderly and children), viral infections, brucellosis, typhoid, TB, drugs (e.g. carbimazole, sulphonamides, chemotherapy).
- **Increased in:** inflammatory conditions (e.g. bacterial infections, trauma, surgery, burns, haemorrhage), disseminated malignancy, infarction, drugs (e.g. steroids), myeloproliferative disorders, myeloid leukaemias.

Lymphocytes
- **Decreased in:** steroid therapy, AIDS, marrow infiltration, post-chemotherapy or radiotherapy, SLE, uraemia, Legionnaire's disease.
- **Increased in:** viral infections (e.g. CMV, rubella), whooping cough, toxoplasmosis, lymphatic leukaemia.

Monocytes
Increased in acute and chronic infections, malignant disease, chronic inflammation.

Eosinophils
Increased in: asthma and allergic disorders, parasitic infections, skin disease (e.g. pemphigus), urticaria, eczema, malignant disease, irradiation, during the convalescent phase of any infection.

Basophils
Increased in: viral infection, urticaria, myxoedema, post-splenectomy, malignancy, haemolysis.

Normal values
- Haemoglobin: 13–17g/dl (men), 12–16g/dl (women).
- White cell count: 4–11 × 10^9/l.
- Neutrophils: 2-7.5 × 10^9/l.
- Lymphocytes: 1.3-3.5 × 10^9/l.

- Eosinophils: $0.04–0.44 \times 10^9$/l.
- Basophils: $0-0.01 \times 10^9$/l.
- Monocytes: $0.2–0.8 \times 10^9$/l.
- Platelets: $150–400 \times 10^9$/l.

Platelets

Spontaneous bleeding is more likely with platelet counts $<20 \times 10^9$/l. Platelet cover is required prior to procedures to raise counts $>50 \times 10^9$/l.

Causes of a decreased platelet count (thrombocytopenia)

- Infection.
- Haemorrhage.
- Disseminated intravascular coagulation.
- Bone marrow failure.
- Vitamin B_{12}/folate deficiency.
- Heparin ('HITS' – heparin-induced thrombocytopenia syndrome).
- Idiopathic thrombocytopenia purpura (ITP).
- Thrombotic thrombocytopenic purpura (TTP).
- Haemolytic uraemic syndrome (HUS).
- Hypersplenism.

Causes of a raised platelet count

- Post-splenectomy.
- Chronic iron deficiency.
- Chronic infections.
- Malignancy.
- Rheumatoid arthritis.
- Essential thrombocythaemia – rare; counts may reach $>1000 \times 10^9$/l.

Cardiac injury markers

The diagnosis of myocardial infarction is defined as a typical rise and fall in troponin, or a more rapid rise and fall in CK-MB with at least one of the following:
- Ischaemic symptoms (chest pain).
- Development of pathological Q waves on ECG.
- ECG S–T elevation or depression.
- Coronary intervention.

Troponins

These are structural protein components of muscle. Troponins T and I are only found in cardiac muscle and are released following myocardial injury. Troponin I rises after 3–6h and peaks at about 20h. At 12h sensitivity is generally good enough to exclude myocardial infarction if no rise in troponin level is seen.

Both troponins remain elevated for a much longer time than CK, AST, or LDH (see below). Troponin I is detectable in blood for up to 5 days and troponin T for 7–10 days following myocardial infarction. Marked elevation in troponin can also occur with sepsis, myocarditis, cardiac failure, cardiac trauma (e.g. surgery, road traffic accidents), coronary artery spasm from cocaine, and pulmonary embolism. As troponins are renally excreted, levels are raised in renal failure.

Cardiac enzymes

Creatinine kinase (CK) is detectable in plasma within hours of myocardial injury. The cardiac specific form (CK-MB) can be measured if there is concurrent skeletal muscle injury. Aspartate transaminase (AST) is released 1–3 days' post-cardiac injury. Both CK and AST peak at 24h and fall over 2–3 days. Lactate dehydrogenase (LDH) is released 2–10h post-injury and peaks at 3 days. Red blood cells contain LDH so any cause of haemolysis can give false positive results.

Brain (or B-type) natri-uretic peptide (BNP)

Cardiomyocytes produce and secrete cardiac natri-uretic peptides. High levels are predominantly associated with heart failure and increase in relation to severity. Various commercial assays are available, each with their own diagnostic range. They are useful as a screening tool for patients presenting with dyspnoea, for prognostication, and for titration of therapy. Levels rise in sepsis (due to myocardial depression), the elderly, in renal failure, and in pulmonary diseases causing right ventricular overload (e.g. pulmonary embolus).

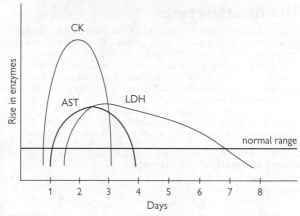

Fig. 8.1 Temporal change in cardiac enzymes. Reproduced with permission from *Critical Care Nursing*, Adam and Osborne (2005), Oxford University Press.

Further reading

Adam SK, Osborne S. (2005) *Critical Care Nursing*. Oxford: Oxford University Press.

Liver function tests

Bilirubin is formed from the breakdown of haemoglobin and is conjugated with glucuronide by the liver. If there is excess bilirubin in the circulation due to haemolysis (or failure of uptake or conjugation), some unconjugated bilirubin remains in the circulation. Unconjugated bilirubin is lipid soluble and does not appear in the urine. Conjugated bilirubin normally passes into the gut where intestinal flora convert it to urobilinogen. Some of this is absorbed and appears in the urine, since it is water-soluble. The rest is converted to stercobilin, which colours the faeces brown. If the common bile duct is blocked, plasma-conjugated bilirubin rises. Some is excreted in the urine making it dark, while less bilirubin passes into the gut making the faeces pale.

Markers of hepatocellular damage
- Alaninine aminotransferase (ALT).
- Aspartate aminotransferase (AST).
- Lactate dehydrogenase (LDH).

ALT is more liver-specific, but is also raised in shock states. AST is elevated in myocardial infarction and skeletal muscle damage. LDH is raised in kidney and blood diseases. Very high values of aminotransferases are suggestive of viral hepatitis or toxic damage.

Markers of obstruction (cholestasis)
- Bilirubin.
- Alkaline phosphatise.
- Gamma-glutamyl transferase (γ-GT).

Jaundice is detected when bilirubin >45μmol/l. Alkaline phosphatase is greatly elevated in obstructive jaundice, but is also released from bone, liver, intestine, and placenta. A raised level in the absence of other signs of liver disease or pregnancy suggests malignant secondary deposits in the liver (or bone), or Paget's disease. A raised γ-GT is a sensitive marker of hepatobiliary disease. Increased synthesis is also induced by alcohol, various drugs (e.g. phenytoin) and toxins, and acute and chronic hepatic inflammation.

Markers of reduced synthetic function
- Albumin.
- Clotting factors.

Plasma albumin and concentrations of the clotting factors II, VII, IX, and X (readily detectable as a prolonged INR or PT) are reduced in long-standing liver disease. Albumin levels are also often low in critical illness due to protein catabolism, capillary leak, decreased synthesis, and dilution with artificial colloids.

Normal values

- Albumin: 35–53g/l.
- Bilirubin: 3–17μmol/l.
- Conjugated bilirubin: 0–6μmol/l.
- Alanine aminotransferase (ALT): 5–50U/l.
- Alkaline phosphatase (ALP): 100–280U/l.
- Aspartate aminotransferase (AST): 11–55U/l.
- γ-glutamyl-transferase (γ-GT): 5–37U/l.
- Lactate dehydrogenase: 230–460U/l.

Coagulation monitoring

Basic coagulation screen

Blood should ideally be taken by venepuncture, rather than via an arterial catheter to avoid dilution and contamination by heparin. Ensure samples are placed in the correct bottles.

The basic screen consists of:
- Platelet count.
- Prothrombin time (PT).
- Activated partial thromboplastin time (APTT).
- Thrombin time (TT).

Prothrombin time: tests the extrinsic system and is the time taken for the patient's citrated blood to clot when tissue factor and calcium are added. Measures deficiencies of factors V, VII, X, prothrombin, and fibrinogen. The international normalized ratio (INR) relates the PT to control and is normally 1.0. It is prolonged in liver disease, vitamin K deficiency, and warfarin anticoagulant therapy.

Activated partial thromboplastin time: evaluates the intrinsic and common pathways. It is prolonged with heparin therapy, DIC, severe fibrinolysis, deficiency of factors VII, IX, XI, or XII in the intrinsic pathway, or deficiency of factors II, V, or X in the common pathway.

Thrombin time: assesses conversion of fibrinogen to fibrin. Prolonged levels are due to inhibition of fibrin formation and indicate the presence of FDPs (see below).

Specific tests

Fibrinogen degradation products (FDPs) and D-dimers: fibrin fragments released by plasmin lysis. Measured in the critically ill to confirm disseminated intravascular coagulation (DIC). A level of 20–40µg/ml is common post-operatively, in sepsis, trauma, renal failure and DVT. Assay of the D-dimer fragment is more specific for fibrinolysis (e.g. in DIC), since it is only released when fibrin is formed.

Activated clotting time: predominantly tests the intrinsic pathway. It is prolonged with heparin therapy, thrombocytopenia, hypothermia, haemodilution, fibrinolysis and high dose aprotinin. The normal range is between 100 and 140s.

Coagulation factor assays: available for all coagulation factors and used to diagnose specific defects. It is the most specific method of controlling low molecular weight heparin therapy as heparins inhibit factor Xa activity.

Normal values

- Platelets: 150–400 × 109/l.
- Prothrombin time: 12.3–16.1s.
- APTT: 27.4–40.3s
- Thrombin time: control +/–3s.
- INR: 1–1.2.

Microbiology

At least 10–15% of critical care patients develop nosocomial (hospital-acquired) infection. Take samples from the suspected site, and from blood, urine, sputum, CSF, and drainage fluids as indicated. In-dwelling intravascular catheters may require removal ± replacement and the tips sent for culture. In some critical care units routine screening (usually for MRSA) is performed, e.g. from axilla and perineum. New techniques allow for more rapid identification of the presence of organisms via antigen testing (e.g. *Pneumococcus, Legionella*) or molecular DNA methods (e.g. PCR)

Taking samples

- Send samples promptly to the laboratory in correct container and medium.
- Always wear gloves when handling or taking specimens.
- Use a sterile technique.
- Correctly label the specimen.
- Ensure date and time of sampling is written on the form.

Sputum

Often contaminated by upper respiratory tract organisms. Samples from intubated patients can be taken into a sputum trap inserted into the suction catheter circuit. Samples can also be taken via blind or directed (bronchoscopic) bronchoalveolar lavage, or using a protected catheter brush. Take blood cultures if pneumonia is suspected. Wear eye protection if a closed circuit catheter system is not used.

Urine

Samples can be taken from the urinary catheter by a small gauge needle through a sampling port, which should be first cleaned using a sterile alcohol wipe. The sample can be examined microscopically for organisms, casts, and crystals, plated onto culture medium with a calibrated loop, and incubated for 18–24h prior to examination. The tips of removed urinary catheters are not sent to the laboratory.

Blood cultures

Clean skin thoroughly with iodine or alcohol and allow to dry. Take 10–20 ml blood, and place in anaerobic and aerobic culture bottles. Take cultures from in-dwelling catheters if catheter-related sepsis is suspected. Interpret positive cultures in conjunction with patient status. Gram-negative or *S. aureus* isolates are usually taken as significant.

Intravascular cannulae tips for culture

Remove the cannula. Insert the end in transport medium and, using sterile scissors, cut off the remainder of the cannula.

Wound swabs

Swab the suspected area and place in transport medium. Swabs can be moistened in sterile normal saline first for dry wound sampling. Pus can also be aspirated from a wound and should be sent immediately to the laboratory.

Virology, serology, and assays

Viral and atypical antigen antibodies
A clotted blood specimen is taken for assay, and it is usual to send acute and convalescent (14 days) serum to determine if antibody titres are rising Single sample titres may be used to determine previous exposure and carrier status.

Viral culture
Most commonly used for CMV (cytomegalovirus). Samples of blood, urine, or bronchial aspirate may be sent for DEAFF testing (detection of early antigen fluorescent foci). Herpes virus infections may be detected by electron microscopy of samples (including pustule fluid) and adenovirus in immunosuppressed patients with a chest infection.

Human immunodeficiency virus (HIV)
HIV-positive status carries lifestyle consequences, and should ideally be assessed with prior counselling and consent. In the critically ill, such consent can rarely be obtained. Unconsented testing may be used where management may change significantly with knowledge of HIV status, or where organ donation is being considered. The viral load and/or CD4 count may be used to assess the likelihood of symptomatology being AIDS-related. The CD4 count falls with acute critical illness. High-risk patients should be considered for testing, e.g. homosexual males, iv drug abusers, haemophiliacs, African origin. Patients or staff who are recipients of a needlestick injury can be treated with anti-retroviral therapies if the donor is known to be HIV positive; unconsented testing is reasonable in this situation.

Hepatitis screening
Serology includes screening for hepatitis A, B, and C. There is a 10% carrier rate of hepatitis B in South East Asians and serology should be sent in all high risk patients, e.g. jaundice, iv drug abusers, homosexuals, prostitutes, those with tattoos or unexplained liver enzyme abnormalities. Hepatitis B surface antigen should be measured in staff who suffer accidental exposure to body fluids, e.g. through needlestick injury. Those who are not immune may be treated with immunoglobulin.

Fungi
Candida and *Aspergillus* can be assessed by culture ± antigen tests. Cryptococcus can be detected by Indian ink stain in biopsy samples.

Antibiotic assays
Usually performed for drugs with a narrow therapeutic range, such as aminoglycosides and vancomycin. It is unusual to request an assay on day 1 of treatment. Thereafter, samples are taken daily prior to giving a dose and at 1h after an intravenous injection or infusion.

Toxicology

- Samples can be taken from blood, urine, vomitus, or gastric lavage (depending on drug or poison ingested).
- Confirm with the biochemistry laboratory or local poisons unit as to which and when body fluid samples should be taken for analysis.
- Samples are taken in order to:
  - identifiy unknown toxic substances (e.g. cyanide, amphetamines, opiates) causing symptomatology and/or pathology (always take a urine sample for analysis);
  - confirm toxic plasma levels and monitor treatment effect, e.g. paracetamol, aspirin;
  - monitor therapeutic drug levels (usually plasma) and avoid toxicity, e.g. digoxin, aminoglycosides, lithium, phenytoin;
  - confirm the presence of a drug for medico-legal reasons, e.g. alcohol, recreational drugs following road traffic accidents/trauma.

Miscellaneous monitoring

Intra-abdominal pressure measurement

Usually measured via an indwelling urethral catheter, but also by:
• Transfemoral catheters in the inferior vena cava.
• Intraperitoneal catheters.
• Gastrostomy tubes.
• Nasogastric tubes.
• Intrarectally.

Measurement of intra-abdominal pressure (IAP), measurement via an urinary catheter

Measure 2–4-hourly according to clinical need. Note that abdominal compartment syndrome (see 📖 Complications following trauma, p. 428) cannot be totally excluded in the presence of a normal IAP, since bladder pressure may not capture elevated abdominal pressure within a localized area (Fig. 9.1).

Positioning of patient

• Place supine so the weight of abdominal contents does not press on bladder.
• If not possible, the position of the first measurement should be documented and subsequent recordings made in the same position.
• The transducer should be zeroed and level with the pubic symphysis.

Recording intra-abdominal pressure via an urinary catheter

• A 2- or 3-way Foley catheter should be *in situ*.
• The procedure is carried out aseptically, using sterile gloves.
• Place a sterile towel beneath the catheter connection.
• Clamp the drainage bag distal to the sampling port.
• Draw up 50ml sterile saline into a catheter syringe.
• Disconnect the drainage bag, inject the saline, and reconnect.
• Insert an 18-gauge needle attached to a transducer into the sampling port of the Foley catheter.
• Release the clamp momentarily until fluid fills the tubing and then reclamp.
• Allow the transducer to equilibrate and record the pressure.
• An alternative method is to insert a 3-way tap between the needle and transducer, and then inject the saline via the tap to avoid repeated disconnection of the drainage bag.
• The same method is used when measuring IAP via a nasogastric tube.

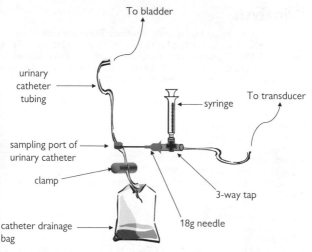

Fig. 9.1 Measurement of intra-abdominal pressure. Reproduced with permission from *Critical Care Nursing*, Adam and Osborne (2005), Oxford University Press.

Table 9.1 Burch's grading system for abdominal compartment syndrome

Grade	Bladder pressure (cmH₂O)	Equivalent pressure (mmHg)	Treatment strategy
I	10–15	7–11	Monitor only
II	15–25	11–18	Treatment based on clinical condition
III	25–30	18–26	Most will require compression
IV	>35	>26	All require decompression

Reproduced with permission from *Critical Care Nursing*, Adam and Osborne (2005), Oxford University Press.

Further information

Adam SK, Osborne S. (2005) *Critical Care Nursing*. Oxford: Oxford University Press.

Urinalysis

Urine can be routinely tested using dipsticks. These are read manually against a reference chart within 15s to 2min of dipping in the urine. Tests include pH, blood, protein, glucose, ketones, specific gravity, and white cells. Specific gravity can also be measured with a gravimeter. Mid-stream urine specimens can be sent to the laboratory for:

- Potassium.
- Sodium.
- Osmolality.
- Urea, creatinine, nitrogen.
- Protein, micro-albumin.
- Myoglobin.
- Neutrophils.
- Drugs and poisons (sent to Poisons Reference Laboratory).
- Antigens, e.g. Legionnaires' disease, *Pneumococcus*.
- Bacteria.
- TB.
- Blood (haematuria).
- Granular casts.
- Malignant cells.
- Some tests (e.g. urine:plasma ratios of urea, creatinine, and osmolality) are performed in conjunction with a blood test. 24h urine collections (with a matched blood sample) can be sent for 24h creatinine clearance, although some critical care units use 'spot' creatinine clearance measurements.

Colour

Certain excretory products can change urine colour from the normal pale straw colour, e.g.:

- **Red:** haemoglobin, blood, or myoglobinuria, rifampicin therapy
- **Orange:** concentrated urine, bile
- **Green/blue:** drugs, e.g. propofol, methylthioninium chloride (methylene blue)
- **Cloudy:** urate, phosphate, white blood cells, bacteria
- **Pale:** excessive diuresis, chronic renal failure.

Lactate

Biochemistry

Pyruvate is the end product of glycolysis, the metabolism of glucose. Most pyruvate is then metabolized to acetyl CoA, the major substrate for the Krebs' cycle that feeds electrons to the electron transport chain for eventual generation of ATP. The remaining pyruvate is in equilibrium with lactate (via the enzyme lactate dehydrogenase). In mitochondrial dysfunction (e.g. hypoxia, sepsis), less pyruvate is used, so more is converted to lactate. Lactate is a buffer so a high blood lactate does not automatically imply a lactic acidosis. In renal replacement therapy the replacement fluid is usually buffered with lactate so blood levels may rise without acidosis being present.

Measurement

Bedside analysers can rapidly measure blood lactate. Venous or arterial blood can be used. A blood sample can also be collected in a heparin fluoride tube (to prevent coagulation) and sent to the laboratory for measurement. The normal arterial blood lactate concentration is <1.5mmol/l.

Lactic acidosis

This occurs when production of lactic acid is in excess of its removal. The major sources are skeletal muscle, brain, gut, and red blood cells. Removal is mainly by metabolism to glucose in the liver and kidney. Liver removal is impaired in cirrhosis and by poor perfusion.

Lactic acidosis is traditionally classified as type A or type B. Type A occurs when inadequate tissue oxygenation causes excess production. A severe and persistent type A lactic acidosis is associated with a poor prognosis. Calculation of DO_2 may confirm inadequate tissue oxygen delivery, but a normal DO_2 does not guarantee adequacy of supply.

Type B occurs when there is no systemic tissue hypoxia, and is usually related to drugs or poisons that interfere with mitochondrial respiration. Examples include some anti-retroviral HIV therapy, metformin, cyanide, and carbon monoxide poisoning..

Adrenaline (epinephrine) therapy can also cause hyperlactataemia by stimulating release of lactate from skeletal muscle. This accelerated 'aerobic' glycolysis often occurs in the absence of tissue hypoxia.. In sepsis, hyperlactataemia is mainly due to increased activity of the muscle Na+ pump and not to tissue hypoxia.

Temperature

Disposable probes or thermistors now supercede the use of mercury thermometers.

Sites of temperature monitoring include mouth, nasopharynx, aural canal, oesophagus, rectum, axilla, skin, and blood.

- Recording temperature of blood in the pulmonary artery (via a thermistor on the tip of a pulmonary artery catheter) is the most accurate measurement of core temperature.
- Rectal temperature recordings can be affected by heat-producing organisms in the bowel, cool blood returning from the legs, and the insulation effect of faeces.
- Axilla temperature is a poor measure of core temperature, but is the best location to measure muscle temperature (e.g. in malignant hyperthermia).
- Recording temperature in the aural canal is quick and simple, but can be affected by wax.
- When recording temperature in the oesophagus the probe must be positioned at the lower oesophagus. This provides a good measure of core temperature in hypothermic patients.
- Skin temperature (in correlation with core temperature) is useful to assess tissue perfusion (e.g. muscle/skin grafts).
- Toe-core temperature differences can be used to assess perfusion. The bigger the difference, the worse the peripheral perfusion. This may be due to a poor cardiac output or to an abnormal peripheral vasculature (e.g. excess constriction, peripheral vascular disease).

Bladder temperature measurement

Core temperature can be monitored by means of a sensor within an indwelling urinary catheter. The catheter, containing a thermistor at its tip, floats in the urine within the bladder and the urine temperature is continuously displayed on a bedside monitor.

Advantages
- Convenient.
- Safe.
- Reliable.
- Provides a good estimate of core temperature.
- Allows continuous measurement of body temperature.

Disadvantages
- Requires a special catheter and monitoring system.
- Additional cost.

Safety and reliability

- All monitoring devices are manufactured to specific standards and recommendations are given for the conditions of their use. It is important that these are adhered to in order to ensure the accuracy of information obtained.
- Most monitoring devices are powered by mains electricity and/or rechargeable battery units. The area surrounding the patient therefore often contains a large number of electrical items. Cables must be treated with care to avoid undue tension. Vital plugs, such as to the ventilator, should be easily identifiable. Care must be taken not to allow spillage of fluid on to plugs and sockets. Position equipment so that leads do not drape across the patient and ensure there is easy access around the bed area.
- Some items of monitoring equipment are heavy and care must be taken when attaching them to items, such as drip stands, in order to avoid breakage or harm to the patient or staff.
- Monitoring items should be placed in such a position that the nurse can see the visual displays at all times.
- If alarm systems are incorporated within the monitoring devices these must be used and the alarm limits set according to the patients condition. Alarm settings should be checked at the beginning of every shift and reviewed if the patient's condition changes.
- It is also imperative to clean monitoring equipment at the beginning of each shift to decrease the spread of bacteria. Micro-organisms can live for days even on cold surfaces.

Respiratory support: mechanical ventilation

Physiology overview: movement of gases I

Respiration supplies oxygen to tissues to support metabolism and removes the waste product of this process – carbon dioxide. It is inter-dependent with the circulation.

There are four components of the process:
- Movement of gases into and out of the body.
- Gas exchange across a membrane.
- Carriage of gases to and from the tissues.
- Metabolic process in the cell to produce energy.

Normal inspiration

Diaphragmatic and intercostal muscles contract pulling the diaphragm down and the anterior chest wall out, which expands the chest cavity. This increases lung volume creating a negative pressure (approximately 3 mmHg), which sucks air into the lung.

Normal expiration

Inspiratory muscles relax and the elastic lung tissues recoil to the neutral position forcing air out. This is a passive process.

Elasticity of lung tissue

This depends on 2 factors:
- **Alveolar surface tension:** this pulls the alveoli closed and resists expansion. Surfactant is secreted to reduce surface tension, but secretion can be affected by acidosis, hypoxia, hyperoxia, atelectasis, pulmonary oedema, acute respiratory distress syndrome (ARDS), etc. Reduced surfactant results in an increase in the work of breathing.
- **Elastic fibres of the lung itself:** these tend to contract and assist in forcing air out of the lung.

Work of breathing

This is the effort involved in moving a specified volume of air into and out of the lung.

Accessory muscles (see Table 10.1) are used to assist breathing during exercise or when work of breathing is increased.

It is affected by:
- Resistance to gas flow in the airways.
- Elasticity of the lung tissue.
- Obstruction to flow.
- Chest wall compliance.

These factors make up the respiratory system compliance.

Table 10.1 Accessory muscles of respiration used by patients in respiratory difficulty

Inspiratory	Expiratory
Pectorals, neck (scalene, sternocleidomastoid), trapezius, external intercostals	Diaphragm, abdominal, internal intercostals

Physiology overview: movement of gases II

Respiratory system compliance

This is the change in volume of the lung divided by the amount of pressure required to produce the volume change.

Large volume changes produced by small pressure changes signify a compliant lung.

Lung compliance consists of static and dynamic compliance.

Static compliance

This is the compliance of the lung itself without the compounding factors of resistance to gas flow and is measured at the end of a known volume inspiration with the airway occluded for 2s to achieve a plateau pressure.

$$Cst_{rs} = \Delta V/P \text{ (end inspiration occluded plateau pressure)}$$

where Cst_{rs} is static compliance of respiratory system, ΔV is tidal volume, and normal range is 60–100ml/cmH$_2$O

Dynamic compliance

This is the whole system compliance, including resistance to gas flow during a breath, and refers to the change in pressure from end inspiration to end expiration:

$$Cdyn_{rs} = \Delta V/(\text{end inspiratory pressure} - \text{end expiratory pressure})$$

where $Cdyn_{rs}$ = dynamic compliance of respiratory system.

In healthy lungs there is little difference between static and dynamic compliance. In patients with airway obstruction, dynamic compliance will decrease rapidly due to resistance to air flow without much change in static compliance (see Tables 10.2 and 10.3).

Table 10.2 Factors affecting compliance

Decreased lung compliance	Increased lung compliance
Pulmonary congestion	Pulmonary oligaemia (decreased blood volume)
Increased pulmonary smooth muscle tone	Decreased pulmonary smooth muscle tone
Increased alveolar surface tension	Augmented surfactant secretion
Pulmonary fibrosis, infiltration, or atelectasis	Destruction of lung tissue (e.g. emphysema)
Pleural fibrosis	

Table 10.3 Definitions of lung volumes for spontaneous respiration

Name	Definition	Range of normal
Tidal volume (VT)	Volume of air moving in and out a normal breath	5–9ml/kg
Minute volume (MV)	Volume of air moving in and out over 1 min (VT × respiratory rate)	5–6l
Vital capacity (VC)	Maximum volume of exhalation after maximum inhalation	3–4.8l
Functional residual capacity (FRC)	Volume of air remaining in the lungs after normal exhalation	1.8–2.4l

Physiology overview: gas exchange I

- This only takes place in the respiratory lobule. In gas exchange areas the barrier between alveolus and alveolar capillary is only 1 cell thick.
- Areas not available for gas exchange are known as dead space.
- Approximately $70m^2$ is provided for gas exchange in the adult lung.
- Physiological dead space varies with ventilation and perfusion of the alveoli so a ratio of dead space (V_D) to tidal volume (V_T) is used ($V_D/V_T = 0.3$ in the normal range).

Gas exchange in the lungs

Diffusion of gases across the alveolar capillary membranes is dependent on differences in gas concentration (or partial pressure) between alveolus and capillary, and is governed by 2 laws.

Dalton's law of partial pressures

Pressure exerted by a mixture of gases in a space is equal to the sum of pressures each gas would exert if occupying the space alone.

Air is a mixture of 3 predominant gases: 79% nitrogen, 20.9% oxygen and 0.03% carbon dioxide.

Boyles law

For a fixed amount of gas kept at a fixed temperature, pressure and volume are inversely proportional (if one increases, the other decreases). Thus, if the volume in which a gas is contained decreases, then the pressure of the gas will increase if the temperature remains constant.

Air at atmospheric pressure = 101kPa. Each gas in air exerts a proportional pressure: 79kPa nitrogen, 21kPa oxygen, 0.03kPa carbon dioxide.

Once it is humidified (after inspiration), air includes water vapour, which at normal body temperature is 6.3kPa. In the alveolus, it is also mixed with carbon dioxide diffusing from the capillary.

The alveolar oxygen level is calculated using the alveolar gas equation:

$$P_AO_2 = F_iO_2 \times 94.8 - P_aCO_2/RQ$$

(where RQ=respiratory quotient estimated at 0.8).

The A–a gradient

This is the alveolar (A) to arterial (a) difference in oxygen and reflects the gas exchange. It is usually 2–3.3kPa and increases with age.

$$\text{A–a gradient} = F_iO_2 \times 94.8 - P_aCO_2/RQ - P_aO_2$$

The P_aO_2/F_iO_2 ratio

This is a reflection of shunting (the ratio of deoxygenated blood to oxygenated after passage through the pulmonary circulation). It is normally >40kPa. A ratio of less than 26kPa reflects intra-pulmonary shunting. It is used to indicate the severity of acute lung injury (see 📖 Physiology overview: movement of gases I, p. 162).

Types of dead space

Anatomical

- Nose, pharynx, trachea, bronchi.
- Adults = 150 ml approximately.

Alveolar

Alveoli that are ventilated, but not perfused with pulmonary blood flow.

Physiological

Sum of anatomical and alveolar dead space.

Physiology overview: gas exchange II

Ventilation/perfusion matching

Efficient gas exchange within the lung (Fig. 10.1) depends on effective matching of ventilated and perfused areas. This can be expressed as a ratio where V = ventilation and Q = perfusion.

- **Dead space:** ventilation good/perfusion poor, i.e. V/Q = >1.
- **Functional lung:** ventilation good/perfusion good, i.e. V/Q = 1.
- **Shunt/perfusion defects:** ventilation poor/perfusion good, i.e. V/Q = <1.

In the normal lung a degree of variation exists and up to 15% can be mismatched (Table 10.4).

Table 10.4 Causes of V/Q mismatch

V/Q >1	V/Q <1 (Shunt)
Pulmonary embolism	Atelectasis
Decreased cardiac output	Consolidation
Extrinsic pressure on pulmonary arteries (tumour, pneumothorax) Pulmonary oedema	Obstructive lung disease (emphysema, bronchitis, asthma)
Destruction of pulmonary vessels	Restrictive lung disease (ARDS, pulmonary and alveolar fibrosis, pneumonia)
Decreased cardiac output	
Obstruction of the pulmonary microcirculation (ARDS)	

The body has 2 intrinsic responses allowing it to adjust to variation in ventilation and perfusion.

Hypoxic pulmonary vasoconstriction

Capillaries in poorly ventilated lung areas (i.e. low pO_2) will vasoconstrict to reduce pulmonary blood flow to the hypoxic region.

Hypocapnic bronchoconstriction

Bronchioles in areas with low pCO_2 in the capillaries will constrict reducing ventilation to the affected areas.

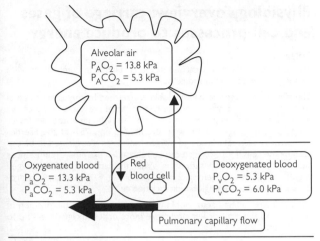

Fig. 10.1 Gas exchange in the lung.

Physiology overview: carriage of gases and cell processes to produce energy

Oxygen

The majority of oxygen is carried in the circulation in combination with haemoglobin in the red blood cells.

The affinity of oxygen to haemoglobin is governed by the environmental partial pressure of oxygen. Thus, at higher partial pressures, more of the haemoglobin binds with oxygen and it is 98–100% saturated. At lower partial pressures, such as those in the tissues, only 75% of the haemoglobin will remain saturated and oxygen molecules are released to be utilized by the cells. More oxygen can be released in extreme circumstances allowing down to 20–30% saturation. When the partial pressure of oxygen is plotted against the haemoglobin saturation, an 'S'-shaped curve is produced. This is the haemoglobin dissociation curve.

Specific factors affect haemoglobin dissociation by shifting the position of the curve to the right or left, and make more or less oxygen available to the tissues.

Factors causing a shift to the Haemoglobin dissociation curve

Shift to the right – more oxygen available to the tissues
- Decreased pH.
- Increased body temperature.
- Increased pCO_2.
- Increased 2,3-DPG.

Shift to the left – less oxygen available to the tissues
- Increased pH.
- Decreased body temperature.
- Decreased pCO_2.
- Decreased 2,3-DPG.

2,3-DPG = 2,3-diphosphoglycerate, a substance produced in the cell during anaerobic respiration (glycolysis).

Carbon dioxide

Carbon dioxide is mostly carried in the red blood cell (93%) as either bicarbonate (70%) or in combination with haemoglobin (23%). A tiny proportion (7%) is carried by the plasma in solution.

Changes in pCO_2 have a direct effect on the carbon dioxide content of the blood and deoxygenated blood will enhance the combination with carbon dioxide, thus increasing uptake in the tissues and decreasing it in the alveoli. This enhances the efficiency of the system.

Cellular energy production

Oxygen diffuses into the mitochondria of the cell, where it combines with glucose, fatty acids, and amino acids to produce energy via the citric acid or Krebs cycle. This energy is stored as a high energy bond linking a third phosphate molecule to adenosine diphosphate (ADP).

Each mmol of oxygen produces 38 mmol of adenosine triphosphate (ATP) that acts as a store of energy, which can be used as needed by the cell.

Arterial blood gas analysis

The measurement of arterial blood gases allows interpretation of the respiratory and metabolic status of the patient.

For details of the sampling procedure see 📖 Blood gas analysis, p. 124.

Respiratory capability

Hypoxaemia, hyperoxaemia, hypercapnia, and hypocapnia can be measured and respiratory support introduced, adjusted, or reduced according to the results.

Metabolic derangement

pH, pCO_2, and derived measurements, such as bicarbonate and base excess (deficit) can be used to interpret causes of acid-base derangement in the body (see Table 10.5).

Table 10.5 Alterations in different types of acidosis and alkalosis

	PH	PCO₂	HCO₃
Acute respiratory acidosis	pH low	pCO_2 high	HCO_3 normal
Acute respiratory alkalosis	pH high	pCO_2 low	HCO_3 normal
Acute metabolic acidosis	pH low	pCO_2 normal or low	HCO_3 low
Acute metabolic alkalosis	pH high	pCO_2 normal	HCO_3 high

Note: there may also be mixed or combined acidosis or alkalosis due to a combination of causes.

Normal blood gas values

- pH 7.35–7.45.
- pCO_2 4.6–6.0kPa.
- pO_2 10.0–13.3kPa.
- HCO_3 22–26mmol/l.
- Base excess: −2 to +2mmol/l.
- O_2 saturation >95%.

Respiration: patient assessment I

The patient should be formally assessed when taking over responsibility for their care and following any major change in the level of respiratory support they are receiving. Ongoing observation should also occur.

Observe

Patient colour

- Abnormal colour can range from pallor and greyness indicating reduced perfusion to frank cyanosis indicating severe hypoxaemia.
- Assess lips and buccal mucosa for central cyanosis. Peripheries can be cyanosed due to poor peripheral circulation and do not indicate low PaO_2.
- Posture can indicate severe breathlessness. Bracing of the shoulder girdle by pushing down on the knees or bed, inability to tolerate lying flat are seen in dyspnoeic patients.

Patient condition

- Sweating or cold clammy skin suggests increased sympathetic tone due to greatly increased effort.
- Altered conscious level or restlessness, and confusion can also indicate that the patient is not coping with the existing level of respiratory support. There may be other causes, e.g. drug toxicity or sepsis, but a respiratory cause should be ruled out before considering alternatives.
- The inability to speak more than a word or two (without other causes, such as endotracheal tube), or to move, suggests severe limitation from breathlessness.

Respiratory pattern and chest wall movement,

- Unequal movement of the chest wall suggests severe underlying dys-function on the immobile side, such as pneumothorax, pleural effusion, and major lobar collapse.
- Poor diaphragmatic or intercostal movement can be due to neurop-athy, myopathy, diaphragmatic splinting, etc.

Use of accessory muscles

Any extra effort required to inhale or exhale will trigger the use of these muscles (see 📖 Physiology overview: movement of gases I, p. 162). These are strong indicators that the patient requires or will require increased levels of respiratory support.

Respiration: patient assessment II

Auscultate

Air entry

Should be equal in right and left, and evident in all lung lobes. Right upper, middle, and lower lobes. Left upper and lower lobes.

Breath sounds

- **Vesicular:** heard over the periphery of the lung.
- **Bronchial:** heard over the trachea.
- **Bronchovesicular:** heard over major airways and most other parts of lung.
- **Added sounds:** fine crackles, coarse crackles, wheezes, rubs.

Palpate

- **Position of the trachea:** normally felt by placing 2 fingers on either side of the sternal notch; displacement to one side is indicative of mediastinal shift away from the affected side (pneumothorax or large pleural effusion) or towards the affected side (large lobar collapse).
- **Skin and soft tissue:** surgical emphysema may be felt with a pneumothorax.

Measure

Respiratory rate

A highly sensitive indicator of respiratory distress and other generalized physical dysfunction. Normal respiratory rate is 12–15 breaths/min. Consistently raised respiratory rate (tachypnoea) is exhausting and if untreated is associated with increased incidence of adverse events, such as cardiac arrest.

Pulse oximetry

A useful continuous monitor of oxygen saturation (see 📖 Pulse oximetry, p. 118). Readings should be correlated with arterial blood gases if there are sudden acute changes.

Arterial blood gases

These give the clearest indication of respiratory function. They should always be interpreted in conjunction with clinical conditions as compensation, for example, through high respiratory rate, may mask the severity of the condition (see 📖 Arterial blood gas analysis, p. 172).

In addition, patient history, diagnosis, care plan, observations, prescription charts, fluid balance chart should all be examined for additional information e.g, fluid overload.

Hypoxaemia and hypoxia

Hypoxaemia

Defined as a low oxygen concentration in the blood:
- <8.0kPa when breathing air.
- <11.0kPa when breathing >0.4 F_iO_2.

Acute compensation can occur to avoid tissue hypoxia, e.g. increasing cardiac output or increasing oxygen extraction by the tissues.

Chronic compensation by increasing red blood cells and haemoglobin levels is seen in COPD or high altitude dwellers.

Causes of hypoxaemia

- **Ventilatory inadequacy:** e.g. mechanical defects including airway obstruction, neuromuscular dysfunction, central nervous system depression.
- **Ventilation/perfusion mismatch:** e.g. pulmonary embolus, poor right cardiac function, ARDS.
- **Shunt:** e.g. atelectasis, pneumonia.
- **Diffusion limitation:** e.g. ARDS, fibrosing alveolitis, pulmonary oedema.

Tissue hypoxia

This is defined as inadequate oxygen to support cell metabolism. It is extremely difficult to monitor directly and hypoxaemia is commonly used as a marker of possible hypoxia.

There are 4 categories of hypoxia.
- **Hypoxic hypoxia:** hypoxaemia results in inadequate oxygen delivery to the cells.
- **Anaemic hypoxia:** arterial oxygen is normal, but oxygen-carrying capacity is inadequate due to either low Hb or dysfunctional Hb (e.g. in carbon monoxide poisoning).
- **Circulatory hypoxia:** oxygen delivery is insufficient to meet cell needs or does not reach the cells due to shunt.
- **Histotoxic hypoxia:** the ability of the cells to utilize oxygen is impaired (e.g. cyanide poisoning, which blocks mitochondrial electron transport).

Oxygen therapy

Oxygen should be administered to any patient in the following situations:
- Respiratory distress (respiratory rate >25 or <8 breaths/min).
- Evidence of hypoxaemia (pO_2 <8 kPa on air).
- Acute events including:
  - acute coronary syndromes;
  - major haemorrhage;
  - pulmonary oedema;
  - pulmonary embolus;
  - seizures;
  - low cardiac output and metabolic acidosis.
- During anaesthesia and the post-anaesthesia recovery period.
- During epidural and PCA delivery.

It constitutes a drug and should only be administered without a prescription in an emergency (see Table 10.6).

All patients who are hypoxaemic require oxygen and the general target oxygen saturation should be >92%. A small proportion (approximately 12%) of patients with acute on chronic pulmonary disease in Type II respiratory failure are dependent on hypoxic drive. They may require a lower target saturation in order to maintain adequate respiration. These patients should be closely monitored during oxygen delivery for signs of increasing drowsiness, and decreased respiratory rate and depth.

Oxygen is a dry gas, which will adversely affect cilial function and sputum clearance. This increases the longer it is used for, and the higher the flow rate it is used at. Ideally, oxygen should be humidified in any patient requiring it for more than 24h. Frequent saline nebulizers are an acceptable alternative for a short period of time in the self-ventilating patient.

Use of high percentage oxygen (>80%) can be associated with nitrogen washout and alveolar collapse as diffusion of most of the gas through to the capillary can occur and little nitrogen is left to maintain intra-alveolar pressure.

Table 10.6 Modes of oxygen delivery

Mode of delivery	Oxygen percentage	Associated problems	Safety priorities	Use
Nasal cannulae	2l/min 23–28% 3l/min 28–30% 4l/min 32–36% 5l/min 40% 6l/min plus (max. 44%)	Limited % O_2 available Inaccurate delivery particularly with high minute volumes Requires patent nasal passages; Mouth-breathing alters the amount of oxygen delivered Drying and uncomfortable for nasal passages. Check O_2 flow rate.	Regular monitoring of respiratory rate and pattern Pulse oximeter to monitor O_2 saturation Positioning of cannulae inside nares.	Low levels of O_2 supplementation for relatively short periods only. Disposable delivery system
Semi-rigid masks	4l/min ~35% 6l/min ~.50% 8l/min ~55% 10l/min ~60% 12l/min ~65%	Inaccurate delivery of O_2, particularly with high minute volumes Limits patient activities such as eating and drinking Drying for patient's mucosa and for secretions Rebreathing may occur	Regular monitoring Respiratory rate and pattern Pulse oximeter to monitor O_2 saturation Check positioning of mask and O_2 flow rate.	Low to medium levels of O_2 supplementation only Disposable delivery system

Continued

Table 10.6 —Cont`d

Mode of delivery	Oxygen percentage	Associated problems	Safety priorities	Use
Venturi-type mask (high-flow system)	With use of appropriate venturi nozzle for each % 2l/min 24% 4l/min 28% 8l/min 35% 10l/min 40 15l/min 60%	Can be drying for patient Regular monitoring of respiratory rate and pattern. If humidification used, an extra attachment is required High inspiratory flow rates may still not achieve required O_2% Limits patient activities, such as eating and drinking	Medium to high levels of O_2 supplementation Use pulse oximeter to monitor O_2. Check positioning of mask and O_2 flow rate	Disposable delivery system.
Humidified oxygen using nebulizer system	Varying rates of flow to deliver 28–60% O_2	Inaccurate delivery of O_2, with high volumes Limits patient activities.	Regular monitoring of respiratory rate and pattern Use pulse oximeter. Check positioning of mask, O_2 flow rate and setting of O_2 percentage on nebulizer system	Low to medium levels of O_2 supplementation Disposable delivery system
Non-rebreathe mask with reservoir bag	90–95% depending on respiratory rate and run at 15l/min of O_2	Reservoir bag should be partially inflated at all times	Ensure reservoir bag is fully inflated before placing on patient	Emergency situations short term use only.

Non-invasive ventilation

- Bi-level positive airway pressure – BiPAP.
- Continuous positive airway pressure – CPAP.

Non-invasive ventilation allows support of respiratory function without the requirement for intubation. It can be delivered by either a tight-fitting face mask, a nasal mask, or a helmet.

Indications for non-invasive ventilation

- Acute exacerbation of COPD.
- Acute pulmonary oedema.
- Specific groups of acute respiratory failure patients where intubation is associated with poor outcomes, e.g. immunocompromised patients, neuromuscular disease, end-stage COPD.
- Facilitation of weaning.
- Post-operative respiratory failure.
- Obstructive sleep apnoea and obesity hypoventilation syndrome.

Contraindications for non-invasive ventilation

- Inability to protect the airway and/or high risk of aspiration.
- Facial surgery or trauma.
- Poor patient tolerance or compliance.
- Claustrophobia.

Commonly, the key to successful NIV is developing trust and confidence between the patient and the nurse. It is well worth spending time on explanation, reassurance. and trialling different set ups so that the patient will tolerate their initial anxiety and allow the NIV to continue.

NIV for weaning is usually a second line intervention once the patient has failed to wean on previous occasions.

The safety of the patient depends on high levels of monitoring. Although seen as less dependent than many patients in critical care, the NIV patient requires constant observation and highly effective nursing support.

Acute pulmonary oedema has been shown to respond to both CPAP and BiPAP providing the patient is haemodynamically stable. This is due to an improved V/Q match and improved cardiac output with reduced work of breathing. The use of CPAP is more generally accepted, although BiPAP may be more effective in patients with high pCO_2.

Table 10.7 Types of non-invasive ventilatory support

Type of support	Set Up	Patient problems
CPAP (delivered by flow generators, NIV ventilators, IPPV ventilator)	Patient explanation	Pressure damage from tight-fitting mask and straps. Protect bridge of nose, ears and chin with hydrocolloid dressing
	Set machine or attach correct valve for agreed level of support – usually 5–10cmH$_2$O	Drying of eyes from gas leaks. Check mask fitting for leaks and pad with hydrocolloid if unable to stop leaks to eyes
	Choose correct size mask	Gastric distension from gas swallowing. Insert NG tube on free drainage
	Connect mask, and straps to machine	Difficulty eating or drinking. Support fluid and nutrition delivery by alternative routes
	Allow patient to try mask without fixing straps	Feelings of claustrophobia. Offer a supportive presence, allow patient opportunities to remove the mask
	Once patient is confident, attach straps	
	Continue to offer support and reassurance until the patient can tolerate it	
NIV (delivered by specific non-invasive ventilators e.g. NiPPY or by IPPV)	Patient explanation	As above
	Set inspiratory pressure at 10–15cmH$_2$O to start and increase to achieve targets	
	Set expiratory pressures at approx 10cmH$_2$O below inspiratory	
	Choose correct type and size of mask for patient	
	Continue as above	

Further information

Brochard L, Mancebo J, Wysocki M, et al. (1995) Noninvasive ventilation for acute exacerbations of chronic obstructive pulmonary disease. *N Engl J Med*, **333**, 817–22.

Nava S, Carbone G, DiBattista N, et al. (2003) Noninvasive ventilation in cardiogenic pulmonary oedema. *Am J Resp Crit Care Med*, **168**, 1432–7.

Intermittent positive pressure ventilation: indications

Although a life-saving intervention, positive pressure ventilation exposes the patient to a large number of potential risks and complications. These include the effects of positive intra-thoracic and intra-pulmonary pressure (barotrauma, decreased venous return) and the increased risks associated with endotracheal intubation. Nurses must be fully aware of these risks and understand how to reduce them in order to protect the patient

Indications for intermittent positive pressure ventilation

• To decrease the work of breathing.
• To reverse life-threatening hypoxaemia.
• To support acute ventilatory failure.

Causes of acute ventilatory failure

• Respiratory centre depression, such as decreased conscious level, intra-cerebral events, sedative, or opiate drugs.
• Mechanical disruption, e.g. flail chest (multiple rib fractures resulting in a free segment of chest wall), diaphragmatic trauma, pneumothorax, pleural effusion.
• Neuromuscular disorders, e.g. acute polyneuropathy, critical illness polyneuromyopathy, myasthenia gravis, spinal cord trauma/pathology, etc.
• Reduced alveolar ventilation due to airway obstruction (foreign body, bronchoconstriction, inflammation, tumour), atelectasis, pneumonia, pulmonary oedema (cardiac failure and ARDS), obesity, fibrotic lung disease.
• Pulmonary vascular disruption, e.g. pulmonary embolus, ARDS, cardiac failure.

Causes of hypoxaemia

• V/Q mismatch, e.g. pulmonary embolus, obstruction of the pulmonary microcirculation (Acute respiratory distress syndrome, see p. 233).
• Shunt, e.g. pulmonary oedema, pneumonia, atelectasis, consolidation, etc.
• Diffusion (gas exchange) limitation, e.g. pulmonary fibrosis, ARDS, pulmonary oedema.

Causes of increased work of breathing

• Airway obstruction.
• Reduced respiratory compliance.
• High CO_2 production (e.g. burns, sepsis, overfeeding).
• Obesity.

Respiratory failure

The majority of patients requiring ventilator support will have some degree of respiratory failure.

Type I respiratory failure

The patient is hypoxaemic, but has normal levels of carbon dioxide, i.e. pO_2 <11kPa on F_iO_2 0.4, with pCO_2 4.5–6.0kPa.

Type II respiratory failure

The patient is both hypoxaemic and hypercapnic, i.e. pO_2 <11kPa on F_iO_2 0.4, or <8.0kPa on air, pCO_2 > 6.5kPa without a primary metabolic acidosis.

Patient indicators of respiratory failure

- Respiratory rate >40 breaths/min or <8breaths/min.
- Deteriorating vital capacity <15ml/kg.

Intermittent positive pressure ventilation: physiological effects

IPPV has significant effects on both respiratory, cardiac, and renal systems. These are principally related to increased intra-thoracic pressure and its effect on normal physiological responses.

Decreased cardiac output and venous return

Increased intra-thoracic pressure reduces venous return (the passive flow of blood from central veins to the right atrium) and increases right ventricular after-load (the resistance to blood flow out of the ventricle by the pulmonary circulation). This reduces right ventricular output and consequently left ventricular output. The use of positive end expiratory pressure (PEEP) means that this occurs throughout the respiratory cycle.

- **Effects:** hypotension, tachycardia, hypovolaemia, decreased urine output.
- **Management:** fluid loading to optimize stroke volume and cardiac output. Inotropes may be necessary if cardiac function is compromised.

Increased incidence of barotrauma

The pressure required to deliver gas to the alveoli through airways which may be resistant to gas flow may cause damage to more compliant areas by over-distension. The damage is caused at higher tidal volumes. This allows gas to escape into the pleura and interstitial tissues, and can result in pneumothorices, pneumomediastinum, and subcutaneous emphysema. Up to 15% of patients develop barotrauma. The problem is particularly severe in conditions with increased airway resistance due to bronchoconstriction such as asthma.

- **Effects:** pneumothorax, pneumomediastinum, subcutaneous emphysema.
- **Management:** tidal volumes near physiological normal, e.g. 6–8ml/kg should be used. Avoid high airway pressures, if necessary by manipulating I:E (inspiratory:expiratory) ratio. Chest drain management of pneumothorax.

Decreased urine output

Response to reduced cardiac output produces release of anti-diuretic hormone, activation of renin-angiotensin-aldosterone (RAA) response and increased salt and water retention.

- **Effects:** oliguria, increased interstitial fluid and generalized peripheral oedema.
- **Management:** fluid filling to optimize stroke volume and cardiac output, careful fluid monitoring.

Intermittent positive pressure ventilation: modes of ventilation

Controlled mechanical ventilation

Pre-set frequency of patient breaths at either a set pressure (pressure controlled) or a set tidal volume (volume-controlled).

Volume-controlled ventilation (set tidal volume) is only used now in conjunction with controlled plateau pressure as the emphasis has shifted to controlling pressure, as well as volume in order to limit potential barotrauma (damage from high airway pressure or volume).

This mode is used when patients are unable to initiate (trigger) breaths due either to sedation, paralysis, or other causes of respiratory centre depression.

The tidal volume of a breath delivered in pressure-controlled ventilation will vary with lung compliance and inspiratory time.

Pressure support ventilation or assist

A pre-set level of inspiratory pressure support is delivered when the patient triggers a breath. The tidal volume of each breath is dependant on lung compliance and respiratory rate, and can be adjusted with the level of pressure support to maintain normal range for the patient.

Assist/control (triggered) mechanical ventilation

The ventilator will respond to patient triggering of a breath with either a pre-set tidal volume or a pre-set level of pressure support breath. In addition, a pre-set back-up rate of breaths will occur if the patient does not trigger at the required rate.

Synchronized intermittent mandatory ventilation

The ventilator delivers a pre-set frequency of breaths, but allows spontaneous breaths to be taken in between. Ventilator breaths are synchronized to these spontaneous breaths.

Choice of mode of ventilation

- CMV is used to provide full ventilator support (when the patient is apnoeic).
- SIMV is used when the patient is able to initiate some breaths, but still requires ventilator assistance at a consistent level to maintain CO_2 removal and oxygenation.
- PSV is used to support the patient's own respiratory efforts allowing increased patient comfort, reduced requirement for sedation, ongoing use of respiratory muscles, and the opportunity to gradually reduce the level of support to facilitate weaning.

Ventilator settings

Respiratory rate (breaths/min, f)
This is usually set at 10–15breaths/min, but may be altered to manipulate the minute volume and/or pCO_2 and pO_2

Tidal volume (ml, V_T)
The aim is for 6–8ml/kg, but this may be altered if there is difficulty optimizing pCO_2 and pO_2

Minute volume (litres, MV or V_E)
This is a product of the tidal volume and respiratory rate and is usually between 2.5 and 12l/min.

Flow rate (litres, V)
This ranges between 40 and 80l/min, and adjusts to ensure VT is reached within available inspiratory time and with optimal airway pressures. Flow pattern can be adjusted from square to either accelerating or decelerating. Square is most common, but decelerating may be beneficial and is always seen in pressure support modes.

Positive end expiratory pressure (cmH_2O)
Commonly, this is set at between 5 and 10cmH_2O, but ideally when the patient is fully ventilated, the setting is determined by the lower inflexion point on the pressure-volume loop.

Airway pressure
In order to reduce barotrauma, it is usual to limit the plateau airway pressure to <35cmH_2O

Pressure support/assist (cmH_2O)
Levels are set according to patient need for assistance and range from 5 to 35cmH_2O. Levels are adjusted according to the tidal volume achieved by the patient with an aim of between 6 and 8 ml/kg depending on pCO_2 and pO_2.

Inspiratory:expiratory ratio
The normal is 1:2, but may vary from 2:1 to 1:4 in order to increase time for inspiration in severe airflow limitation, e.g. asthma or to assist expiration by lengthening expiratory time and avoid air trapping.

Trigger/sensitivity
- This can be either flow-based or pressure based, and is vital in reducing the delay between the initiation of a breath and the ventilator response and thus the patient's work of breathing.
- Flow-based triggers require the patient to reduce a constant base flow by inhaling at a rate of a minimum of 1l/min, which is very sensitive.
- Pressure-based triggers require the patient to generate a negative pressure of −1 to −10cmH_2O to initiate the breath.

The ventilator settings are summarized in Table 10.8.

Table 10.8 Ventilator settings

Initial settings for ventilator	Parameters	Typical pt (70kg)
RR	10–15	10–15breaths/min
VT	6–8ml/kg	420–560ml
PEEP	3–10cmH$_2$O	5cmH$_2$O
Peak airway pressure	≤35cmH$_2$O	≤35cmH$_2$O
I:E ratio	1:2	1:2
Oxygen (adjusted to blood gas results)	0.4–0.6 F$_i$O$_2$	0.4–0.6 F$_i$O$_2$

Pressure–volume relationships

- Pressure–volume loops can be viewed in graphics screens on most modern ventilators.
- The pressure–volume relationship in a ventilator breath consists of 3 stages:
  - initial increase in pressure with little change in volume;
  - linear increase in volume as pressure increases;
  - pressure increase with no further volume increase.
- Information from this can be used to inform ventilator settings, such as PEEP (positive end expiratory pressure) and upper airway pressure limits.

Inflexion points – inspiratory

These signify the change between each stage of the ventilator breath (Fig. 10.2).

Lower inflexion point

The lower inflexion point occurs between stages 1 and 2, and is the point at which airway resistance is overcome, allowing alveolar opening. In a patient who is fully ventilated, and making little or no respiratory effort the lower inflexion point is the point at which lower airways would close on expiration. PEEP should be therefore be set at this level to avoid gas trapping.

Upper inflexion point

The upper inflexion point occurs between stages 2 and 3, and is the point at which lung capacity for the breath has been reached. It can be used to adjust settings for maximum inspiratory pressure.

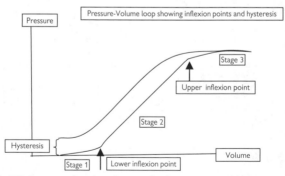

Fig. 10.2 Pressure–volume loop showing inflexion points and hysteresis. Reproduced with permission from *Oxford Handbook of Critical Care* 2nd edition, Singer and Webb (2005).

Further information

Singer M and Webb AR (2005). *Oxford Handbook of Critical Care*, 2nd edn. Oxford: Oxford University Press.

Troubleshooting

The patient is highly vulnerable to a number of problems whilst dependent on a mechanical ventilator. The critical care nurse is responsible for the patient's safety, and it is his/her responsibility to ensure that any problems are recognized as soon as possible and dealt with in an effective manner.

A guide to recognition and management of the more common problems is given here (Table 10.9), but the nurse should be aware that there may be other causes of problems not listed here.

If there is any doubt about the functioning of the ventilator and the patient is deteriorating the nurses should immediately:
• Call for help.
• Manually ventilate the patient using a manual ventilation bag on 100% oxygen.
• Review the patient for indicators of what is causing the problem.

Table 10.9 Troubleshooting problems in the ventilated patient

High airway pressure	
Manifested by:	Airway pressure alarm sounds, persistent rise in peak airway pressure, evidence of patient distress, haemodynamic instability
Causes:(a) *Life-threatening* (i.e. investigate and rule out/treat at once)	ET (or ventilator tubing) obstruction, pneumothorax, severe bronchospasm.
(b) *Other*	Build-up of secretions in airway
	Patient breathing out of synchronization with ventilator 'fighting')
	Patient coughing
	Increased peak airway pressure resulting from V_T set too high for patient, or inspiratory time set too short, or addition of PEEP
	Displacement of the ET tube
	(a) *downwards* – causing coughing from irritation of the carina, or slipping down the right main bronchus and meeting smaller airways with increased resistance
	(b) *upwards* – causing cuff herniation through the larynx, resulting in patient discomfort and agitation.

Table 10.9 Troubleshooting problems in the ventilated patient—Cont`d

High airway pressure

Intervention	1. If patient is severely compromised remove from ventilator, and manually ventilate using rebreathe bag and 100% oxygen. Assess lung compliance (the degree of resistance to inspiration) and symmetry of inflation while bagging. Call for senior and medical help
	2. Perform suction to clear any secretions and to determine whether tube is patent. If secretions are very thick review humidification and instill 2–3ml normal saline down ET tube prior to suctioning. Repeat as necessary
	3. If the cause is complete obstruction of the ET tube, emergency re-intubation will be necessary. If there is no one immediately available to re-intubate it is possible to ventilate the patient following extubation using a Guedel airway and tight-fitting facemask with manual ventilation. It is important to have the patient's neck resting on one pillow and to lift the jaw forwards to maintain a patent airway. If trained and proficient in its use, a laryngeal mask airway is an alternative to either re-intubation or facemask bagging
	4. Auscultate lungs for signs of wheezing, reduction in air entry, and altered breath sounds
	5. If the cause is a pneumothorax and there is cardiovascular compromise, immediate insertion of a chest drain or large needle will be necessary (by medical staff) to allow relief of tension
	6. If the patient is stable, attempt to ascertain the cause of increased airway pressure
	7. Reassure and attempt to alleviate any cause of distress if the patient is restless and distressed by ventilation ('fighting'). This is suggested by tachypnoea, breathing out of synchronization with the ventilator, and continually coughing or gagging
	8. Check blood gases if restlessness and distress continues and/or peripheral oxygen saturation remains low. Increase F_iO_2 and consult with medical staff
	9. If the patient is restless and unable to settle on the ventilator, but otherwise cardiovascularly stable with appropriate blood gases, review sedation and inform senior or medical staff if an increase ± paralysis is indicated
	10. Review ventilator settings and discuss with senior or medical staff if settings seem inappropriate or addition of PEEP appears to have caused a problem

Continued

Table 10.9 Troubleshooting problems in the ventilated patient—Cont'd

Low airway pressure	
Manifested by	Sounds of air leak, decreased expired minute volume (MV), low airway pressure reading
Causes:	
Life-threatening:	Disconnection or major leak from the ventilator, burst cuff on endotracheal/tracheostomy tube. Leak in the ventilator circuits, loss of seal on cuff, bronchopleural fistula (with massive air leak through chest drain), ventilator dysfunction
Intervention	1. Check the patient is attached to the ventilator
	2. Check connections on ventilator tubing for leaks, tears, or cracks
	3. Check cuff pressure to ensure a seal is present. Use cuff pressure manometer to check cuff pressure is less than 30mmHg. If the leak continues inflate cuff further if necessary
	4. Check inspired tidal volume to ensure the ventilator is delivering its set amount
	5. Check ventilator function
	6. Check levels set for pressure alarm limits are appropriate
	7. If low airway pressure continues and the tidal volume is not being delivered the ET tube or the ventilator may need changing. Manually ventilate the patient and inform senior nursing or medical staff

Low minute volume	
Manifested by:	Low MV alarm sounding, MV read-out shows less than set MV, audible cuff leak, patient may appear distressed and haemodynamically compromised, oxygen saturation may drop and the patient may appear cyanosed
Causes: (a)Life-threatening:	Disconnection from the ventilator, inappropriate ventilator settings (i.e. flow rate may be too low to allow set volume in time allocated by set respiratory rate), hole in ventilator tubing
(b)Other:	Leak caused by tubing connections working loose, loss of seal on cuff, presence of bronchopleural fistula with chest drain in situ

Table 10.9 Troubleshooting problems in the ventilated patient—Cont'd

Low minute volume	
Intervention	1. Unless the cause of low MV is immediately apparent, manually ventilate patient.
	2. Check ventilator tubing from machine to patient, testing connections, and looking for holes
	3. Review ventilator settings to ensure MV is capable of being delivered and that ventilator is not malfunctioning.
	4. Auscultate the trachea to detect any leak around the cuff. Refill cuff as before.
	5. Monitor air leak through chest drain if present. If increased inform medical staff. Ventilation may have to be increased or altered to allow for leak.

High minute volume	
Manifested by	Sounding of high MV alarms, patient making respiratory effort
Causes: (a) Life-threatening:	Possible ventilator malfunction
(b) Other	Patient making respiratory effort which is excessive, inappropriate ventilator settings
Interventions	1. Check causes of patient's tachypnoea such as pain, hypoxia, hypercapnia
	2. Review ventilator settings with senior and/or medical staff

Hypoxaemia	
Manifested by	Peripheral O_2 saturation <90%, arterial blood gases show fall in pO_2 to below 8–10kPa, patient is restless (unless heavily sedated ± paralysed), tachycardic, possibly hypotensive, and cyanosed

Continued

Table 10.9 Troubleshooting problems in the ventilated patient—Cont'd

Hypoxaemia

Causes (a)Life-threatening	Pneumothorax, pulmonary embolus, sputum plug, or other body obstructing major airway, severe haemodynamic compromise, severe bronchospasm, severe pulmonary oedema, ventilator malfunction
(b)Other	Build-up of thick secretions, increase in severity of disease, atelectasis, bronchospasm, repositioning of patient causing increase in shunt, leak in ventilator tubing, patient 'fighting' ventilator, pulmonary oedema
Interventions	1. If hypoxaemia is severe and/or causing haemodynamic compromise ventilate patient on 100% oxygen. Call for help
	2. Check ventilator is delivering set ventilation and that alarm limits are appropriate
	3. Check arterial blood gases and ensure that pulse oximeter is picking up a good signal
	4. Auscultate chest for air entry and abnormal breath sounds, depending on findings, suction and/or chest physiotherapy may be necessary. Observe symmetry of lung movement and consider pneumothorax
	5. Ascertain cause of hypoxaemia — reposition patient if recently placed on side, in consultation with medical staff consider need for chest X-ray, review haemodynamic causes such as decreased cardiac output. Review need for further sedation
	6. In consultation with medical staff, ventilator settings such as FiO_2, tidal volume, I:E ratio, etc., may be altered

Hypercapnia

Manifested by	$pCO_2 > 6.0kPa$, patient appears restless and agitated with tachypnoea if on weaning modes or possibly showing signs of respiratory effort if on controlled ventilation
	Note. Habitual CO_2 retainers (chronic COPD, etc.) may tolerate or even require much higher levels of CO_2 to maintain normal pH values as renal compensation will have adjusted for levels of bicarbonate. In patients with severe pulmonary disease, such as ARDS where there is risk of further lung damage with the high airway pressures necessary to reduce pCO_2, it may be *preferable* to tolerate high levels of CO_2 providing acidosis is adequately compensated ('permissive hypercapnia')
Causes: (a)Life-threatening	No urgently life-threatening causes, but long-term uncorrected hypercapnia may cause severe metabolic problems
(b)Other	Inadequate MV either from patient if in weaning modes or ventilator settings. Compensation for metabolic alkalosis, carbohydrate overload, or increased CO_2 related to increased metabolic rate, air trapping (intrinsic or autoPEEP)

Table 10.9 Troubleshooting problems in the ventilated patient—Cont'd

Hypercapnia	
Interventions	1. Ensure the patient is receiving the set mv or if weaning, that the patient is achieving the MV required
	2. Check air entry and perform suction to discount any sputum plugging or obstruction
	3. Review ventilator settings with medical staff and alter MV if necessary. A decrease in ventilation may be necessary if the patient is air-trapping

Autopeep (intrinsic PEEP, air-trapping)	
Manifested by	Failure of alveolar pressure to return to zero at the end of exhalation
	Increased resistance to airflow and increased work of breathing
Cause	Incomplete/impeded exhalation either as a result of high MV (>10 l/min), or in respiratory or cardiac disease, particularly chronic airway limitation
Interventions	1. Ensure low-compressible volume ventilator tubing is used
	2. Review ventilator settings with medical staff and decrease MV by decreasing respiratory rate or alter inspiratory flow rate to decrease inspiratory time and increase expiratory time
	3. Reduce metabolic workload to reduce respiratory demand

Improving oxygenation in the ventilated patient

In severe acute lung pathology (ARDS, etc.), simply increasing the oxygen may be inadequate to support the patient's oxygen requirements. Alternative interventions may also be needed, including the following.

Positive end expiratory pressure

- PEEP is applied to maintain alveolar opening and prevent collapse. It is commonly set at between 3 and $5cmH_2O$, but may need to be increased when alveolar resistance is increased and the patient is hypoxaemic. PEEP will increase FRC by improving V/Q matching and prevent collapse of recruited alveoli.
- PEEP is usually increased by small increments ($3–5cmH_2O$) in response to hypoxaemia and in relation to the F_iO_2.
- Response to alteration of PEEP is monitored using blood gas analysis
- Pressure volume loops can be used to identify the lower inflexion point and to determine the optimal PEEP setting.

Prone positioning

Placing patients in the prone position improves oxygenation in some patients (termed 'responders') and although the mechanism is still not established, this is now used as an adjunct to maintain levels of oxygen in hypoxaemic patients requiring high F_iO_2.

Although oxygenation may be improved there is no evidence of benefit on outcome. Not all patients can be turned prone and the risk-benefit of any manoeuvre must be evaluated (see 📖 Care of a patient on intermittent positive pressure ventilation: positioning, p. 220).

Nitric oxide (NO)

Inhaled NO crosses the alveolar membrane, and acts locally on the pulmonary vasculature, dilating vessels, and increasing blood flow. This improves ventilation/perfusion (V/Q) matching and, therefore, gas exchange as blood flow is only increased to the ventilated areas. As soon as it enters the blood, NO is bound to haemoglobin and has no further systemic (i.e. hypotensive) effect.

Nitric oxide gas is added to the gas delivery of the ventilator or in the inspiratory limb, volumes are measured in parts per million (ppm) by a monitor. Optimal delivery levels are identified by titrating the NO against either pO_2 or SpO_2. Levels should be re-titrated at least once a shift. Withdrawal of NO should be slow as there may be rebound pulmonary hypertension and hypoxaemia.

Although significant increases in oxygenation are seen in up to 60% of patients with inhaled NO this is not associated with an improvement in overall mortality.

Safe use of nitric oxide

- Monitoring of exhaled nitrogen dioxide levels (toxic substance produced when NO combines with oxygen). Levels >0.005 ppm are rare
  and only levels >5 ppm are considered dangerous.
- Avoid high levels of condensation or water pooling in ventilator
  circuits by using HME filters as nitrogen dioxide in solution produces
  nitric acid.
- Monitor methaemoglobin levels: >5% total haemoglobin is significant.
  This is formed when NO combines with haemoglobin.

Managing hypercapnia in severe pulmonary disease

In patients with severe pulmonary disease, such as ARDS, where there is risk of further lung damage with the high airway pressures necessary to reduce pCO_2, it may be *preferable* to tolerate high levels of CO_2 providing acidosis is adequately compensated ('permissive hypercapnia').

Permissive hypercapnia

Rather than increase the likelihood of barotrauma by increasing the volume of the breath. The patient's pCO_2 is allowed to rise up to 10 KPa or more, providing that pH can be maintained at >7.2. As a high CO_2 level is a very strong respiratory stimulant, this can only be done with well sedated patients

Tracheal gas (oxygen) insufflation

Insufflating a continuous flow of oxygen via a narrow catheter close to the carina via an endotracheal tube is occasionally used to reduce hypercapnia. The mechanism for action is believed to be washout of CO_2 in the anatomic dead space during end-expiration.

Gas flows should be limited to less than 6l/min, otherwise increased airway pressures and tidal volumes may be damaging. The gas flow must be warmed and humidified as it is passing directly into the trachea.

High frequency ventilation

High-frequency ventilation (HFV) incorporates techniques using ventilation frequencies greater than 60–2000breaths/min and tidal volumes of between 1 and 5ml/kg. This is useful where the lungs are very noncompliant or there is a bronchopleural fistula causing large leaks of gas (and loss of tidal volume) from normal ventilation.

High frequency oscillation

A rapidly oscillating gas flow is created by a device that acts like a woofer on a loudspeaker, producing a high frequency rapid change in direction of gas flow. Most of the experience with this has been in the paediatric population, but recent work has been carried out in adults with severe ARDS, suggesting it may be beneficial.

Oscillation can be applied externally or via the endotracheal tube.

High frequency jet ventilation

High-pressure air and oxygen are blended, and supplied through a noncompliant injection (jet) system to the patient via an open (uncuffed) circuit. The driving pressure of this gas can be adjusted to alter the rate of flow from the maximum (2.5atm) down to zero. Added (warmed and humidified) gas is entrained from an additional circuit via a T-piece attached to the endotracheal tube. The entrainment circuit should provide at least 30 1/min of flow. Highly efficient humidification (usually via a hotplate vaporizer humidifier) is necessary due to the high flows of otherwise dry gas. The usual frequency set is between 100 and 200breaths/min delivering tidal volumes of 2–5ml/kg.

In an entrainment system, the tidal volume delivered by the ventilator increases with driving pressure and decreases with respiratory frequency. It remains the same with alterations in I:E ratio.

Caring for the patient on intermittent positive pressure ventilation

Endotracheal tubes

Delivery of effective positive pressure ventilation requires a closed system in order to prevent the escape of gas. Endotracheal tubes facilitate this using an inflatable cuff. This also provides some (although not complete) protection from aspiration of gastric secretions, blood, etc.

Indications for intubation

- To protect or maintain a patent airway.
- To facilitate IPPV.
- To enable delivery of high concentrations of oxygen.
- To facilitate removal of pulmonary secretions.

Most adult patients have oral endotracheal (mouth to trachea) tubes. Although nasal intubation is thought to be more comfortable, it requires smaller tube sizes, carries a risk of sinusitis, and cannot be used with coagulopathy, maxilla-facial trauma, and basal skull fracture.

However, nasal (nose to trachea) intubation is more common in children.

Types of tubes

Single-patient use tubes made from PVC (polyvinyl chloride) or silicone are most commonly used. These have high volume, low pressure cuffs to reduce the likelihood of trauma to the tracheal mucosa.

Special tubes are available, such as adjustable flange and reinforced tubes for complex airway management, and double lumen tubes (a lumen in the right and left main bronchus) for asynchronous ventilation.

Cuff management

The pressure in the cuff of the tube should be checked routinely using a cuff pressure manometer. High pressures will result in tissue damage as the cuff pressure should not exceed 30mmHg (capillary occlusion pressure). This should only occur as a temporary measure to ensure effective ventilation continues until an alternative tube can be placed.

Securing the tube

Traumatic extubation, tube displacement, loss of cuff seal, and cuff herniation through vocal cords can all occur if the tube is not adequately secured. Unplanned extubation occurs in up to 19% of patients with the ensuing high risk of complications.

Cotton tapes are commonly used, but may be less effective than commercial ties and there may be an increased risk of pressure damage.

Size of tubes

- Adult male patients: size 8–9mm internal diameter, cut to 23cm length (end of tube should be approx. 3–5cm above the carina).
- Adult female patients: size 7–8mm internal diameter, cut to 21cm length.
- Smaller sizes are available for narrowed airways, e.g. oedema, stenosis, etc., and larger sizes for enlarged tracheas.

Complications associated with endotracheal tubes

- Tracheal stenosis, ulceration and necrosis (usually related to pressure damage from cuff).
- Tracheomalacia (degeneration of the cartilaginous rings).
- Damage to vocal cords (on insertion or with mishandling of the tube).
- Increased risk of ventilator associated pneumonia.
- Pressure damage to lips, gums, etc., due to tube ties

Intubation

Wherever possible this should be a planned orderly procedure, but there will always be emergency (crash) intubations. In either situation, safety is the bottom line. This depends on trained, competent staff, who work as a team, access to the right fully-functioning equipment which is in the right place, and back-up from senior staff when necessary.

Safety priorities (preparation)
- Check all equipment to ensure function (e.g. manual ventilation bag, suction, etc.).
- Attach the ventilator to the gas source and run self-test.
- Ensure iv access is patent and reliable.
- Ensure emergency drugs and fluids are to hand.
- Check ventilator settings are appropriate for the patient and that inspiratory oxygen concentration is initially high.

Preparing the patient
- Explain what is going to happen if the patient is aware and there is time. If possible, mention the temporary loss of speech associated with the tube.
- Pre-oxygenation via face mask for at least 5min.

Procedure
- Check all equipment is to hand.
- Check tube is cut to size and cuff patency tested (usually done by whoever is intubating).
- Ensure continuous monitoring of ECG, SpO_2, RR, and blood pressure.
- Position patient supine with pillow under occiput or, if orthopnoea is too severe, be prepared to lay the patient flat as soon as induction drugs are given.
- Intubation position is neck flexed and head extended.

Under anaesthetist's instructions
- Deliver iv drugs.
- Carry out cricoid pressure.

Post-intubation
- Inflate cuff to ensure seal, attach catheter mount and HME.
- Secure the tube.
- Check air entry and attach ventilator.
- Carry out full set of respiratory and cardiac observations.
- Arrange a chest X-ray to confirm correct tube placement.
- After about 15min take an ABG to confirm ventilator settings are appropriate.

Complications of intubation
- **Haemodynamic instability:** vasodilatation, hypotension, arrhythmias.
- **Tube malposition:** endobronchial intubation or failure to intubate.
- **Trauma:** haemorrhage, damage to vocal cords.
- **Reaction to anaesthetic drugs:** hyperkalaemia, hyperthermia.

Cricoid pressure

- Used in situations where there is risk of reflux of gastrointestinal contents (emergency intubation without time for fasting).
- Pressure is exerted on the cricoid cartilage of the trachea to compress the pharyngeal airway and prevent reflux of gastric contents.

Equipment for intubation

- Laryngoscopes (light checked and working): 1 curved, 1 straight laryngoscope blade.
- Endotracheal tube: selection of sizes.
- Lubricant: e.g. KY jelly.
- Magill's forceps.
- Bougie (introducer)/Stylet.
- 10ml syringe filled with air.
- Artery forceps.
- Tube tapes or holder.
- Catheter mount.
- HME (heat moisture exchanger): if using.
- Cuff pressure manometer.
- Manual ventilation bag and oxygen supply.
- Drugs for intubation (induction agent, sedative, muscle relaxant).
- Capnograph.
- Emergency trolley for back-up.
- Suction.
- Ventilator.

Maintaining a patent airway

Normal physiological processes for warming and humidifying air passing into the lungs are by-passed by endotracheal or tracheostomy tubes.

This causes:
- Increased viscosity of mucus (causing drying and encrusting in the airway).
- Depressed ciliary function.
- Micro-atelectasis from small airway obstruction by mucus.

In addition:
- The ability to cough is limited by the tube itself and the sedation the patient receives to facilitate the presence of the tube.
- There is loss of natural periodic sigh during IPPV, which reduces lung expansion and may increase atelectasis.
- Dehydration will reduce the moisture content of mucus.

Accumulation of secretions causes blockage of minor airways leading to atelectasis and ultimately collapse of lobar segments. This will increase shunt (see 📖 Physiology overview: gas exchange II, p. 168) and affect the patient's ability to maintain oxygenation.

Sputum clearance requires

- Adequate humidification.
- Suctioning and bronchial hygiene.
- Chest physiotherapy.
- Adequate systemic hydration.

Humidification

The optimal method of humidification should

- Deliver inspired gas to the trachea at 32–36 °C with a water content of 33–43g/m^3.
- Be simple and easy to use.
- Adapt to a variety of methods of ventilation and oxygen therapy.
- Avoid increasing airway resistance or reducing compliance.
- Reduce the risk of infection.

Types of humidifiers

Heat moisture exchanger (HME)

These are filters that are hygroscopic (attract water), on the patient side, and hydrophobic (repel water), on the ventilator side. The exhaled gas from the patient deposits water and heat onto the filter, which is then picked up by the inhaled gas from the ventilator. They also have filtering properties for small bacteria and viruses, which reduce infection risks. HMEs are light and disposable.

Limitations are a fixed level of humidification, which may be insufficient at high gas flows, and they may increase resistance to air flow in the circuit if allowed to become too wet or sputum impregnated.

Nebulizers

- The simplest devices deliver aerosolized water droplets produced either by a jet of gas passed through a film of fluid or by creating a fine spray from suction from a reservoir.
- More effective nebulizers use a spinning disc to create droplets by centrifugal force or an ultrasonic frequency vibrating tranducer. These can reach supersaturation of gas without being limited by temperature.
- Droplets need to be smaller than 1μm to reach the alveoli, those greater than 7μm are deposited in the upper airways.
- Nebulizers can deliver topical medication, as well as humidification.
- Limitations are increased infection risk and possible over-hydration with supersaturation of gas. They can also increase resistance to air flow.

Hot water bath humidifiers

Gas is driven over or through a heated water bath. Adequate humidity can only be achieved at water temperatures between 45° and 60°C. Heated wires in the circuit can maintain gas temperature and saturation by preventing heat loss, and therefore preventing water condensation within the tubes.

Reliable temperature control is vital both to ensure patient safety and to guarantee humidification. Closed circuit systems mean that infection is less likely, although it may occur in the warm moist environment if there is condensation within the tubes.

Cold water humidifiers

Gas from an oxygen flow meter passes through a venturi system into a cold water reservoir. Only partial humidification is achieved.

Instillation of normal saline

Boluses of normal saline instilled directly into the trachea during suctioning are unlikely to have much direct humidification effect. Some groups consider their use deleterious, invoking bronchospasm. However, they elicit a cough from the patient, which can be useful in clearing secretions and continue to be used when there is no obvious problem for the patient.

Further information

Kuriakose A. (2008) Using the synergy model as best practice in endotracheal tube suctioning of critically ill patients. *Dimens Crit Care Nurs* **27**, 10–15.

Suctioning

Suctioning is an essential component for maintaining patency of the airway. It is performed intermittently when evidence of secretions in the large airways can be heard (coarse crackles, coughing, wheeze). It is also used as part of chest physiotherapy.

It is not pleasant for the patient, and has been described as feeling like choking or losing your breath. Patients should be prepared for it and reassured that it will be short-lived.

Use of closed suction systems has been the subject of considerable debate, although thought to be less likely to cause desaturation and haemodynamic instability, recent reviews of evidence suggest this may be clinically insignificant, and are associated with no significant reduction of ventilator associated pneumonia and increased likelihood of colonization.

Safety principles for suctioning

- Set suction level at less than 26.6kPa (200mmHg/260cmH$_2$O) to minimize trauma.
- Aseptic or non-touch technique using clean gloves.
- Ensure use of the correct size of catheter (see Table 11.1).
- Suction catheter should only be inserted to just above the carina to reduce trauma. Insertion should stop if any resistance is felt.
- Suction is applied only during withdrawal of the catheter, it should be continuous during this time.
- Insertion and withdrawal of the catheter should not take longer than 15s.
- The patient, their ECG, and their SpO$_2$ should be observed throughout the procedure.
- No more than 3 suctions passes should be carried out during one suctioning episode.
- If an open suction system is used, wear goggles or face visor, as well as aprons and gloves.
- If a closed system is used, check for patency of the catheter and sleeve, rinse system with saline after use, check catheter is always fully withdrawn from the ET tube after use.

Precautions suctioning borderline hypoxaemic patients

Increased levels of oxygen should be given for 2min prior to suctioning (pre-oxygenation).

Occasionally, post-suction hyperinflation may be needed to reduce the risk of atelectasis.

Suctioning can be risky and has been associated with:

- Decreased mixed venous saturation.
- Decreased P_aO_2.
- Arrhythmias (associated with vagal stimulation and hypoxaemia).
- Micro-atelectasis.
- Haemodynamic instability.
- Increased intracranial pressure.
- Bronchoconstriction.
- Trauma to the mucosa.

Determining the size of suction catheter used

- Suction catheters are sized in French gauge (FG) or Charriere (CH).
- This is a measure of external diameter. 1 FG = 1/3mm.
- Suction catheters should not be more than ½ the internal diameter of the ET tube.

Suction catheter (FG)	External diameter (mm)	For use with ET tube size (mm)
8	2.6	≥6
10	3.2	≥7
12	4.0	≥8
14	4.6	≥9
16	5.0	≥10

Proposed advantages of closed suction systems

- Decreased level of contamination by organisms.
- Reduced episodes of desaturation during suction.
- Reduced incidence of splash contamination of the eyes.
- No loss of PEEP due to breaking the ventilator circuit.

Further information

Jongerden I, Rovers M, Grypdonck M, Bonten M. (2007) Open and closed endotracheal suction systems in mechanically ventilated intensive care patients: a meta-analysis. *Crit Care Med* **35**, 260–70.

Extubation

Preparation of the patient includes explaining the procedure and securing their co-operation during tube removal.

Emergency equipment and a member of staff with the ability to re-intubate should be readily available.

The patient's RR, S_pO_2, and ECG, should be monitored during extubation, and for the next few hours afterwards to ensure respiratory distress or post-extubation laryngeal oedema does not occur.

Short-term ventilation: indications for extubation

- Haemodynamic stability.
- Awake and able to cough/clear secretions.
- Shallow breathing index: f/V_T (respiratory rate /tidal volume) ≤105.
- $FiO_2 < 0.4$ with ABGs within normal range for patient.

Principles of extubation

- A minimum of 2 members of staff should be present.
- The patient is usually most comfortable in the sitting position. He/she should be given an explanation of the procedure.
- The airway and oropharynx should be cleared of secretions.
- One person cuts the tapes (or undoes the commercial tube holder) deflates the cuff, and holds the tube, whilst the other will suction and withdraw the tube with suction ongoing if secretions are copious. Withdrawal should take place on inspiration as the vocal cords attempt to oppose on exhalation.
- The patient will need assistance to clear any further secretions by coughing, and should then be offered a mouthwash or oral toilet.
- Ongoing oxygen should be provided via facemask or NIV, depending on the patient's condition.

Potential complications

Post-extubation laryngeal oedema can occur (more commonly if the patient has had repeated intubations). Signs of airway obstruction (stridor, dyspnoea, fatigue) should be investigated usually via naso-endoscopy. Treatment is commonly steroids (dexamethasone) to relieve inflammation.

Extubation

Removing an endotracheal tube is a very easy procedure; however, like all endotracheal intubation, extubation needs to be planned and carried out appropriately. Extubation can be done on an awake or anaesthetized patient. Before removing the tube, the patient must be well-oxygenated and their stomach emptied of air or food.

Anaesthetized child, null trache-ostomy

Complications

Tracheostomy

A tracheostomy is an opening in the anterior wall of the trachea providing direct access to the airway. It is usually positioned in the mid-line between the 1st and 2nd tracheal rings for percutaneous, and between the 3rd and 4th rings for surgical tracheotomy. It is performed in patients who require longer-term ventilatory support, have acute upper airway obstruction or trauma, or who require permanent alternative airway access.

Percutaneous dilational tracheotomy
- A rapid procedure that can be performed in the ICU, avoiding the need to transfer to theatre. The patient is usually already intubated and sedated.
- Preparation includes explanation and consent, as well as correction of any coagulopathy. It is a full aseptic procedure with lidocaine and adrenaline skin infiltration to anaesthetize and reduce bleeding.
- After a midline skin crease incision about 1–1.5cm long, blunt dissection exposes the tracheal wall. A guide wire is inserted through a needle placed between two tracheal rings over which a dilator to the appropriate size is placed. The trachostomy tube is then placed over the dilator. An alternative technique uses a forceps dilator and the tracheostomy tube is placed through the forceps.
- It is usual to monitor end-tidal carbon dioxide during the procedure to ensure ventilation is adequate.
- Percutaneous tracheotomy has been shown to be as safe as surgical.

Surgical tracheotomy
A more involved procedure requiring a full operating theatre environment. Usually required for difficult procedures and for those patients requiring permanent tracheostomies.

Complications
- **Early:** haemorrhage, paratracheal placement, pneumothorax and subcutaneous and mediastinal emphysema, cricoid cartilage damage.
- **Late:** tube displacement, stomal infection, tracheal stenosis.
- Rarely, tracheoesophageal fistula or erosion of neighbouring blood vessels may occur due to pressure necrosis or damage from excessive tube movement due to patient agitation.

Table 11.1 Types of tracheostomy tubes

Tube type	Use
Single lumen, cuffed	Short-term ventilation 5–7 days
Double lumen with inner cannula, cuffed	Longer-term ventilation
Double lumen with inner cannula and fenestration, cuffed	Diverts passage of air through vocal cords. With cuff deflated and one-way valve over end of tube spontaneously ventilating patient can speak
Single lumen, uncuffed	Very long-term when mechanical ventilation is not required
Adjustable flange	Allows point of entry into trachea to be adjusted to accommodate for variations in depth of subcutaneous tissue
Minitracheostomy (4.0mm cuffless tube placed through cricothyroid membrane)	Clearance for retained secretions
	Emergency lower airway access

Tracheostomy tube sizes
- 26–36 FG or size 8–12mm external diameter.
- Different manufacturers use different sizing.

Further information
Freeman BD, Isabella K, Lin N, et al. (2000) A meta-analysis of prospective trials comparing percutaneous and surgical tracheostomy in critically ill patients. *Chest* **118**, 1412–18.

Care of the patient with tracheostomy tube

Tracheostomy tubes are more comfortable, reduce the risk of vocal cord damage, allow access to the patient's mouth for thorough oral care and when the patient is weaning are thought to reduce dead space, and work of breathing. The patient's need for sedation will also be reduced.

Safety priorities

Tracheal dilators, a replacement tube, and a tube one size smaller should be kept at the bedside in case of displacement or complete obstruction. These should accompany the patient at all times.

Care of the stoma

A dry keyhole dressing should cover the stoma, and it should be cleaned with an aseptic technique, using normal saline 2–3 times daily or more frequently if necessary. The stoma should be inspected for signs of infection or bleeding.

If secretions from the stoma are copious, the skin may need protection with a hydrocolloid wafer and the secretions suctioned away as needed.

Care of tracheal inner cannulae

Removable inner cannulae should be replaced 8-hourly with a temporary cannula and cleaned. Sterile water should be used with either a sponge, small brush, or tape run through the tube.

Changing the tracheostomy tube

- A mature fistula takes about 5–7 days to form and tubes should not be changed before this time except in an emergency.
- Tubes with inner cannulae, which can be removed and cleaned, are less likely to require changing as they will not become encrusted with secretions over time. If they are made from polyurethane or silicone they can be left in place for several weeks.
- Nurses trained in the technique can undertake tube changes, but there should always be medical back-up available and an assistant.
- The procedure should be explained to the patient and the equipment assembled. The patient should be well-oxygenated, and have both mouth and trachea suctioned by the assistant.
- The new tracheostomy tube cuff should be checked by inflating with a syringe and the introducer should be slightly withdrawn and replaced to check that it is easily removed.
- The stoma site is cleaned with saline, and the tapes or fixation device cut. The assistant holds the old tube in place until the cuff is deflated and then it is removed.
- The new tube is inserted, the introducer withdrawn and the cuff inflated.
- If the patient is ventilated the ventilator is reattached and air entry checked, and the new tube is then secured.

Restrictions with a tracheostomy

Bypass of the patient's larynx will:
- Reduce the effectiveness of the cough.
- Limit physiological PEEP.
- Remove the ability to speak.
- Make swallowing difficult.
- Bypass normal humidification and warming mechanisms.

Use of Passy-Muir valves with tracheostomies

Passy-Muir valves are one-way valves designed to be used in both ventilated and spontaneously breathing patients. They must only be used with the cuff deflated. The valve opens to allow gas flow through the tracheostomy into the lungs during inspiration, but closes on expiration. Expired gas is redirected up through the tube fenestration or round the deflated cuff flowing through the vocal cords. This allows the patient to speak, facilitates swallowing, and may reduce the work of breathing.

Contraindications to use of Passy-Muir valve

- Unconscious or comatose patient.
- Inflated or foam-filled tracheostomy tube cuff.
- Severe airway obstruction.
- Severe risk of aspiration.
- Greatly reduced lung elasticity.
- Unmanageable thick secretions.
- Sleeping patient.
- The device is not designed for use with endotracheal tubes.

Decannulation of tracheal tubes

Removal of a tracheostomy tube will increase dead space, with associated increased work of breathing of up to 30%. For this reason, the patient's ability to cope with this increase should be carefully assessed prior to decannulation. In some long-term tracheostomized patients (4–6 weeks or more) it may be better to reduce the size of the tracheostomy tube before removal.

The patient should have been able to breathe for >24h with the cuff deflated and the cannula capped off (ideally, this should be a fenestrated tube).

Readiness for decannulation

- No ongoing requirement for IPPV that cannot be provided by NIV.
- Adequate cough.
- No physiologically significant upper airway lesion, e.g. tissue over-granulation or stenosis.

Decannulation

- Explain what is going to happen to the patient. Assemble equipment similar to that for extubation, except that a mouthwash may be unnecessary and an occlusive dressing for the stoma will be needed.
- Use similar principles to those for extubation, with the addition of cleaning of the tracheostomy site with normal saline before extubation.
- The patient should be monitored closely for the next 24h after decannulation. The occlusive dressing should be tested for patency by asking the patient to cough.
- The stoma site should close spontaneously over 7–14 days and should be re-dressed on a daily basis.
- Sputum clearance should be facilitated with regular saline nebulizers and deep breathing exercises.

Care of a patient on intermittent positive pressure ventilation: positioning

Right and left lateral positioning

- Matching of lung ventilation with perfusion (V/Q) is important in supporting gas exchange.
- In the lateral position the dependant lung will receive more blood flow during IPPV. With unilateral lung damage or disease, the 'good' lung should be placed in the dependant position to match increased perfusion with ventilation.
- In addition, movement of secretions is assisted by gravity from the upper lung, and alternating left and right lateral positions will facilitate movement of secretions into the main airways where it can be removed by suction.

Semi-recumbent positioning

Supine body positioning has been associated with a significantly increased risk of ventilator-associated pneumonia, thought to be due to aspiration. Patients should therefore be nursed at 30–45° to the horizontal to reduce the likelihood of aspiration of stomach contents.

A secondary advantage to this positioning is the alteration in the position of the diaphragm, which reduces resistance to inspiration, increasing depth of breathing and reducing the likelihood of basal atelectasis.

Prone positioning

This technique is used in severe acute respiratory distress syndrome (ARDS) to improve gas exchange. It is thought to improve oxygenation in some patients (responders) by reducing compression atelectasis in dependant regions, improving V/Q matching, reducing alveolar overdistension, and increasing lung recruitment. However, no improvement in outcome has been associated with this improvement in oxygenation.

The manoeuvre is risky and not all patients benefit; therefore, the risk/benefit ratio for each patient must be considered before using the technique.

In general, it should not be considered unless the patient has a $P_aO_2 <$ 8.5kPa, on $F_iO_2 \geq 0.6$ with PEEP $\geq 10cmH_2O$ with maximal optimization of support

Contraindications

- Absolute contraindications are severe head, spinal, or abdominal injuries and severe haemodynamic instability.
- Relative contraindications include frequent seizures, raised ICP, multiple trauma, pregnancy, and severely distended abdomen.

Problems associated with prone position
- Facial and conjunctival oedema.
- Pressure ulcers on knees, shoulders, iliac crests, and face.
- Limited access to endotracheal/tracheostomy tubes.
- No immediate access for cardiopulmonary resuscitation.

Technique for prone positioning

- Safe prone positioning will require two personnel on either side of the patient and one at the head, who is purely responsible for the patient's head and airway.
- The movement is done in two stages from back to lateral and then over to prone.
- The patient is moved as far over to one side of the bed as possible and the arm on the opposite side (onto which the patient will be rolled) is tucked under the hip. The other arm is arranged over the chest initially and the patient is rolled onto their side. Pillows are placed under the chest/shoulders and pelvis, and the patient is lowered gently onto their front with both arms at the side and their head turned to one side. One arm is flexed up with the head rotated away from it. The whole bed is tilted up to 30° in a reverse Trendelenberg.
- Optimal length of time in the prone position and frequency of turns is not known and should be based on the patient's response. If improvement in oxygenation continues, the patient can remain prone for up to 18h at a time, although the head and arms will require 2-hourly repositioning to prevent pressure damage.

From Balas (2000).

Further reading

Balas, MC. (2000) Prone positioning of patients with acute respiratory distress syndrome: applying research to practice. *Crit Care Nurs* **20**, 24–36.

Gattinoni L, Tognoni G, Pesenti A, et al. (2001) Effect of prone positioning on the survival of patients with acute respiratory failure. *N Engl J Med* **345**, 568–73.

General care of the patient on a ventilator

Stress and anxiety

Most patients on IPPV have greatly increased levels of anxiety and stress, which are compounded by their inability to communicate. It is important that the nurse recognizes symptoms of anxiety and stress, and responds to them.

The most common stressors reported by critical care patients are noise levels, continuous lighting, crowding with unfamiliar people, restriction of mobility, and social isolation. These must be addressed by flexing the demands of treatment as much as possible to allow alleviation of these factors (see 🕮 Stressors in critical care, p. 44).

The most important responses are to naturalize lighting wherever possible, ensure differentiation of day from night, reduce noise levels, respect and protect the patient's privacy, and encourage/support ongoing involvement of family and loved ones.

Factors contributing to psychological problems

- Discomfort.
- Fear.
- Loss of control.
- Disorientation.
- Disease pathology.

Sedation

Most patients on IPPV require some form of sedation, initially in order to tolerate their endotracheal tube. Further details can be found in 🕮 Sedation, p. 54.

Nutrition

Alternative forms of nutritional support are necessary when the patient is intubated. The effects of malnutrition on the critically ill patient are severe and efforts should be made to establish appropriate levels of intake as soon as possible. Two groups are particularly vulnerable. Further details are available in 🕮 Nutrition: assessment, p. 374.

- Patients exhibiting the septic response (i.e. fever, high levels of urinary nitrogen excretion, high metabolic rate), do not utilize nutrition effectively to regenerate depleted muscle mass.
- Malnourished patients have an increased risk of developing pneumonia and other complications, due to the associated dysfunction of the immune system and the possible limitation of surfactant production seen with fatty acid deficiency.

Nutrition for weaning from ventilation
- Over-feeding of carbohydrate causes the body to lay down fat stores. This process produces considerably more CO_2 than that produced by the breakdown of food for energy. This will require an increased minute volume and respiratory workload to excrete the excess CO_2.
- Depletion of important minerals and trace elements, such as zinc, magnesium, and phosphate, also have a deleterious effect on respiratory muscle function. Repletion of muscle mass is not possible without these minerals.

Immobility and muscle atrophy
Lack of use of muscles, such as the diaphragm and intrathoracic muscles, for respiration will lead to atrophy. It is important to move to patient-initiated ventilation modes as soon as possible in order to prevent this.

Weaning

The vast majority of patients have little difficulty weaning from mechanical ventilation once the disease process is resolved. However, a small number of patients will take considerably longer due to ongoing ventilator dependence.

Providing the central nervous system respiratory drive is functional, the ability to wean the patient will be a balance between load imposed on the respiratory muscles and the capacity of the muscles to handle it.

Determining readiness for weaning

The decision to wean is made following assessment of physiological and physical status. Protocolized weaning tools have a strong level of evidence to support their effectiveness. A daily screening tool should be initiated by nursing or physiotherapy staff, allowing patients who are ready to be identified and a spontaneous breathing trial (SBT) commenced.

If the patient passes the SBT, then they can be extubated. If they fail the criteria, then the patient should be placed back on mechanical ventilation, and the cause identified and treated. They should be re-screened the following day.

A protocol using these tools resulted in 88% of patients being extubated.

Preparing a patient for a spontaneous breathing trial

Weaning should start in the early part of the day (when the patient is less tired) with a clear explanation of the procedure. The patient should be helped into a sitting position to allow expansion of lung bases and the endotracheal/tracheal tube is suctioned to clear the airway. The nurse should remain with the patient and closely observe the respiratory rate, ECG, pulse oximeter, and blood pressure as the level of support is removed or reduced, and during the spontaneous breathing trial.

Spontaneous breathing trial

The patient is placed on a T-piece or CPAP of 5cmH$_2$O for between 30 and 120min. If the patient is on a T-piece for >30 min, CPAP should be applied to compensate for loss of laryngeal PEEP. During the trial, if the patient exhibits any of the criteria for failure (see 📖 Daily screening tool, p. 225) they are considered to have failed the trial and should continue on ventilatory support.

Patients who have been ventilated for longer than a week or who fail more than 3 consecutive spontaneous breathing trials may require a more staged approach to weaning (see 📖 Weaning the long-term ventilated patient, p. 226).

Daily screening tool

Each patient should be screened for readiness for weaning on a daily basis. Weaning should be considered and a spontaneous breathing trial carried out if the following criteria are met:
- P/F ratio > 200mmHg (or 26kPa).
- PEEP <5cmH$_2$O.
- Adequate cough during suctioning.
- $f/V_T \leq$ 105ml/min (measured with CPAP of 5cmH$_2$O).
- Requires no or low-dose vasopressor or inotrope infusions.

Where f = frequency or rate of breathing and V_T = tidal volume (in litres) P = PO$_2$, F = FiO$_2$.

Spontaneous breathing trial

The patient is placed on a T-piece or CPAP of 5cmH$_2$O, and monitored closely for between 30 and 120 min.

If any of the following criteria are met, the trial is considered to have failed:
- Respiratory rate >35 for >5min.
- Oxygen saturation <90% for >5min.
- Heart rate increased or decreased by >20% for >5min.
- Systolic BP >180 or <90mmHg for at least 1min.
- Increased anxiety, agitation, or diaphoresis are present for > 5min.

See also 📖 Extubation, p. 212.

Further information
MacIntyre N. (2007) Discontinuing mechanical ventilatory support. *Chest* **132**, 1049–56.

Weaning the long-term ventilated patient

When patients have been ventilated for longer than about a week, there may be a need for a staged reduction of ventilator support to allow respiratory muscle bulk and stamina to be re-built.

Weaning plans need to be individualized and should be reviewed over a period of time, rather than changed on a daily basis.

Assessment of factors likely to prevent weaning

As a first step, the patient should be reviewed for the factors listed in the box 'Factors likely to prevent weaning', which should be resolved or optimized prior to commencing weaning.

Techniques of longer-term weaning

- Research supports the use of either pressure support weaning or multiple daily T-piece weans as the most effective methods of weaning, as opposed to SIMV. Recent additional work in COPD patients supports the use of NIV to wean. Protocolized or programmed reductions in levels of support or alternatively, programmed increases in time spent on T-piece also seem to be more successful.
- Rest days to allow the patient to concentrate on other aspects of rehabilitation, such as building leg muscles, should be built into the weaning programme.
- There are many contributing factors to weaning failure both physiological and psychological, and these all need to be considered.
- A multiprofessional approach gives the patient the best opportunity for success, with weekly review meetings incorporating all the contributing professions to ensure that all aspects of care are enhanced.
- Use of positive feedback is vital for the patient, either in the form of a progress chart, which focuses only on positive achievement or utilizing biofeedback by allowing the patient to see their own respiratory rate or oxygen levels.
- Psychological support plays an important part in success, and family and friends can be hugely influential in maintaining the patient's drive and motivation to continue.

Professionals who contribute to long term weaning

- Nurses.
- Physiotherapists.
- Dietitians.
- Doctors.
- Speech and Language therapists.
- Occupational therapists.

Additional support
- Patient's family and friends.
- Counsellors/Spiritual advisers.
- Other previous long-term intensive care patients.

Factors likely to prevent weaning

- Sepsis.
- Increased CO_2 production.
- Electrolyte/fluid imbalance.
- Decreased magnesium and phosphate levels.
- Pain.
- Haemodynamic instability.
- Metabolic alkalosis.
- Extreme malnutrition.
- Unresolved respiratory problems.
- Cardiac failure.
- High intra-abdominal pressure.
- Sedation and other causes of reduced conscious level.

Factors contributing to weaning failure

Physiological

- **Increased respiratory workload:** e.g. airway resistance, atelectasis, ET tube.
- **Increased ventilatory requirements:** e.g. pyrexia, shivering, increased activity.
- **Reduced ventilatory drive:** e.g. sedatives, suppressed hypoxic drive, metabolic alkalosis.
- **Poor oxygenation:** e.g. V/Q mismatch, anaemia.
- **Limited cardiac response to weaning effort:** e.g. heart failure.
- **Muscle weakness/fatigue:** e.g. over-worked respiratory muscles, poor nutrition leading to muscle depletion, myopathies.

Psychological

- **Poor motivation to succeed:** e.g. depression, hopelessness.
- **Increased dependency:** e.g. on the ventilator, learned helplessness due to loss of control.
- **Inability to understand what is happening:** e.g. delirium, delusions, cognitive dysfunction.
- **Personal impacting factors:** e.g. pain, anxiety, fear.

Environmental

- Lack of sensory stimulation.
- Sleep deprivation.

Further information

Macintyre N, et al. (2001) Evidence-based guidelines for weaning and discontinuing ventilatory support: a collective task force facilitated by the American College of Chest Physicians; the American Association for Respiratory Care; and the American College of Critical Care Medicine. *Chest* **120**, 375S–95S.

Pneumothorax, tension pneumothorax, and bronchopleural fistulae

A pneumothorax is the presence of air between the visceral and parietal pleura. It occurs when trauma or a spontaneous rupture creates a hole between the alveolar or bronchial wall and the pleura, allowing air to escape into the pleural space. Severity of symptoms depend on the size and underlying respiratory function, and include dyspnoea, hypoxaemia, and pain.

On assessment, there may be decreased breath sounds, unequal chest movement, and hyper-resonance over the area when percussed.

CXR should confirm the presence of a pneumothorax.

Tension pneumothorax

A tension pneumothorax can develop when the rupture in the alveolar wall acts as a one-way valve. Thus, air escapes into the pleural space on inspiration, but cannot return into the lung on expiration. It is more common when the patient is on IPPV. Increased pressure within the pleural space occurs, collapsing the lung on the affected side and ultimately displacing the mediastinal structures towards the unaffected lung. The clinical effects of this are life-threatening and immediate.

Clinical effects of tension pneumothorax
- Tachycardia and a rise in blood pressure, followed by hypotension as cardiac output decreases (due to ↑ intrathoracic pressure which impedes venous return and compresses the heart).
- Cyanosis, respiratory distress, and agitation with rapid fall in O_2 saturation.
- On IPPV, airway pressures increase dramatically, and expired MV may fall.
- Left untreated, cardiovascular collapse and cardiac arrest will occur.

On assessment, the patient will have unilateral chest movement. Air entry and breath sounds will be greatly decreased on the affected side. There will be a displaced apex beat and hyper-resonance on percussion. The trachea may be shifted from the midline towards the unaffected side.

Bronchopleural fistula

A fistula connecting lung and pleural space will produce the same effect as a pneumothorax, but is less likely to close spontaneously and may require surgical intervention.

Intervention

- If hypoxaemic, increase inspired oxygen.
- If the pneumothorax is not life-threatening, diagnosis and position is confirmed by CXR, and an underwater seal chest drain inserted.

- A tension pneumothorax is an emergency situation and help must be sought immediately for:
  - relief of tension by percutaneous insertion of a large gauge needle or a 12/14g iv cannula in the second intercostal space, mid-clavicular line (patients on IPPV will not suck air in through the needle or cannula unless they are making spontaneous breathing efforts).
- insertion of chest drain;
- bronchopleural fistulae may take weeks to heal and require ongoing chest drainage with −5kPa suction;
- if air leak is compromising ventilation, high frequency jet or asymmetric lung ventilation may be required;
- in addition, HMEs may be ineffective and alternative forms of humidification may be necessary.

Pneumonia

- Pneumonia is an inflammatory process caused by bacterial, viral, fungal, protozoan, and occasionally chemical (e.g. gastric aspiration) factors.
- It is classified into lobar, bronchial, and atypical.
- On assessment, the patient will have fever, cough, dyspnoea, and may complain of pain. Commonly, the cough will be productive with purulent secretions, but not always. On auscultation there will be reduced breath sounds and bronchial breathing, often accompanied by coarse crackles.
- CXR may show consolidation, cavitation, or effusion associated with the area of the infection.
- Treatment depends on aetiology and infecting agent, but all patients require similar support and management.
- Hospital-associated pneumonia is defined as pneumonia occurring either after the first 48h of hospital admission or in intubated patients.

Ventilator-associated pneumonia (VAP)

VAP is a newly-acquired pneumonia in a patient who has been ventilated ≥ 48h. Aspiration of bacteria colonizing the oropharynx or upper GI tract is thought to be the main route for pneumonia in intubated patients as the endotracheal tube holds the vocal cords open, facilitating aspiration. The incidence in critical care is around 17%, and it carries a significant risk for morbidity and mortality. Prevention is vital.

Prevention of VAP
Key components are:
- Semi-recumbent (45° head up) positioning.
- Rigorous oral hygiene.
- Use of HME bacterial filters for humidification.

Other important factors are thought to include reducing/holding sedation daily, and preventing peptic ulcer and deep vein thrombosis in these patients.

Management
- Antibiotic therapy.
- Oxygen therapy, CPAP, and IPPV may all be necessary to maintain pO_2.
- Chest physiotherapy and bronchial hygiene to clear secretions.
- Postural drainage and position changes.
- Adequate nutrition to prevent complications associated with malnutrition (see Nutrition: assessment, p. 374).
- Prevention of further infection.

Further information
Kola A, Eckmanns T, Gastmeier P. (2005) Efficacy of heat and moisture exchangers in preventing ventilator-associated pneumonia: meta-analysis of randomized controlled trials. *Intens Care Med* **31**, 5–11.

Nutrition
Patients with COPD are usu
ment of appetite, dyspnoea c
support should be started ea

During weaning, these patier
excess CO_2 production relat
taken to ensure that carbohy

Further information
National Institute for Clinical Excellen
    Guideline 12. NICE, London. (www.

Acute asthma I

Asthma is an acute, reversible airway restriction caused by bronchospasm in response to a range of stimuli. These include allergens, infections, and exercise. Bronchospasm invokes smooth muscle constriction mucosal oedema and excessive mucus production.

Assessment

The patient may be distressed, tachypnoeic, tachycardic, and dyspnoeic, with polyphonic wheeze (expiratory ± inspiratory) and use of accessory muscles. They will be unable to say more than a few words with one breath. In severe situations, the patient may be unable to speak, cyanosed and the chest may be silent due to little/no air flow.

Management

Airway and breathing
- If unable to speak or obtunded, immediate intubation will be necessary.
- Give the concentration of oxygen required to maintain pO_2.
- An ABG should be taken to assess levels of pCO_2 and pO_2. Intubation and ventilation should occur if pCO_2 is rising and/or pO_2 is falling.
- Ongoing monitoring of S_pO_2, respiratory rate, and pattern, should be carried out with regular ABGs.

Circulation
Patients should be monitored closely (ECG, BP). Signs of circulatory instability (tachycardia >150bpm, arrhythmias, low BP, chest pain, etc.) should be treated immediately.

Reduction of bronchospasm and inflammation
- Bronchodilators (ß$_2$-agonists e.g. salbutamol) are usually inhaled, but may be given iv.
- Steroids, such as prednisolone or iv hydrocortisone are used to reduce hypersensitivity, although this takes a number of hours to begin working. Beclometasone may also be inhaled.
- Aminophylline can be given iv to relax bronchial smooth muscle.
- Anticholinergics, such as ipratropium bromide, may be inhaled to relax smooth muscle.
- Magnesium sulphate iv can also be used to relax smooth muscle.
- In severe cases, adrenaline (epinephrine) can be used either subcutaneously, by nebulizer, or inserted down the endotracheal tube.

Support of respiratory function
- Humidification and fluid hydration to avoid mucus plugging.
- Physiotherapy and bronchoscopy, as necessary. CPAP may be useful.

Sedatives
Should only be given prior to ventilation as they can reduce the respiratory drive causing hypoventilation and precipitating respiratory failure.

Antibiotics
Only given if there are obvious signs of infection (fever, increased white cell count).

Chronic obst

COPD includes chror
asthma. Most patients
sema. Acute exacerbati
also be related to atm
anaesthetics). Inappropi
therapy can precipitate

Management
This is similar to asthm
most cases, infection is
antibiotics should be gi

Support of respiratory
Caution with oxygen th
dependent on hypoxic
retention of high leve
oxygen (greater than 2£
systems. Arterial blood
evidence of increasing
be relative to the pati
than that of the normal
• Non-invasive ventilat
  effective in these pat
• Physiotherapy shoulc
• A respiratory stimula
  if NIV is not available
  with deteriorating cc

Mechanical ventilation
The decision to intub
carefully considered w
If possible, it should b
time well in advance o
ventilation is difficult, a
afterwards.

If there is a reversible
treatable infection, the
has taken place. Howe
uing deterioration in
life without prospect
quality of life deteriora

Ventilation should ain
reduce an elevated P_aC

Weaning
Weaning can be a pro
tory reserve and nutri
support and gradual in

Pulmonary embolus (PE)

PE is the occlusion of a pulmonary artery by a thrombus. The embolus is most commonly thrown off from a deep vein thrombosis of the pelvic or leg veins. Severity of effect is directly related to the size of the embolus and, thus, the size of the vessel that has been blocked.

Other sources of emboli include amniotic fluid embolus and fat embolus after long bone trauma.

Symptoms

These are tachypnoea, tachycardia, dyspnoea, and pleuritic chest pain. There may also be haemoptysis.

Diagnosis is made on clinical presentation (including a raised CVP), CXR (reduced blood flow 'oligaemia' to an area of lung, evidence of pulmonary infarction, classically a wedge-shaped shadow), ECG (right axis deviation, S1, Q3, T3 configuration, right ventricular strain pattern, partial right bundle branch block, see 📖 Chapter 5, pp. 91–116), hypoxaemia, and exclusion of other likely causes. If the patient is stable, spiral CT scan with contrast pulmonary angiography and V/Q scans may be performed.

Management

• High flow oxygen to maintain $S_pO_2 \geq 90$–95%, CPAP, and IPPV as necessary.
• Fluid challenges to optimize right heart function.
• Anticoagulation using low molecular weight heparin.
• Thrombolytic therapy if cardiovascular compromise.
• Pulmonary embolectomy if patient is moribund.
• Prevention of any further deep vein thrombosis using elastic support stockings, exercises, and mobilization.

Table 11.2 Anticoagulant and thrombolytic regimens

	Dose	Frequency
Low molecular weight heparin regimes		
Dalteparin	200units/kg	Every 24h
Enoxaparin	150units/kg	Every 24h
Tinzaparin	175units/kg	Every 24h
Thrombolytic regimens		
Alteplase	100mg	Once over 90min then heparin infusion
Streptokinase	500 000units × 1 100 000units/h	Over 30 min then for 24 h

Cardiac disorders

The cardiovascular system

This consists of:
- **The pulmonary circulation:** pulmonary artery, veins, and capillaries.
- **The systemic circulation:** the aorta, arteries, veins, and capillaries of the rest of the body (supplied by the left ventricle).

Blood flow through the heart
- Venous blood returns to the right atrium via inferior and superior venae cavae.
- Atria force blood into ventricles just prior to ventricular contraction.
- The pressure created at the beginning of ventricular contraction closes valves between the atria and ventricles (mitral and tricuspid).
- Ventricular contraction forces blood from right ventricle (RV) into pulmonary artery and from left ventricle (LV) into aorta.
- The LV is more globular and muscular than the right due to the pressure disparity between the pulmonary and systemic circulation.

Pressure changes during a cardiac cycle
Left ventricle
- During systole, peak pressure is ~120–160mmHg (rises with age).
- In diastole, pressure falls to thoracic cavity pressure of ~0mmHg.
- LV pressure changes from 120 to 0mmHg during the cardiac cycle.

Right ventricle
- During systole, peak pressure is ~25mmHg (the same volume of blood is ejected as the left ventricle, but at a lower pressure).
- In diastole, pressure falls to thoracic cavity pressure of ~0mmHg
- The RV pressure thus changes from 25 to 0mmHg.

Aorta
- During systole, peak pressure is ~120mmHg (same as LV).
- During diastole, aortic pressure is maintained by the elastic recoil of arterial walls and distal resistance. Pressure falls to ~80mmHg.
- Aortic pressure thus changes from 120 to 80mmHg.

Pulmonary artery
- During systole peak pressure is ~25mmHg (same as RV).
- During diastole pressure falls to ~8mmHg.
- Pulmonary artery pressure thus changes from 25 to 8mmHg.

Atrial pressure changes
- These are more complex due to bulging of the tricuspid and mitral valves during ventricular systole, and downward movement of the atrioventricular ring following opening of the pulmonary and aortic valves.
- Atrial pressure increases (due to the upward return of the atrioventricular ring and filling from the venae cavae) until the mitral valves open again and atrial contraction occurs.

The transport role of the cardiovascular system
- Oxygen from lungs to tissues.
- Carbon dioxide from tissues to lungs.
- Nutrients from digestive tract and storage organs to tissues.

- Metabolic waste from tissues to kidneys.
- Hormones and mediators to distant sites of action.

Anatomy and physiology

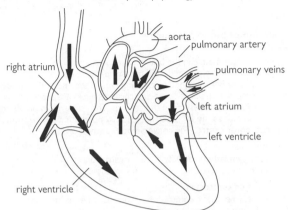

Fig. 12.1 Diagram of a cross-section of the heart showing direction of flow.
Reproduced with permission from *Critical Care Nursing*, Adam and Osborne (2005),
Oxford University Press.

Further information

Adam SK, Osborne S. (2005) *Critical Care Nursing*. Oxford: Oxford University Press.

Blood pressure and flow

Blood pressure (BP)
Arterial BP is the product of cardiac output and peripheral vascular resistance.

Regulation of blood pressure
Neural control
- The vasomotor centre in the brainstem controls vasomotor tone and heart rate via the sympathetic and parasympathetic nervous systems. Tone is primarily maintained by ongoing sympathetic nervous outflow.
- Baroreceptors in the aortic arch and carotid sinuses are sensitive to stretch exerted by pressure in the arteries. They transmit impulses that increase in rate as the BP rises and inhibit sympathetic outflow from the vasomotor centre. The converse occurs when BP falls.

Vasomotor tone
- Increased sympathetic activity = vasoconstriction.
- Decreased sympathetic activity = vasodilatation.

Heart rate and contractility
- Increased sympathetic stimulation → increased heart rate + increased force of contraction.
- Decreased sympathetic stimulation → decreased heart rate + decreased force of contraction.
- Increased parasympathetic stimulation → decreased heart rate + decreased force of contraction.

Capillary fluid shift mechanism
- Important when blood volume is too low or too high.
- Increased blood volume raises systemic pressure and hydrostatic pressure in the capillaries. This increases the shift of fluid across capillary membranes into the interstitial space.
- Decreased blood volume lowers capillary hydrostatic pressure and allows oncotic pressure (exerted by plasma proteins) to pull fluid by osmosis from the interstitial space into the capillaries.
- This response takes between 10min and several hours to adjust BP towards normal.

Renal excretory and hormonal mechanisms [renin-angiotensin-aldosterone (RAA)] mechanism
- Important for long-term control of BP and circulatory volume.
- Formation of urine is regulated by pressure in the renal arteries.
- The renin-angiotensin system responds to falls in BP that reduce renal perfusion by secreting angiotensin I, which is converted to angiotensin II (a potent vasoconstrictor). This increases BP and stimulates the adrenal cortex to secrete aldosterone. Aldosterone increases re-absorption of sodium and water from renal distal tubules and collecting ducts. BP then rises as the circulating volume increases.

Blood flow

- Depends on the contractile force of the ventricle and the difference between the pressure generated by the heart and the pressure at the end of the vessel (i.e. the difference between mean arterial pressure (MAP) and central venous pressure (CVP).
- Arterioles regulate blood flow. Any alteration in their diameter can produce major changes in blood flow. If arteriolar pressure is high due to vasoconstriction, blood flow may fall due to the increased resistance the heart has to pump against. The converse holds for vasodilation.
- Factors affecting flow include vessel diameter and length, and blood viscosity – these form the resistance to blood flow.
- Poiseuille's law describes this:

    Blood flow = [pressure $\times$ (diameter)^4]/length $\times$ viscosity

- The smooth muscle within the arteriole wall provides its tone. It responds to local tissue requirements, e.g. oxygen, carbon dioxide, nutrients, electrolytes, and metabolic waste (autoregulation).
- Sympathetic nerves moderate the state of vasoconstriction of arteries, veins and arterioles (autonomic control) by transmitting a continuous stream of impulses that maintain vasomotor tone. Vasoconstriction is produced by increased sympathetic impulses and vasodilatation by reduced sympathetic impulses.
- Autonomic control governs distribution of blood flow to the regions of the body. Factors affecting autonomic control include body temperature, exercise, and changes in blood volume.

Table 12.1 Stimuli for autoregulation in various organs

Organ	Stimulus for autoregulation
Heart and most body tissues	Lack of oxygen
Kidneys	Concentration of electrolytes and metabolic waste
	Lack of oxygen
Brain	Lack of oxygen
	High carbon dioxide levels

Determinants of cardiac performance I

Cardiac output (CO)
This is the amount of blood ejected from the left ventricle in 1min.
- CO is the product of stroke volume and heart rate.
- Manipulation of either SV or HR can affect cardiac output.
- Normal range is 4–6l/min.
- CO can be adjusted to body size ('cardiac index', CI) by dividing it by the body surface area (BSA). Normal range is 2.5–4.0l/min/m^2.

Heart rate
- An elevated heart rate (HR) can compromise cardiac output by:
  - increasing oxygen consumption by the myocardium;
  - reducing diastolic time, and thus perfusion of the coronary arteries;
  - shortening the ventricular filling phase of the cardiac cycle, causing a decreased blood volume to be pumped on the next contraction.
- A decreased HR may raise CO due to a longer filling time. With diseased hearts the myocardium may be so depressed that it cannot contract long enough to eject a bigger volume, causing a fall in CO.
- Other factors affecting heart rate include body temperature, thyroid, and adrenal function, psychological status, and arrhythmias.
- Healthy hearts tolerate rates between 30 and 170bpm for relatively long periods, but compromised cardiac function will reduce this tolerance

Stroke volume (SV)
The amount of blood ejected by the LV during one contraction, it is the difference between end-diastolic (EDV) and end systolic (ESV) volume. Normal range is 60–100ml. SV can be expressed as a percentage of end-diastolic volume, i.e. the 'ejection fraction' (EF). It is dependent on:
- Myocardial muscle contractility.
- Preload (the volume of blood filling the ventricle).
- Afterload (the resistance to blood flow from the ventricle).
- Heart rate (tachycardia reduces the time for diastolic filling).
- Normal EF is between 60 and 75%.

Preload
This is the degree of stretch of the muscle fibres at the end of diastole.
- The more blood in the ventricle, the greater the stretch, and thus the greater the force of contraction (Starling's law).
- It is a self-regulating system allowing the force of contraction to equal the volume of blood required to be ejected from the ventricle.
- There is an optimal range of stretch beyond which force of contraction is reduced, rather than increased (see Table 12.2).
- Preload is difficult to measure at the bedside; the pressures required to fill the ventricles are indirect guides only.
- CVP equates to the RV end diastolic (filling) pressure. Pulmonary artery wedge pressure equates to LV end diastolic (filling) pressure.

Table 12.2 Factors influencing ventricular preload

Decreased preload	*Volume loss:* haemorrhage, vomiting, oliguria
	Vasodilatation: pyrexia, drugs (e.g. nitrates), septicaemia, neurogenic shock, anaphylactic shock
	Tachycardia (potentially insufficient diastolic filling time)
	Impeded venous return (e.g. high intrathoracic pressure, pericardial tamponade, pulmonary embolus)
Increased preload	*Volume gain:* renal failure, excess blood products, excess iv fluids
	Vasoconstriction: hypothermia, drugs (e.g. adrenaline (epinephrine), dopamine >5 mcg/kg/min, noradrenaline (norepinephrine)), heart failure, pain, anxiety
	Bradycardia

Reproduced with permission from *Critical Care Nursing*, Adam and Osborne (2005), Oxford University Press.

Further information

Adam SK, Osborne S. (2005) *Critical Care Nursing*. Oxford: Oxford University Press.

Determinants of cardiac performance II

Afterload

This is the resistance to outflow of blood that must be overcome by the ventricles during systole:
- The most important factor determining afterload is resistance.
- Pulmonary vascular resistance (PVR) dictates RV afterload and the systemic vascular resistance (SVR) dictates LV afterload. Resistance is derived from cardiac output (CO), right atrial pressure (RAP), pulmonary artery wedge pressure (PAWP), mean pulmonary artery pressure (MPAP) and mean arterial pressure (MAP).

$$SVR = [(MAP - RAP) \times 80 \text{dyn s/cm}^5]/CO$$

$$PVR = [(MPAP - PAWP) \times 80 \text{dyn s/cm}^5]/CO$$

- normal range of SVR is 800–1200dyn s/cm^5;
- normal range of PVR is 50–200dyn s/cm^5.
- Afterload has an inverse effect on ventricular function. As resistance to ejection increases, so does the workload of the ventricle. A dysfunctional ventricle may not be able to maintain or increase the stroke volume against a high resistance and cardiac output may fall with excess vasoconstriction.
- In the presence of peripheral vasodilatation, the heart has less resistance to pump against so cardiac output usually increases.
- Factors affecting afterload are shown in Table 12.3.
- Causes of increased RV afterload include pulmonary embolus and pulmonary hypertension.
- Causes of increased LV afterload include aortic valve stenosis and systemic hypertension.

Table 12.3 Factors affecting afterload

Increased afterload	Vasoconstricting drugs (e.g. noradrenaline (norepinephrine))
	Anxiety
	Hypovolaemia
	Hypothermia
	Cardiogenic shock
	Atherosclerosis
Decreased afterload	Vasodilating drugs (e.g. nitrates, hydralazine, sodium nitroprusside)
	Anaphylactic shock
	Septicaemia
	Hyperthermia
	Neurogenic shock

Reproduced with permission from *Critical Care Nursing*, Adam and Osborne (2005), Oxford University Press.

Contractility

The ability to shorten heart muscle fibres (i.e. contraction) without altering their length or preload:

- The force of contraction of myocardial muscle cells alters in response to neural stimuli and levels of circulating catecholamines.
- Catecholamines bind to ß$_1$-adrenergic receptors on the myocardial membrane. This increases cyclic AMP and protein kinase A levels, triggering an increase in intracellular levels of calcium and an increase in contraction. This is energy-dependent so a failing heart with critical levels of ischaemia may be further compromised.
- Factors affecting contractility are shown in Table 12.4.

Table 12.4 Factors affecting contractility

Increased contractility	Positive inotropic drugs
	Endogenous catecholamines
	Hypervolaemia
	Hyperthyroidism
Decreased contractility	Negative inotropic drugs
	Functional loss of myocardium
	Anaerobic metabolism (intracellular acidosis)
	Hypoglycaemia
	Hypomagnesaemia
	Hypoxia

Reproduced with permission from *Critical Care Nursing*, Adam and Osborne (2005), Oxford University Press.

Further information

Adam SK, Osborne S. (2005) *Critical Care Nursing*. Oxford: Oxford University Press.

Oxygen delivery and consumption

Ensuring that tissues are well supplied with oxygen is an important therapeutic target in order to prevent tissue hypoxia, and subsequent organ dysfunction and failure.

Oxygen delivery (DO_2)

- This is the amount of oxygen delivered to the tissues by the blood.
- It depends on blood flow and the amount of O_2 carried in the blood.
- Blood flow is measured by cardiac output (CO) and the amount of oxygen carried is determined by the haemoglobin (Hb) concentration and the arterial oxygen saturation (S_aO_2).
- Oxygen delivery (DO_2) is calculated as:

  $$DO_2 \text{ (ml/min)} = CO \times (1.34 \times Hb \times S_aO_2) \times 10$$

  - a small amount of O_2 is carried dissolved in plasma, but this is a minimal at normal atmospheric pressure (normobaric) levels.
- Normal DO_2 for the resting adult is approximately 1000ml/min.
- O_2 is extracted by the tissues from arterial blood, leaving an O_2 reserve carried back to the heart and lungs in the venous blood. If demand by the tissues increases, this reserve will decrease if oxygen supply does not also increase to meet this increased demand.

Physiological mechanisms of increasing oxygen delivery

The cardiac and respiratory systems can increase the delivery of oxygen to the tissues when demand increases (e.g. during exercise):

- Respiratory effort increases to augment O_2 uptake and remove CO_2.
- Venous return (and thus preload) is increased.
- Heart rate and contractility are increased by adrenergic stimulation.

Oxygen consumption (VO_2)

- This is the amount of O_2 consumed by the tissues over one minute
- It is calculated by measuring the arteriovenous oxygen difference (i.e. the difference in oxygen content between arterial and venous blood):

  i.e. $VO_2 \text{ (ml/min)} = CO \times (1.34 \times Hb \times [S_aO_2 - S_vO_2]) \times 10$

  - the normal range is 220–250ml/min.
- Blood taken from the pulmonary artery is considered true 'mixed venous' blood; the percentage oxygen saturation of this blood is termed the mixed venous oxygen saturation (S_vO_2). This is not directly measurable unless the patient has a pulmonary artery catheter *in situ*. Venous blood taken from a central venous catheter (central venous oxygen saturation – $S_{cv}O_2$) is sometimes used to approximate for mixed venous saturation and although there is a difference in absolute value there is close tracking across a range of haemodynamics
- Normal S_vO_2 is 70–75%. If increased oxygen extraction occurs it may drop well below 50%. This signifies a serious disturbance in the oxygen supply-demand relationship.

Oxygen extraction ratio (O_2ER)

The oxygen extraction ratio (O_2ER) is the amount of oxygen extracted by the peripheral tissues divided by the amount of oxygen delivered. This can be calculated by taking a sample of venous blood from the pulmonary artery and a sample from an arterial line. The oxygen saturation of both are measured precisely using a co-oximeter.

$$O_2ER = [arterial - venous\ O_2\ saturation]/arterial\ O_2\ saturation$$

- The normal value in an adult is about 25%.
- Factors increasing the O_2 extraction ratio are:
  - decreased cardiac output;
  - increased oxygen consumption (when not accompanied by a matched increase in oxygen delivery);
  - anaemia;
  - decreased arterial oxygenation.
- DO_2 and VO_2 can be adjusted for the patient's size by dividing them by the body surface area to produce the oxygen delivery index (DO_2I) and the oxygen consumption index (VO_2I).

Table 12.5 Interventions to improve oxygen delivery

System	Manipulation	Rationale	Intervention
Cardiovascular	Optimize preload	Blood flow to the tissues will be increased	Serial fluid challenges until no further increase in SV (Starling curve)
	Reduce afterload (if possible)		Reduce afterload (e.g. with nitrates) to normalize SVR
	Increase contractility		Inotropes to increase cardiac output (e.g. dobutamine, dopexamine, epinephrine
	Increase heart rate (if bradycardic)		
Blood	Maintain Hb level within normal limits	The oxygen carrying capacity of the blood will be maximized	Transfuse to keep Hb above a certain threshold e.g. 8g/dl
Respiratory	Maintain arterial oxygen saturation >95%	The blood reaching the tissues will be adequately oxygenated	Increase inspired oxygen to maintain S_aO_2
	Respiratory support if patient is fatigued or hypoxaemic	The work of breathing may in itself increase oxygen demand	Hyperoxygenate prior to suction procedures if necessary

Reproduced with permission from *Critical Care Nursing*, Adam and Osborne (2005), Oxford University Press.

Further information

Adam SK, Osborne S. (2005) *Critical Care Nursing*. Oxford: Oxford University Press.
Rivers E, Anders D, and Powell D. (2001) Central venous oxygen saturation monitoring in the critically ill patient. *Curr Opin Crit Care* **7**, 204–11.

Pacing

This is a therapeutic stimulation of myocardial contraction using a small electrical current. It may be temporary (using an external pulse generator) or permanent (using an implanted pulse generator). There are two types of pacing electrode:

- **Unipolar:** has only one conducting wire and electrode; electrical current returns to the pacemaker via body fluids.
- **Bipolar:** has two conducting wires and two electrodes. The impulse passes down one wire to the distal electrode, and the circuit is completed via the second electrode and wire back to the pacemaker

Pacing routes

Transvenous endocardial

- A bipolar electrode wire is passed down a vein to the endocardial surface of the septal region of the right ventricle.
- The wire usually has an inflatable balloon at its tip to aid flotation during 'blind' placement.
- The position is checked by ECG monitoring. Right atrial stimulation produces large P waves and right ventricular stimulation produces widened QRS complexes occurring at the rate set on the pacing box. A pacing spike on the ECG is seen before each stimulated complex.
- The voltage threshold should be checked for good electrode placement (see later).
- Positioning a wire without a balloon is usually performed under X-ray imaging.

Epicardial

Electrodes are sutured on the pericardial surface during surgery. One or two electrodes are used. If only one is used, a skin surface electrode is used to complete the circuit.

External (transcutaneous)

- Large adhesive pads are placed on the patient's chest and back.
- Three ECG electrodes are also connected from the external pacer to the usual positions on the patient's chest.
- Current is passed between the skin electrodes inducing a paced heartbeat.
- This is the preferred method of pacing in an emergency.

Transoesophageal

An electrode is placed in the patient's oesophagus. It is a difficult and unreliable method to use in an emergency.

Modes of pacing

Most temporary pacemakers are only capable of single-chamber demand or fixed rate pacing. More advanced models can synchronize pacing in dual chambers (atrium and ventricle).

Fixed rate

- The heart is stimulated at a fixed rate per minute and will not alter in response to any intrinsic activity.

- It is only used if there is no underlying rhythm as arrhythmias may result if the pacing beat occurs close to the patient's own beat.

Demand
- An impulse is initiated if a pre-set interval elapses without an intrinsic stimulation of the ventricle.
- The interval is determined by the rate at which the pacemaker is set (e.g. a setting of 60bpm will only initiate pacing if the patient's rate falls <60bpm).

Synchronous
Electrodes are placed in the right atrium and ventricle, and allow synchronization of the stimulus in both chambers. A sensing electrode in the atria will sense an atrial contraction and stimulate a ventricular beat via the pacing electrode in the ventricle.

AV sequential
Stimulation of both atria and ventricle with a set interval between them. This allows optimal atrial filling before ventricular contraction.

Pacing threshold
- The minimum level of current needed to consistently pace the heart.
- Measured when the pacemaker is first attached; it should be <1.0mA.
- Check the threshold daily, or if any change occurs in the rhythm.
- Set the pacemaker current at 2–3 times above the threshold to allow for gradual worsening in threshold due to fibrosis at the electrode tip.

Overdrive pacing for tachycardia
- The pacing rate is set 10–15bpm above the rate of the tachycardia and may suppress ventricular or atrial tachycardias.
- Used for terminating paroxysmal SVT, atrial flutter, and ventricular tachycardia (it is ineffective for atrial fibrillation or sinus tachycardia).

Care of the patient with a pacemaker
- Securely fix connections between pacemaker and patient.
- Monitor the patient with temporary pacing using the ECG lead, which gives the clearest display of the pacing spike.
- Any failure of pacing will cause an absence of the spike without a following QRS complex (battery failure can be a cause).
- Absence of a QRS following a pacing spike is known as 'failure to capture'. It can be due to an increase in threshold or displacement of the pacing electrode. The delivered current may need to be increased or the wire repositioned.

Hypotension

A patient is usually considered hypotensive if MAP falls <60mmHg (or higher if the patient was previously hypertensive) or is associated with clinical symptoms of organ hypoperfusion. The aim of treatment is to:

- Establish and treat the cause.
- Maintain tissue oxygenation by increasing cardiac output, Hb, and /or arterial oxygen saturation (if appropriate).
- Maintain tissue perfusion by increasing the systemic blood pressure if there is evidence of compromise, e.g. oliguria.

Causes of hypotension

Hypovolaemia

Causes include haemorrhage, fluid loss, pooling of fluid in extravascular spaces, inadequate fluid intake, and vasodilatation.

- Immediate treatment is by rapid administration of fluid (crystalloid, colloid, blood, or blood products as appropriate).
- If the circulation does not respond promptly to fluid, further monitoring is necessary to guide the need for more fluid and/or drugs.
- Give repeated fluid challenges over 5min until CVP rises by ≥3mmHg 5–10min after a 200ml challenge. If mean BP <60mmHg despite a rise in CVP ≥3 mmHg and tissue hypoperfusion persists, drug therapy is indicated, ideally with cardiac output monitoring.
- A <10% response in stroke volume to a rapid 200ml fluid challenge suggests the patient is well filled (or, occasionally, that fluid losses such as major haemorrhage ≥ the rate of replacement). If hypoperfusion is still present, vasoactive drugs will be required.

Cardiogenic

Causes include cardiac failure, tachy/brady-arrhythmias, valvular stenosis/incompetence.

- Ensure patient is adequately volume resuscitated to exclude co-existing hypovolaemia.
- Initial treatment is with inotropic drugs if hypotensive.
- Reducing afterload (without excessively dropping blood pressure) is an important means of improving cardiac efficiency, since peripheral resistance and hence left ventricular work is decreased.
- A vasodilator (e.g. glyceryl trinitrate) may be carefully infused and titrated to response.
- Ensure intravascular volume is maintained if vasodilators are given.

Obstructive

Causes include cardiac tamponade, pulmonary embolism, and tension pneumothorax.

- The cause must be identified and promptly treated in order to restore blood pressure and adequate organ perfusion.
- Consider if CVP is raised and pulsus paradoxus (exaggeration of normal respiratory swing in blood pressure) is present
- Pulsus paradoxus may not be present if tidal volumes are low.

Inflammatory

Causes include sepsis, burns, trauma, and pancreatitis.

- The insult stimulates a generalized and exaggerated inflammatory response, resulting in loss of peripheral tone, and increased capillary leak. The resultant vasodilatation, relative hypovolaemia, loss of vascular tone (hyporeactivity), and possible myocardial depression from circulating toxins and mediators may cause hypotension.
- Fluid resuscitation is usually the immediate, first-line treatment.
- For severe hypotension, empiric inotropic (e.g. adrenaline (epinephrine)) or vasopressor (e.g. noradrenaline (norepinephrine)) drugs may also be needed, while adequate haemodynamic monitoring is being applied.
- Large volumes of fluid may be required; infusions should continue until no further improvement in stroke volume is seen. Volume overload should be avoided.
- If hypotension related to a high cardiac output persists after adequate fluid resuscitation, vasopressors will be required – high doses are often necessary. Noradrenaline (norepinephrine) is predominantly used for as it is an effective vasoconstrictor. Alternatives include dopamine and vasopressin/terlipressin.
- If myocardial dysfunction is present and afterload is raised, then adrenaline (epinephrine), dobutamine, or milrinone may be of benefit as they increase myocardial contractility. Dobutamine and milrinone may cause hypotension due to their vasodilatory effects.

Anaphylactic reactions

See ⬚ Chapter 20, pp. 471–486 for treatment of hypotension caused by anaphylaxis. In brief, fluid and pressors (often adrenaline (epinephrine)) are given in combination with corticosteroids, and an antihistamine, plus removal/cessation of the triggering agent.

Other causes

- Hypoadrenalism.
- Hypopituitarism.
- Poisoning.
- Side effect of drug therapy.

Manifestations of organ hypoperfusion

- Oliguria.
- Cool peripheries, skin pallor.
- Confusion, altered consciousness, syncope, agitation.
- Metabolic acidosis.
- Compensatory tachycardia.

Table 12.6 Hypotension: haemodynamic parameters.

Cause of hypotension	CO	PAWP	SVR
Hypovolaemia	↓	↓	↑
Cardiogenic	↓	↑ or →←—	↑
Inflammatory	↑	↓	↓
Obstructive	↓	↑ or →←—	
Anaphylactic	↑	↓	↓↑

↑, Increased; ↓, decreased; →←—, unchanged.

Reproduced with permission from *Critical Care Nursing*, Adam and Osborne (2005), Oxford University Press.

Further information

Adam SK, Osborne S. (2005) *Critical Care Nursing*. Oxford: Oxford University Press.

Hypertension

A sustained, raised BP above that considered normal for the patient's age. Chronic antihypertensive therapy is normally begun if the resting diastolic pressure is consistently above 90–95mmHg. Acute treatment may be started at lower pressures for specific conditions, e.g. dissecting aortic aneurysm, eclampsia, hypertensive encephalopathy. There are two types of hypertension:

- **Primary (or essential):** where the cause is unknown.
- **Secondary:** there is an identifiable cause.

Causes of secondary hypertension

- **Endocrine:** e.g. phaeocromocytoma, primary hyperaldosteronism, Cushing's syndrome, acromegaly.
- **Renal:** e.g. chronic glomerulonephritis, chronic pyelonephritis, renal artery stenosis, polycystic disease.
- **Pregnancy-induced** (pre-eclampsia/eclampsia).
- **Intracranial haemorrhage**.
- **Co-arctation of the aorta**.
- **Vasculitic conditions**, e.g. polyarteritis nodosa, SLE.
- **Drug-related:** e.g. withdrawal of antihypertensive drugs, monoamine oxidase inhibitor antidepressants taken with tyramine-containing foods, some recreational drugs.
- Consider compounding factors, such as pain and distress.

Manifestations of hypertensive emergency

- **Neurological:** headaches, dizziness, transient ischaemic attacks, focal disturbances, confusion, fits, coma (hypertensive encephalopathy), stroke.
- **Cardiovascular:** palpitations, heart failure, angina, myocardial infarction.
- **Renal:** renal failure, proteinuria.
- **Other:** retinopathy.

Disorders causing an acute hypertensive crisis

- Malignant hypertension.
- Phaeochromocytoma.
- Pre-eclampsia/eclampsia.
- Any cause of raised intracranial pressure.
- Drug-related (e.g. withdrawal of clonidine).
- Idiopathic.

Management of an acute hypertensive crisis

- The aim is to reduce BP urgently, but smoothly, without a sudden fall over 12–24h. This may need to be faster, e.g. if the patient has heart failure or encephalopathy. Over-aggressive reduction of BP should be avoided as this may cause poor organ perfusion, including stroke.
- A mean BP of approximately 120–130mmHg may be an appropriate initial target, although this depends on the underlying condition). If the cause of a raised BP is a raised ICP, the BP is usually allowed to remain

high (but not excessive) to maintain an adequate cerebral perfusion pressure (see neurological chapter).
- Continuous BP monitoring is essential.
- The choice of hypotensive drug will depend on the cause of hypertension and the urgency of treatment.
- The most commonly used drugs in critical care are intravenous glyceryl trinitrate, sodium nitroprusside (produces a rapid effect and can be finely controlled), labetalol, and hydralazine – all given by iv infusion. If the patient is not suffering a hypertensive emergency, oral or nasogastric therapy may be considered with smooth reduction of BP to an acceptable level over 24–48h.
- The drug dosage should be titrated against response.

Malignant encephalopathy

Caused by uncontrolled hypertension from any cause. Occurs in chronically hypertensive patients when an acute BP elevation increases cerebral perfusion resulting in exudation of fluid into the brain. Arteriolar damage and necrosis occur, leading to cerebral oedema, ischaemia, and papilloedema.

Clinical features
- Headache.
- Confusion.
- Seizures.
- Nausea and vomiting.

Management
Antihypertensive therapy (often labetalol) with careful reduction to target BP over 6–12h.

Assessment of the patient with chest pain

History

Details should include: type of pain, length of history, precipitating factors, social history (e.g. smoking, alcohol, diabetes, hyperlipidaemia, drugs (medical and recreational such as cocaine), and family history.

Physical assessment

Further details are given in 📖 Chapter 5 and 📖 Chapter 6. See also Table 12.7.

Table 12.7 Physical assessment in the patient with a cardiac disorder

	Observation	Note particularly if:
Skin	Colour, touch	Pale, cyanosed, mottled, cold, clammy, hot, presence of ankle oedema
Respiration	Rate, depth	Tachypnoeic, dyspnoeic, using accessory muscles, orthopnoeic (breathless lying flat)
Pulse	Feel, rate	Thready, full volume, bounding tachycardia, irregular
Pain	Site, duration, severity	Associated with movement, respiration, at rest, position, eating
Other		Oliguria, nausea, vomiting, presence of cough possibly due to pulmonary oedema. Anxious, restless

Reproduced with permission from *Critical Care Nursing*, Adam and Osborne (2005), Oxford University Press.

Causes of chest pain

- Acute coronary syndrome (angina).
- Myocardial infarction.
- Pericarditis.
- Oesophagitis.
- Gastritis and peptic ulceration.
- Pancreatitis.
- Pneumonia.
- Pulmonary embolism.
- Pleurisy.
- Acute aortic dissection.
- Chest wall, e.g. intercostal myalgia, costochondritis, shingles.

Types of chest pain

This may help differentiate pain of cardiac from non-cardiac origins.

- **Stable angina:** typically constricting, retrosternal, radiating to the arms (predominantly left), neck, or jaw. Often occurs in response to stimuli that increase the oxygen demand of the heart (e.g. exercise).
- **Unstable angina:** as in stable angina, but the periods of pain are prolonged, may occur at rest, and may have no precipitating factors.
- **Myocardial infarction:** typically crushing, severe retrosternal pain, which may extend to left arm, neck, jaw, or back. Often accompanied by nausea, vomiting, or sweating. The onset of pain is not always associated with exertion and is not relieved by rest. Some patients, however, may have little or no pain, e.g. diabetics.
- **Pericarditis:** usually sharp, retrosternal, and more painful on inspiration. Often worse on lying flat, relieved when sitting up and leaning forward.
- **Pleuritic pain:** sharp, localized, worse on inspiration, and coughing.
- **Pulmonary embolism:** usually pleuritic in nature, and may be associated with haemoptysis and/or dyspnoea.
- **Oesophageal pain:** usually associated with or eased by food, and worse on lying flat. May be relieved by nitrates. Oesophageal rupture is usually preceded by vomiting.
- **Aortic dissection:** 'tearing', rather than crushing, often felt in the back.
- **Musculoskeletal pain:** usually identified by the effect of movement and position. The chest wall may be tender to touch at the specific location.

Investigations

- 12-lead ECG.
- Chest X-ray.
- Blood tests including: (i) troponin and cardiac enzymes; (ii) urea and electrolytes; (iii) glucose (may be elevated in myocardial infarction); (iv) haemoglobin; (v) clotting studies (if anticoagulant therapy has been administered or myocardial ischaemia affecting a young person); (vi) cholesterol and triglyceride levels; (vii) arterial blood gas analysis if acidosis or hypoxaemia are present; (viii) other specific tests as indicated, e.g. digoxin levels, cocaine levels.
- Special tests as indicated, e.g. echocardiography, angiography, CT chest ± abdomen.

Haemodynamic monitoring

Adequate monitoring is essential to allow assessment of cardiac function. The extent of monitoring will depend on the patient's condition, but will include a minimum of ECG monitoring and blood pressure. CVP, pulmonary artery pressure and oxygen saturation may be indicated. Urine output will provide a guide to renal perfusion. Full details of invasive and non-invasive monitoring are given in the cardiovascular monitoring chapter.

Further information

Adam SK, Osborne S. (2005) *Critical Care Nursing*. Oxford: Oxford University Press.

Acute coronary syndromes (ACS)

These are a range of symptoms associated with chest pain. If myocardial injury is associated with ACS then this is termed myocardial infarction. ACS is divided into those with clear myocardial injury on ECG (ST elevation is evident) known as ST elevation myocardial infarction (STEMI) and those without ST elevation, but with biochemical markers (NSTEMI), or unstable angina (UA) if no biochemical markers are evident.

Myocardial infarction

A region of myocardium becomes irreversibly necrosed due to thrombo-embolic occlusion of the coronary artery supplying that area of heart muscle, direct trauma, or electrocution.

Risk factors

- Smoking.
- Hyperlipidaemia.
- Hypertension.
- Diabetes.
- Obesity, age, family history, environmental, and geographical factors.

Physical assessment and investigations

See 📖 Assessment of the patient with chest pain, p. 256, and 📖 Chapter 8, p. 144 for details of cardiac enzymes. Troponin may be elevated due to other causes, e.g. pulmonary embolism.

12-lead ECG changes

Initial convex ST elevation and T wave inversion (implying injury and ischaemia) usually seen in leads adjacent to the infarcted area. This is a STEMI. If no ST elevation present, this is defined as a NSTEMI. Leads opposite the area show inverse changes. Pathological Q waves then develop, although this can vary from minutes to days. Some 20% of patients present with no ST segment elevation, nor clearly identifiable Q waves. Co-existing left bundle branch block may obscure ECG signs of acute MI. Serial ECG ± cardiac enzyme estimations should be taken over 3 days to confirm an acute MI.

Initial management

- Assess patient (see 📖 Assessment of the patient with chest pain, p. 256).
- Administer oxygen to maintain S_aO_2 95–98%.
- Give 2–4 puffs of GTN spray or one GTN tablet SL, and 150mg aspirin.
- Continuous ECG monitoring, pulse oximetry, regular BP recording.
- Wide bore peripheral iv access.
- Opiate (e.g. diamorphine 2.5–5mg) + anti-emetic if in pain or distress.
- Blood samples for investigations, chest X-ray, ECG.
- Perform immediate percutaneous intervention (PCI). If not available or contraindicated, give thrombolytic agent (unless also contraindicated) plus heparin (see 📖 Thrombolytic therapy, p. 262).
- Commence beta-blocker (unless contraindicated).

- Manage complications (e.g. cardiac arrest, pulmonary oedema, cardiogenic shock, haemodynamically compromising arrhythmias).
- Relief of anxiety and distress, provide appropriate information.
- Bedrest for first 24h.
- Gold standard management is rapid reperfusion of coronaries with either primary percutaneous coronary intervention or thrombolysis. PCI has been shown to have better outcomes.

Angina pectoris

Usually caused by critical narrowing of one or more coronary arteries leading to a myocardial oxygen debt and ischaemia during periods of increased demand (e.g. exercise). Unstable angina (pain at rest or on minimal exertion) indicates severe stenosis of the artery and there is a major risk of infarction. Other causes of angina include:

- Severe anaemia.
- Aortic stenosis.
- Hypertrophic cardiomyopathy.
- Coronary artery spasm (Prinzmetal angina).
- Arrhythmias that compromise cardiac output.

Physical assessment and investigations

See 🕮 Assessment of the patient with chest pain, p. 256. Cardiac enzyme estimation over several days will show no serial rise and further investigations will be necessary (e.g. exercise ECG, dobutamine stress test, thallium scanning, angiography).

12-lead ECG

The ECG may reveal ST segment elevation and T wave flattening. It may be normal outside an attack and should be repeated during pain.

Management

Unstable angina warrants hospital admission, aggressive medical treatment, and investigation with a view to coronary revascularization (e.g. balloon angioplasty ± stent insertion, coronary bypass surgery).

- Administer oxygen to maintain S_aO_2 95–98%.
- Wide bore peripheral iv access.
- Correct any hypotension and tissue hypoperfusion.
- Glyceryl trinitrate 0.3mg SL or 0.4–0.8mg by buccal spray, followed by intravenous nitrate infusion.
- 75–150mg aspirin (for antiplatelet aggregation effect).
- Continuous ECG monitoring, pulse oximetry, regular BP recording.
- Consider beta blocker unless contraindicated.
- Low molecular weight heparin + clopidogrel (unless contraindicated).
- Blood tests, chest X-ray, ECG.
- Consider GlycoProtein IIb IIIa inhibitor (such as iv eptifibatide) if at high risk of MI.
- Bedrest if symptoms are severe or persist.
- Relief of anxiety, appropriate information.

Thrombolytic therapy

The pharmacological lysis (breakdown) of blood clots in order to arrest a disease process or reduce its complications. Its use is beneficial in:
• Myocardial infarction.
• Massive pulmonary embolus.
• Thromboembolic stroke.
• Acute limb ischaemia due to thrombus, embolus.

Contraindications to thrombolysis

Absolute contraindications
• Bleeding disorders.
• Active bleeding.
• Neurosurgery/cerebrovascular accidents within 2 months.
• Intracranial neoplasm/aneurysm.
• Serious trauma/major surgery within 10 days.
• Aortic dissection.

Relative contraindications
• Diabetic retinopathy.
• Untreated hypertension.
• Traumatic or prolonged CPR.
• Recent obstetric delivery.
• Recent puncture of major vessel.
• Warfarin therapy.

Thrombolytic drugs

• All thrombolytic agents work by activating plasminogen, which removes the fibrin mesh of the clot (fibrinolysis). This allows the clot to become soluble and is then subject to further proteolysis by other enzymes. Blood flow is then restored to the occluded vessel.
• Apart from streptokinase all thrombolytic agents are administered with heparin (unfractionated or low molecular weight) for 24–48h. Heparin does not reduce the size of the clot, but prevents its enlargement or the re-occlusion of the vessel.
• They are given iv, but can be given intra-arterially during angiography.
• Two types of thrombolytic drugs are available – those naturally occurring (e.g. streptokinase and urokinase) and drugs produced by recombinant therapy (e.g. tissue plasminogen activator – rTPA).
• Some centres consider rTPA or equivalents as first line therapy for patients <45 years with a large anterior MI presenting <4h and in cardiogenic shock. rTPA should not be used more than 6 hrs after the onset of symptoms in patients >75 years old (due to the risk of CVA) and in the absence of ECG changes.
• Arterial and/or central venous cannulation should not be delayed following commencement of thrombolysis if clinically indicated.
• Considerable haemorrhage can occur and this can be reversed by stopping the infusion, giving fresh frozen plasma and tranexamic acid (10mg/kg repeated after 6–8 h).

- If given for acute myocardial infarction reperfusion arrhythmias are common. Usually, these are benign, but temporary cessation of the infusion may be necessary.
- Allergic or anaphylactic reactions to streptokinase can occur (rash, hypotension), and are treated by stopping the infusion and giving hydrocortisone 200mg iv, chlorphenamine 10mg iv and ranitidine 50mg iv. Support the circulation if necessary before restarting thrombolytic therapy – rTPA can be given instead.

Acute heart failure/cardiogenic shock

This is the inability of the heart to supply adequate amounts of O_2 and nutrients to meet the body's metabolic needs. Features of low cardiac output are related to inadequate forward blood flow plus retrograde venous congestion. Some pathologies causing excess metabolic demands (e.g. thyrotoxic crisis) result in high-output cardiac failure. Decreased cardiac output and tissue hypoperfusion ± hypotension in the presence of adequate circulating volume is known as cardiogenic shock.

Major causes
- Myocardial infarction.
- Drugs (e.g. overdose of beta-blockers or verapamil).
- Arrhythmias (tachy/brady).
- Valve dysfunction.
- Sepsis.
- Cardiomyopathy/myocarditis.
- Trauma causing myocardial contusion.
- Pericardial tamponade.
- Constrictive pericarditis (e.g. TB).
- Severe anaemia.
- Pulmonary embolus.
- Hypertensive emergency.
- High output failure, e.g. thyrotoxic crisis, beri-beri.

Clinical features
General
Low cardiac output, stroke volume, and tissue hypoperfusion causing:
- Muscle fatigue (including respiratory muscles).
- Oliguria, raised urea and creatinine.
- Confusion, agitation, drowsiness, coma.
- Cool peripheries, cyanosis, pallor, sweating.
- Dyspnoea, tachycardia, hypoxaemia, low arterial and venous SO_2.
- Metabolic acidosis, raised lactate.

In right heart failure
Increased venous congestion causing:
- Peripheral oedema.
- Hepatic congestion, splanchnic ischaemia.
- Raised CVP.

In left heart failure
Increased pulmonary hydrostatic pressure causing:
- Pulmonary oedema, wheeze.
- Pleural effusion ± cardiomegaly.
- Raised PAWP.

Investigations

See 📖 Assessment of the patient with chest pain, p. 256. In addition, B-type natriuretic peptide (BNP) may be measured (see 📖 Chapter 8, pp. 135–152). Chest X-ray may show pulmonary oedema, and echocardiography will show regional or global wall motion abnormality ± valve abnormalities ± tamponade.

Management

- If possible, identify and treat the cause (e.g. arrhythmia).
- High flow oxygen to maintain S_aO_2 95–98%. Monitor blood gases. Consider early non-invasive ventilatory support (CPAP, BiPAP). Endotracheal intubation and mechanical ventilation may be needed to reduce work of breathing, improve gas exchange, and ease distress.
- Continuous haemodynamic monitoring. The extent of monitoring depends on the severity of failure. At a minimum, this includes ECG, BP, and pulse oximetry, but in severe cases will require monitoring of cardiac output.
- Pre- and afterload reduction by iv infusion of nitrates (give nitrates SL or via spray, while the infusion is being prepared). Titrate infusion rapidly to target level. Tolerance to nitrates develops by about 24h, necessitating a higher dose to achieve a similar effect.
- Within 24h commence ACE inhibition (unless contraindicated), starting at low doses and increasing to appropriate long-term dose.
- Diuretics (e.g. furosemide) are rarely needed initially unless the cause of heart failure is intravascular fluid overload, which will be managed by afterload reduction. They may be indicated for acute-on-chronic heart failure, especially if the patient usually takes diuretics. Do not give diuretics if the patient is hypovolaemic.
- Hypotension may be due in part to left ventricular underfilling. This may be related to hypovolaemia, obstruction (e.g. tamponade, PE, mitral stenosis) or right heart failure. If hypovolaemia is suspected cautious filling with 100–200ml fluid challenges should be given to optimize stroke volume. No rise in SV, and/or a rise in PAWP or CVP ≥3mmHg post-fluid suggests optimal filling has been achieved. Monitor urine output.
- Give iv opiate, e.g. diamorphine 2.5mg, for pain or agitation.
- If vasoconstriction or hypotension persists, and there is evidence of tissue hypoperfusion, inotropes should be considered (e.g. adrenaline (epinephrine), dobutamine, milrinone). All have additional vasodilator or vasoconstrictor effects so BP may be considerably affected. Only give the dose that is absolutely necessary to maintain adequate organ perfusion as these drugs all increase myocardial oxygen demand. Mixed venous oxygen saturation is a guide to the ability to meet the body's oxygen demands. In severe heart failure this can drop markedly. A therapeutic target is to keep S_vO_2 >60%.
- Intra-aortic balloon counter pulsation or ventricular assist devices can augment cardiac output, reduce cardiac work, and improve perfusion. Surgery may be required if heart failure is due to an anatomical problem, e.g. tight aortic stenosis, acute ventricular septal defect.

Pericarditis and pericardial tamponade

Pericarditis

Inflammation of the pericardium typified by sharp chest pain radiating to the neck, arm or back. It is relieved by sitting forward and worsens or lying down, inspiration or coughing. A friction rub is often heard on auscultation. ECG often shows ST elevation in all leads.

Causes

- Infection – viral (e.g. coxsackie), bacterial, TB, or fungal.
- Myocardial infarction.
- Malignancy.
- Radiotherapy.
- Trauma.
- Uraemia.
- Connective tissue disorders (e.g. SLE).
- Idiopathic.
- Side effect of drug therapy (isoniazid, ciclosporine, hydralazine).
- Post-cardiac surgery.

Management

- Non-steroidal anti-inflammatory agents (e.g. indometacin).
- Treat cause if possible.
- Occasionally surgery is required if constrictive pericarditis causes haemodynamic compromises.

Complications

- Pericardial effusion and possible cardiac tamponade.
- Constrictive pericarditis.

Pericardial tamponade

This is an accumulation of fluid (blood, effusion) or air into the pericardial space, which can result in reduced ventricular filling and subsequent haemodynamic compromise. Features include dyspnoea, tachycardia, tachypnoea, cool, clammy extremities, and signs of tissue hypoperfusion.

Causes

- Infection.
- Post-myocardial infarction.
- Drugs (hydralazine, isoniazid).
- Post-cardiac surgery.
- Aortic dissection.
- Connective tissue disorders (e.g. rheumatoid arthritis).
- Trauma.
- Malignancy.
- Radiation therapy.
- Iatrogenic (e.g. after sternal biopsy, central line insertion).
- Uraemia.
- Idiopathic.

Management

Significant effusions require drainage (pericardiocentesis) either by open surgery or percutaneously. The percutaneous approach can be carried out under echocardiography, fluoroscopically or performed 'blind', although this is risky and should only be carried out in emergencies by an expert operator.

'Blind' pericardocentesis

- The patient is positioned semi-supine.
- Under local anaesthetic, a long 18-gauge needle connected to a syringe is introduced by the side of the xiphisternum under the costal margin and advanced in the direction of the scapula. An ECG V lead is attached to the needle to detect myocardial penetration (ST segment changes or multiple ventricular ectopics may be seen).
- The catheter may be transduced to check it is not in the right ventricle (it will show the classic right ventricular waveform).
- When fluid is aspirated the catheter should be advanced no further.
- A 3-way tap is attached and drainage performed.
- Alternatively, a guide wire may be advanced through the cannula into the pericardial space, the cannula is removed, and a pigtail catheter placed over the guide wire.
- Blood may be aspirated (haemopericardium), particularly following trauma, cardiac surgery or malignancy.
- Specimens should be sent for culture and cytology.

Infective endocarditis (IE)

An infection of the endocardial surface of the heart, usually involving ≥1 of the heart valves. Organisms adhere to the surface of the valve, and invade and destroy the valvular leaflets. Vegetations may develop, which prevent the valves from functioning properly. Fragments can break off producing emboli in the brain, gut, limbs, etc. The commonest infecting organisms are *Streptococcus viridans* and *Staphylococcus aureus*. Others include enterococci, *Coxiella burnetti*, and fungi. Prosthetic valves can also be affected.

IE can lead to intractable heart failure and myocardial abscesses. Two major types exist – acute and subacute. Acute IE frequently involves normal valves and is rapidly progressive. Subacute IE typically affects abnormal valves and its course may extend over many months.

Risk factors

- Invasive procedures (e.g. iv cannulation, pacing wires, surgery).
- Cancer (especially colorectal).
- Diabetes.
- Dental manipulation.
- iv Drug abuse (right heart valves are usually affected).
- Alcoholism.
- Renal failure.
- Urinary tract infection.

Features

- Pyrexia.
- Features of heart failure (see 📖 Acute heart failure/cardiogenic shock, p. 264).
- Thrombo-emboli (e.g. stroke).
- Immunological sequelae (e.g. glomerulonephritis).
- Vascular [e.g. acute limb ischaemia, haemorrhagic lesions on palms and soles of feet, on nails (splinter haemorrhages) and in conjunctiva].
- Distal abscesses, e.g. in brain.
- Heart murmurs.
- Arrhythmias.
- Repeatedly positive serial blood cultures or relapse on discontinuing antibiotics.
- Vegetations seen on valves on echocardiography.
- Signs of chronic illness (e.g. clubbing, splenomegaly, weight loss).

Management

- High dose iv antibiotics (often for 6 weeks).
- Treatment of specific complications (e.g. heart failure, arrhythmias).
- Surgery may be required (e.g. valve replacement or repair, drainage of myocardial abscesses).
- Education and preventative measures. National guidelines no longer recommend routine prophylaxis for surgical or dental procedures in risk groups.

Further information

NICE (2008) *Prophylaxis against infective endocarditis: NICE guidelines.* NICE, London.

Cardiomyopathy and myocarditis

Cardiomyopathy

This is disease of the heart muscle itself. There are three main types.

Dilated

- The commonest form, with an enlarged heart cavity and weakened heart muscle, which can lead to failure and arrhythmias.
- As blood flows more slowly through the heart, mural thrombi may form with the potential for systemic emboli.
- Causes include chronic ischaemia infection, sepsis, autoimmune processes, excess alcohol, recreational drug abuse, exposure to drugs or chemicals, excess catecholamines (Takotsubo syndrome) from severe stress (including anxiety) or a phaeochromocytoma.

Hypertrophic

- Ventricular muscle mass is increased.
- In one form, hypertrophic obstructive cardiomyopathy (HOCM), the septum enlarges and obstructs flow from the left ventricle. The thickened septal wall can distort the mitral valve, causing it to leak.
- Sudden death can occur from arrhythmias or outflow obstruction.
- The patient may complain of chest pain, dyspnoea, syncopal attacks, or palpitations.
- An increase in sympathetic activity can cause hypertension.
- It is mainly an inherited disease and usually affects young adults.

Restrictive

- The myocardium becomes excessively rigid and it is harder for the ventricles to fill between heartbeats.
- The commonest cause in the UK is amyloid, which causes abnormal protein deposits in the myocardium. In the tropics, it is mainly due to idiopathic fibrosis.

Management

- Perform 12-lead ECG and echocardiography. Biopsy is occasionally performed.
- Treat heart failure or angina if present.
- Treat arrhythmias (cardioversion or an implantable defibrillator may be necessary).
- Treat hypertension.
- Anticoagulate.
- Surgery may be required, e.g. alcohol ablation or excision of excess muscle in HOCM, heart transplantation.
- Counselling and education.
- Screen family members.

Myocarditis

Inflammation and consequent weakening of the myocardium.

Causes

- Infection (bacterial, viral, protozoal, fungal, parasitic).
- Immunological (e.g. rejection after heart transplant).

- Auto-antigens (e.g. systemic vasculitis).
- Toxic (e.g. drugs, toxins such as snake venom, heavy metals).
- Physical agents (e.g. electrocution, radiation, hyperpyrexia).

Clinical features

- Chest pain (stabbing).
- Congestive heart failure.
- Palpitations (secondary to arrhythmias).
- Sudden death (particularly in young adults).
- Fever.
- Pericarditis and endocarditis ('pancarditis') may co-exist.

Investigations

- ECG – diffuse T wave inversion, possible saddle shape ST segment elevation.
- Elevated inflammatory markers, e.g. CRP, ESR.
- Elevated troponin.
- Definitive diagnosis is by myocardial biopsy.

Management

- Antibiotics.
- NSAIDs.
- Supportive treatment (e.g. of heart failure).
- The role of steroids is hotly debated.
- Severe heart failure may require ventricular assist device insertion and, sometimes, transplantation.

Anti-arrhythmic drugs I

These can be categorized into four classes, determined by their action on the electrophysiological mechanisms of the myocardial cells.

Class I
- Class 1A drugs lengthen the effective refractory period by inhibiting fast Na^+ currents and, hence, reduce the speed or prolong the duration of the action potential.
- Class 1B drugs inhibit the fast Na^+ current, while shortening action potential duration. They selectively affect diseased or ischaemic tissue and are thought to promote conduction block, interrupting re-entry.
- Class 1C drugs powerfully inhibit His-Purkinje conduction with QRS widening, inhibit fast Na^+ channels with depression of the action potential, and also shorten action potential in the His-Purkinje fibres.

Class II
Include ß-adrenergic antagonists, which inhibit myocardial ß-receptors and reduce the rate of pacemaker discharge.

Class III
These lengthen action potential duration and, thus, the effective refractory period. They homogenize the pattern of the action potential throughout the heart with relatively little negative inotropic effect.

Class IV
Inhibit slow channel-dependent conduction (calcium) via the AV node.

Amiodarone
- Complex drug, shares properties of all classes of anti-arrhythmics.
- Lengthens the effective refractory period by prolonging the duration of the action potential.
- Has a powerful Class 1 effect, inhibiting sodium channels.
- Non-competitively blocks alpha- and beta-adrenergic receptors.
- A calcium antagonist effect may be responsible for the bradycardia and AV nodal inhibition sometimes associated with its use.

Indications
- Ventricular tachyarrhythmias.
- Recurrence of paroxysmal atrial fibrillation or flutter.
- Wolff–Parkinson–White arrhythmias.

Dosage
- In life-threatening arrhythmias 150–300mg over 3 mins then iv infusion of 15mg/kg/24h via a central vein. Reduce thereafter to 10mg/kg/24h for 3–7 days, then maintain at 5mg/kg/24h. The loading dose is essential because of the slow onset of full action.
- For less dangerous arrhythmias, 300mg is infused over 1h (via central line) followed by a further 900mg over the next 23h. The daily dose is reduced thereafter.

Side effects
- Pneumonitis (at high doses) potentially leading to pulmonary fibrosis.
- Torsade de pointes may result from QT prolongation plus hypokalaemia.

- Hypothyroidism as it can inhibit the conversion of T_4 to T_3.
- Phlebitis if infused peripherally, nausea.
- Prolongs prothrombin time (may cause bleeding if on warfarin).
- Potentiates the effect of digoxin.

Lidocaine (lignocaine)

- A class IB agent that acts on the ischaemic myocardium.
- More effective in the presence of a high plasma potassium level.

Indications

- Emergency treatment of ventricular arrhythmias.
- Suppression of ventricular arrhythmias associated with myocardial infarction and ischaemia.

Dosage

- Initial loading dose of 100mg iv followed by an infusion of 1–4mg/min. This is gradually reduced over 24–48h.
- Decrease dose in the elderly where toxicity can develop rapidly.

Side effects

- Drowsiness, speech disturbances, dizziness at high infusion rates.
- Seizures, agitation, coma at toxic levels.
- Clearance via the liver may be reduced if receiving cimetidine or propanolol. Drugs that reduce hepatic enzymes (e.g. barbiturates, phenytoin, rifampicin) may increase dosage requirements.

Magnesium sulphate

Low serum or intracellular Mg^{2+} levels are associated with an increased risk of arrhythmias. Infusions of Mg^{2+} are therapeutically effective although the precise mechanism has not been identified.

Indications

Recurrent (or resistant) ventricular arrhythmias and atrial fibrillation have been terminated with iv magnesium.

Dosage

- The optimal dosage and frequency has not yet been determined.
- An often-used dosage is 10–20mmol $MgSO_4$ given over 5–10min in emergency or over 1h otherwise followed by a further 20–40mmol over 5–10h.

Side effects

- Sweating and sensation of heat with rapid iv injection.
- Monitor serum magnesium levels. Keep below 2.7mmol/l as higher levels are associated with bradycardia, prolonged PR interval, and AV block. Monitor closely in patients with renal failure as magnesium is excreted via the kidneys.

Anti-arrhythmic drugs II

Adenosine
- Opens potassium channels and inhibits sino-atrial and atrioventricular nodes.
- Opening of potassium channels produces an indirect calcium antagonist effect due to a change in polarity away from that required to open the voltage-gated calcium channels.

Indications
- Paroxysmal supraventricular tachycardia.
- Re-entrant tachycardias via the AV node.
- Useful diagnostic test to distinguish between VT and SVT with aberrant conduction.
- Occasionally effective in some types of VT.
- A rapid bolus of 3–6mg initially. If not effective in 1–2min a further iv bolus of 12mg is given. If no effect the 12mg bolus can be repeated once. The effect will last no longer than 10–30s.

Side effects
- Dyspnoea due to bronchoconstriction.
- Flushing and headache due to vasodilatory effects.
- Transient new rhythms may occur at the time of chemical conversion. Occasionally, the induced heart block may be prolonged.
- Should not be generally used in patients with asthma, second or third degree heart block or sick sinus syndrome. Reduce the dose if the patient is taking dipyridamole due to the inhibitory effect of dipyridamole on adenosine breakdown.
- Caffeine and theophylline will competitively antagonize adenosine.

Verapamil
- Inhibits the action potential of the upper and middle nodal regions where depolarization is calcium-mediated.
- Can terminate tachycardias of re-entry origin believed to be the cause of most paroxysmal supraventricular tachycardias.
- Increases nodal block and the effective refractory period of the AV node.
- Reduces the ventricular rate of atrial fibrillation or flutter.

Indications
Used in supraventricular tachycardias and chronic atrial fibrillation, where myocardial depression is not a problem.

Dosage
- A slow bolus of 2.5mg iv over at least a minute and can be repeated up to a maximum of 20mg.
- Calcium gluconate or chloride (5–10ml 10% solution) should be available for rapid administration (or pretreatment) if there is a negative inotropic effect associated with the bolus.

Side effects
- Hypotension and bradycardia.
- Flushing, headaches, and dizziness due to vasodilatory effects.
- Facial, epigastric, or gingival pain.
- Hepatotoxicity and transient mental confusion.
- It should not be generally given to patients with AV nodal disease, sick sinus syndrome, or myocardial depression.
- Should not be given to patients treated with beta-adrenergic blockers or other anti-arrhythmics.

Beta-adrenergic blockers

There are two types of beta receptor: β_1 and β_2.
- β_1-receptors are found in the sino-atrial node and myocardium, and influence contractility and heart rate.
- β_2-receptors are found in the arterioles of the heart, liver, and skeletal muscle, and in the smooth muscle of the bronchioles and cause vasodilation.

Beta blockers (e.g. atenolol, sotolol, esmolol) are useful for treating supraventricular tachycardias. They act by blocking the effects of catecholamines at the β_1-receptors. This causes:
- Decreased sinus rate.
- Decreased conduction velocity (which can block re-entry mechanisms).
- Inhibition of aberrant pacemaker activity.

Drugs used in the treatment of low cardiac output and/or hypotension

Noradrenaline (norepinephrine)

- Acts predominantly on alpha-adrenergic receptors.
- Increases BP by increasing peripheral resistance. Cardiac output usually falls as a result.
- Hepatic, renal, and splanchnic flows fall, but coronary blood flow may increase due to the increase in diastolic pressure.
- Decreases insulin secretion causing a rise in blood glucose.
- Given by iv infusion via a central vein.
- Dosage is titrated to response starting at 0.01 microgram/kg/min.
- Side effects include arrhythmias, chest pain, and headache.
- As with all catecholamines, has numerous covert effects including immunomodulation, decrease in metabolic efficiency, increased cardiac work, thrombogenicity, and stimulating bacterial growth.

Adrenaline (epinephrine)

- Acts on both alpha- and beta-receptors.
- Low doses produce predominantly beta (inotropic) effects, higher doses produce more alpha (vasoconstricting) effects.
- Increases heart rate, cardiac output, blood pressure, and myocardial oxygen consumption.
- When given as an iv bolus it causes a rapid rise in systolic blood pressure by increasing the strength of ventricular contraction, increasing heart rate, and causing constriction of the arterioles of the skin, mucosa, and splanchnic areas.
- When given as an infusion, there may be a decrease in peripheral resistance due to its action on beta-2 receptors of skeletal muscle. This vasodilator effect may predominate, and any increase in BP is due to cardiac stimulation and an increase in cardiac output.
- Peripheral resistance may rise or be unaltered due to a greater ratio of alpha-to-beta activity in different vascular areas.
- Renal blood flow can fall by up to 40%.
- Increases blood glucose as it decreases insulin secretion, but increases glucagon secretion and the rate of glycogenolysis.
- Bronchodilates, but tends to increase the viscosity of secretions.
- May cause a profound metabolic acidosis due to accelerated aerobic glycolysis, rather than secondary to ischaemia.
- Must administer infusions via a central vein as extravasation can cause local necrosis.
- Dosage is titrated to response starting at 0.01 microgram/kg/min by continuous infusion or 0.05–1mg for bolus dose.

Milrinone

- Positive inotrope and vasodilator with some chronotropic activity.
- Used for short-term iv treatment of patients with acute decompensated heart failure.
- Increases myocardial contractility and improves diastolic function.

- Side-effects include supraventricular and ventricular arrhythmias. It produces a slight shortening of AV node conduction time causing a potential increase in ventricular rate in patients with atrial flutter/ fibrillation, which is not controlled by digoxin. Hypotension, headache, hypokalaemia, nausea, and vomiting may also occur. Its long half-life may cause prolonged excessive vasodilatation and hypotension.

Dobutamine

- A positive inotrope and mild chronotrope.
- It directly stimulates the β_1-receptors, and increases heart rate and stroke volume. SVR and LVED pressure also decrease as it has some β_2 vasodilator properties.

Indications

To increase cardiac output in patients with low output states (e.g. myocardial infarction, cardiogenic shock).

Dosage

- Continuous iv infusion (peripheral or central vein) 2.5–40 micrograms/ kg/min.
- Titrate according to response.

Side effects

- Tachycardia, arrhythmias.
- Hypotension.
- Headache.
- Increases AV conduction (patients in AF may develop fast ventricular rates).
- Use with care in patients with myocardial infarction as increased heart rate may precipitate angina and intensify ischaemia.
- If infused for longer than 72h larger doses may be required to maintain the same effect.

Drugs used in the treatment of hypertension

Glyceryl trinitrate

- Nitrates cause vasodilation, and affect both venous and arterial beds.
- Causes cerebral vasodilation and may increase intracranial pressure.
- Can be given via a peripheral vein as an infusion or as a bolus.
- Dosage is 5–200 micrograms/min. Tolerance (tachyphylaxis) can develop within 24h, requiring an increase in dose to achieve the same effect.
- Side effects include headache, tachycardia, and nausea.

Sodium nitroprusside

- Acts directly on arterial vascular smooth muscle causing vasodilation.
- Cardiac output usually increases (due to a decrease in SVR).
- May cause cerebral vasodilation and a rise in intracranial pressure.
- It is given as an iv infusion (due to short duration of action) via a dedicated cannula; it must be protected from light.
- Invasive BP monitoring is essential as the BP may fall profoundly.
- Dosage is 0.5–1.5 micrograms/kg/min initially, increasing up to 8µg/kg/min according to response.
- When metabolized, it forms cyanide ions and has the potential to cause cyanide toxicity. This is suggested by an unexplained metabolic acidosis). Ideally, it should not be given for more than 24–36h.
- Side-effects include palpitations, headache, dizziness, nausea.

Hydralazine

- Causes peripheral vasodilation, a decrease in SVR and an increase in cardiac output. There may also be tachycardia.
- Administer 10–40mg as diluted, slow, iv bolus; may be repeated after 30 mins, or as an infusion (200–300 micrograms/min initially).
- It is incompatible with dextrose solutions.
- Side-effects include nausea, headache, palpitations, and flushing.

Phentolamine

- Blocks alpha-adrenergic receptors causing vasodilation.
- Increases respiratory tract secretions, gut motility and insulin release.
- Give as a 2.5mg slow iv bolus repeated if necessary or infusion (5–60mg over 30 min then 0.1–2mg/min).
- Side-effects include tachycardia, dizziness, nausea, diarrhoea.

Labetolol

- Acts by blocking both alpha- and beta-adrenergic receptors.
- It lowers SVR but there is little change in cardiac output.
- Give as repeated slow iv boluses starting at 20 mg up to a miximum of 300mg/24h or as an infusion (up to 160mg/h). For urgent treatment 50mg iv can be given over at least 1min, repeated at 5min intervals up to a total of 200mg.
- Side-effects include headache, rashes, and nausea.

Propanolol, metoprolol, atenolol

- Beta-adrenergic antagonists, they are negatively inotropic, reduce heart rate, and increase peripheral resistance.
- Side-effects include bradycardia, bronchospasm, an impaired response to hypoglycaemia, precipitation of heart failure and heart block, and exacerbation of peripheral vascular disease.

Esmolol

- Short-acting beta-adrenergic blocker.
- Will decrease cardiac output and slow heart rate.
- As it has a short half-life (9min), it is given by continuous infusion (50–200 micrograms/kg/min).
- Side-effects include bronchospasm, bradycardia, nausea, vomiting.

Captopril, enalapril, ramipril, etc.

- Angiotensin-converting enzyme (ACE) inhibitors acting on the renin-angiotensin-aldosterone system causing venous & arterial vasodilation.
- They lower BP by:
  - inhibiting conversion of angiotensin to angiotensin II (a powerful vasoconstrictor);
  - inducing natriuresis by reducing the secretion of aldosterone and increasing renal vasodilation;
  - increasing peripheral vasodilation by stimulating synthesis and release of prostaglandins.
- Captopril can cause severe hypotension so an initial test dose of 6.25mg is given to assess its effect (usually seen within 15min). In hypertension, the usual treatment range is 12.5–50mg twice daily. In the treatment of heart failure it can be up to 150mg daily.
- Renal function must be monitored as they are renally excreted.
- Side-effects include hyperkalaemia, angioedema, cough, and altered immune function (neutropenia, skin rashes).

Electrical cardioversion

A process to convert an arrhythmia to sinus rhythm using electrical defibrillation. The defibrillator may be monophasic or a newer biphasic model that requires approximately half the energy setting. When QRS complexes are present, the shock must be properly timed (synchronized) so that it does not occur during the T wave or ventricular tachycardia may be triggered. Cardioversion may be an elective procedure under sedation or general anaesthetic in patients who are acutely unwell due to an arrhythmia, or as an emergency if the arrhythmia is life-threatening and the patient is already unconscious.

Indications for use
- Decompensated atrial fibrillation with rapid ventricular rate.
- Supraventricular tachycardia.
- Ventricular tachyarrhythmias.
- Ventricular fibrillation.

Method for synchronized defibrillation
- Attach ECG electrodes to patient.
- Obtain a clear trace on the monitor (usually in lead II).
- Place pre-gelled defibrillation pads on the patient.
- Turn on the defibrillator.
- Select the energy level (see Table 12.8)
- Turn the defibrillator onto 'synchronized' mode.
- A marker will appear on the monitor showing each QRS complex.
- Charge the defibrillator.
- Ensure no-one is in contact with the bed frame or patient.
- Discharge (shock) – there may be a 1–2s delay as the machine synchronizes the shock to the patient's rhythm.
- Check the rhythm after each shock.
- If converted to sinus rhythm stop. If no change in rhythm, increase energy (see below) and repeat.
- Perform a 12-lead ECG.

Table 12.8 Defibrillator energy levels

Arrhythmia	Monophasic defibrillator	Biphasic defibrillator
Atrial fibrillation, V_T or V_F	200J	120–150J
Atrial flutter, paroxysmal SVT	100J repeat if needed ± escalation to 360J	70–120J repeat if needed ± escalation to 200J

Cardiac arrest and cardiopulmonary resucitation

Cardiac arrest

Cardiac arrest is defined as the absence or severe reduction of cardiac output resulting in inadequate perfusion of vital organs. It is associated with the following arrhythmias:

- Ventricular fibrillation or tachycardia (VF/VT).
- Pulseless electrical activity (PEA).
- Asystole.

Cardiac arrest in hospital is associated with only 17.6% survival to home discharge and should be prevented by early recognition of acute deterioration wherever possible. Shockable rhythms (VF/VT) have a better survival rate with up to 42% of patients leaving hospital. However, most in-hospital arrests are related to pulseless electrical activity or asystole with only 6% surviving to hospital discharge.

Clinical signs of cardiac arrest

- Absence of pulse (felt over 10s).
- Loss of consciousness.
- Minimal or absent respirations.

Monitoring signs of cardiac arrest

ECG trace exhibiting arrhythmia and loss of arterial waveform. NB. Always check the patient; if they are awake and alert it is unlikely to be an arrest.

Initial management

- This should follow national and international guidelines, such as those of the European Resuscitation Council. Although patients in critical care will commonly already be intubated and ventilated, the principles remain the same.
- Confirm cardiac arrest and summon help.
- Check/establish a patent airway – if the patient is already intubated confirm the airway is patent.
- Confirm ventilation is effective and increase inspired oxygen to 100%, if there is any doubt about the ventilator, manually ventilate the patient with a self-inflating bag attached to a high-flow oxygen supply NB. Ensure removal of oxygen supply if bagging during defibrillation.
- Commence cardiac compressions at a rate of 100/min – these should be uninterrupted for breaths if the patient is intubated.
- Follow the advanced life support algorithm opposite.
- Cardiac arrest should be managed by a team with an advanced life support-trained team leader (commonly the senior doctor present), anaesthetist, and minimum of 2 nurses to ensure an effective response.
- Timings, interventions, drug doses, and patient response should be recorded.

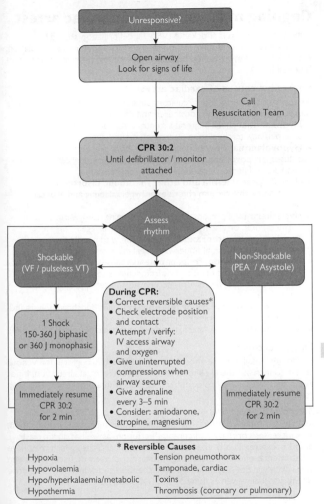

Fig. 12.2 Adult advanced life support algorithm. Reproduced with kind permission of the Resuscitation Council UK (www.resus.org.uk).

Ongoing management of cardiac arrest

If the arrest rhythm is shockable (VF/VT), defibrillation should be carried out immediately. This achieves a 70% return of spontaneous circulation. However, for many patients this is not the case and ongoing management is needed.

Reversible causes of cardiac arrest

As soon as breathing and circulatory support are established, reversible causes of arrest should be considered and corrected where possible:

- **Hypoxaemia:** check bilateral air entry (NB. consider pneumothorax), tube patency, tracheal tube placement, oxygen supply.
- **Hypovolaemia:** ensure adequate, wide-bore iv access, deliver fluid boluses if hypovolaemia suspected, determine potential causes of fluid loss such as haemorrhage and intervene appropriately.
- **Hypo/hyperkalaemia and other metabolic disorders:** check blood gases, give calcium chloride for hyperkalaemia and hypocalcaemia.
- **Hypothermia:** if present, institute re-warming using warm air devices, warmed fluids, or warm gastric and/or bladder lavage.
- **Tension pneumothorax:** decompression with needle thoracocentesis followed by formal underwater seal drain once stable.
- **Cardiac tamponade:** consider potential causes, perform echocardiogram if available, and needle pericardiocentesis to decompress.
- **Toxins:** send samples for drug screen; administer appropriate antidotes.
- **Thrombosis (coronary or pulmonary):** consider thrombolysis and/or cardiothoracic/radiological intervention.
- **Anaphylaxis** (see 📖 Anaphylactic and anaphalactoid reactions, p. 484).

Drug treatment

Wherever possible these should be administered through central venous access to increase the likelihood of reaching the central circulation. If not available, use a large-bore peripheral cannula with a high-flow saline flush to improve uptake.

Adrenaline (epinephrine)

Its vasoconstrictor α effects are predominant in supporting resuscitation. This increases coronary and cerebral perfusion, as well as aortic diastolic blood pressure. The β effects also increase heart rate, which may have a detrimental effect by increasing myocardial oxygen demand. It is given immediately in PEA/asystole or before the third shock in VF/VT. The dose is 1mg iv, usually given as 10ml of 1:10 000 solution.

Atropine

Given for asystole or PEA with a heart rate <60bpm. Atropine blocks the vagus nerve, increases sinus node automaticity and reduces atrioventricular conduction time. The dose is 3mg iv given once only.

Amiodarone

Used for refractory VF/VT and given before the 4th shock. The action potential is prolonged equalizing the length of repolarization in all myocardial cells and increasing the refractory period. It has negative inotropic effects. The initial dose is 300mg in 20ml of 5% glucose given over 5min. It should be given centrally as it is irritant to the veins.

Magnesium

Suppresses myocardial irritability. It can be used for stabilizing torsades de pointes, and both ventricular and supraventricular arrhythmias. The dose is 10–20mmol as magnesium sulphate over 1–2 hrs given as a bolus in arrest situations or over 10min in peri-arrest.

Calcium

Recommended for use only in specific circumstances where hypocalcaemia or overdose of calcium-channel blocker is thought responsible for the arrest. The dose is 10ml of 10% calcium chloride.

Thrombolytics

Given when pulmonary embolus is the suspected cause of arrest, it may take up to 60min to work The dose for tenecteplase is 500–600mcg/kg iv over 10s and alteplase (rt-PA) 10mg iv over 1–2min followed by iv infusion of 90mg over 2h. Heparin needs to be given thereafter.

Sodium bicarbonate

Use is only recommended for life-threatening hyperkalaemia, tricyclic overdose, and to be considered with severe metabolic acidosis (pH <7.1). The dose is 50mmol (50ml of 8.4% solution).

Management of post-cardiac arrest

The goals following return of spontaneous circulation are to support normal cerebral function, maintain a stable cardiac rhythm, restore adequate organ perfusion, and provide good rehabilitation to support quality of life and recovery.

Short periods of arrest may not require more than careful monitoring and circulatory support, but longer periods may result in cerebral injury.

Management should include:

- **Mechanical ventilation and sedation:** maintenance of normocapnia is important in limiting further cerebral damage. Sedation reduces cerebral metabolic rate. Optimal duration is unknown, but many ICUs arbitrarily awaken the patient at 24h to assess function.
- Maintenance of adequate cardiac output and normotension.
- Adequate oxygenation to avoid further hypoxaemia.

Mild therapeutic hypothermia post-cardiac arrest

- Post-arrest cooling has been associated with improved survival and a higher rate of neurological recovery.
- The patient is cooled if still unconscious after return of a spontaneous circulation. A central body temperature of 32–34°C is maintained for 24h following the arrest.
- Methods of cooling vary from water-filled body wraps to extracorporeal cooling involving venous access. Some techniques use cooled boluses of iv fluids with good effect.
- Accurate temperature monitoring is vital and shivering may require control with muscle relaxants.
- Patients with bleeding, cardiogenic shock, and severe sepsis should be considered for exclusion.
- Potential complications of therapeutic hypothermia include coagulopathy, arrhythmias, pneumonia, and sepsis.

Neurological care

Neurological observations

The Glasgow Coma Scale (GCS) is still the most extensively used and widely evaluated tool for assessing neurological function in the acute phase of brain injury (Table 13.1).

The 15-point GCS should be used and information conveyed with a breakdown of the scores in each category (e.g. E = 4, V = 5, M = 6).

Points to remember

- Eye opening to speech should not be interpreted as obeying commands (patient may be responding to the stimulus of voice, rather than the actual command).
- A patient with an endotracheal (ET) tube or tracheostomy may demonstrate orientation by mouthing or writing words.
- For patients unable to obey commands, motor activity must be assessed by applying central painful stimulus. Pressure should be applied to the supra-orbital nerve (by pressing pad of thumb against the brow ridge at inner aspect of brow). If pressure to supra-orbital nerve is contraindicated – due to eye swelling or orbital fractures use trapezius pinch (although less effective and not statistically validated).
- If there is no response to central stimulus, then peripheral stimulus should be applied. Upper limb response only is recorded since leg movement may be a spinal reflex and, therefore, not a true reflection of neurological status.

Prior to the commencement of ICP monitoring in a sedated, ventilated patient pupil responses are the only indicator of neurological deterioration, and should be checked frequently in the acute phase and changes acted upon immediately. Fixed and dilated pupils are a late sign of raised intracranial pressure. Sedatives and NMBAs will not affect pupil reaction.

Table 13.1 Glasgow Coma Scale

Eye opening: arousal mechanisms in brainstem

Spontaneous	4	Observed before approaching or speaking to patient
To speech	3	Response to calling patient's name
To pain	2	Response to peripheral painful stimulus (pressure to side of finger)
None	1	No eye opening (ensure stimulus adequate)

Verbal response: comprehension/transmission of information

Orientated	5	Knows time, place, personal identity
Confused	4	Talking in sentences but disorientated to time and place
Inappropriate words	3	Occasional words rather than sentences
Incomprehensible sounds	2	Grunts or groans
None	1	No verbal response (for intubated or tracheostomy patients enter 'T')

Motor response: functional state of the brain as a whole

Obeys commands	6	Ask patient to lift up arms, stick out tongue, squeeze hand (beware of hand grasp reflex in comatose patient)
Localizing	5	Attempt to remove noxious painful stimulus (purposeful movement)
Flexing	4	Elbow bends and hand moves upwards in normal movement
Abnormal flexion	3	Elbow bends, but is accompanied by spastic flexion of wrist
Extension	2	Straightening of elbow accompanied by spastic flexion of wrist
None	1	No motor response (ensure stimulus adequate)

- **Limb responses:** difference in responsiveness in one limb compared with the other indicates focal brain damage.
- **Pupillary response:** pupillary pathways relatively resistant to metabolic insult therefore presence or absence of light reflex is single most important sign potentially distinguishing structural from metabolic coma:
  - pupils assessed for size, shape, equality, reaction to light;
  - sedatives and NMBAs do not affect pupil reaction.
  - Bilateral fixed and dilated pupils in patient with score of 14 or 15 suggests recent occurrence of seizure.

General principles in the care of neuroscience patients

- Many of the guiding principles in the care of neuroscience patients are the same for each condition and have been dealt with here in a general systems overview. Initial assessment should follow established ABCDE principles.
- Specific parameters and interventions are included under the headings for that condition.
- The effective management of all neuroscience patients relies on a multidisciplinary approach.

Neurology

The ability to effectively monitor and detect changes in a patient's condition is crucial to outcome.

GCS ≥ 9
- See TBI and SAH for specific management.
- A drop in GCS or development of new focal deficit requires immediate medical review, and possible repeat CT scan and increased frequency of observation.
- Frequency of observations should be relevant to the patient's condition, CT findings, and the risk of complications.

GCS ≤ 8
- Requires sedation, intubation, and ventilation for airway protection and (if applicable) control of raised ICP (optimizing arterial blood gases).
- Sedation and intubation should also be considered if fluctuating or significantly deteriorating conscious level even if not in coma (GCS ≤ 8) or to manage an extremely agitated patient.
- Once sedated and prior to the insertion of ICP monitoring, pupil changes are the only indicator of neurological deterioration and should be checked at least hourly (pupil reaction is not affected by sedatives or NMBAs).

Seizures
Seizures are seen as result of cortical disruption from trauma, presence of blood or infection.
- 1st seizure treated with benzodiazepines as per local policy. Anticonvulsant therapy normally prescribed after 2nd seizure, but consult with neurosurgeon/neurologist (phenytoin drug of choice).
- Generalized convulsive seizures must be controlled due to increased demands on cerebral metabolism, risk of injury to patient and potential loss of airway. In immediate post-ictal (post seizure) period conscious level may be slow to recover and pupil changes and limb weakness may be seen.
- Administer oxygen therapy and maintain safe environment.
- Seizures are difficult to detect in patients receiving NMBAs (may be signalled by bilateral pupillary dilatation, tachycardia, and small increase in arterial pressure).
- Metabolic causes for seizure must be excluded.
- Possibility of sub-clinical seizures should be considered if the patient remains unresponsive after cessation of sedative agents and may require EEG.
- If the patient is a known epileptic consult with neurologist regarding long-term medication.

Cranial nerve dysfunction

Cranial nerve dysfunction can occur in all neuroscience patients as a result of direct injury to the nerve, or as a result of infection or inflammation. Cranial nerve dysfunction may have implications not only for nursing care, but also for airway management and weaning from mechanical ventilation. Speech and language therapist (SALT) referrals should be made early for these patients Observe for any signs of:

• Inability to cope with oral secretions, drooling, or pooling of secretions in side or back of mouth.
• Gurgling or 'wet' voice.
• Poor or absent cough or gag.
• Facial asymmetry/droop.
• Inability to open or close eye.

Sympathetic storming and agitation

After the acute phase of brain injury patients may experience either sympathetic storming or agitation. Agitation may be seen in various neurological conditions, while sympathetic storming is seen predominantly after severe traumatic brain injury and is due to autonomic hyper-reflexia. Both sympathetic storming and agitation make it difficult to wean patients from sedation and ventilation.

Sympathetic storming and agitation

Sympathetic storming

Episodic and exaggerated response occurring spontaneously or to stimulus
Resolves over time but may take weeks
Should be managed in the short term as symptoms can be severe and may exacerbate brain injury

GCS ≤ 8
(Motor score ≤ 4)

Symptoms
Tachycardia
Tachypnoea
Diaphoresis
Hypertension
Abnormal movement of limbs
Arching of back

Treatment
Consider **beta blocker** or **clonidine** infusion titrated until symptom control

Consider weaning after 24–48 h 'storming free'

Avoid over-stimulation

May require individual patient parameters to avoid over-treatment with sedation

Early mobilization/tilt table

Agitation

Disturbed behaviour seen as an early symptom in patients with PTA

Resolves with return of ability to retrieve and store information

In longer term usually due to personality changes

GCS ≥ 9
(Motor score 5–6)

Symptoms
Confusion
Restlessness and agitation
Limited awareness
Disturbed perception of environment
Inability to learn new tasks

Treatment
For acute or rapid control use **lorazepam** or **haloperidol**

To facilitate weaning from sedation and ventilation consider **risperidone** NG or **clonidine** infusion prior to ceasing sedation

Avoid using sedation/analgesia to treat agitation (but exclude pain as cause)
Exclude other causes, e.g. UTI or metabolic disturbances

Early mobilization
Minimise sensory stimulation
Promote normal sleep pattern

13.1 Algorithm 1. Sympathetic storming and agitation.

Respiratory

Respiratory complications are common in neuroscience patients, and advanced respiratory support is often required for airway control and to prevent secondary brain injury.

Patients with GCS ≤ 8 at any time are at risk of developing aspiration pneumonia. Aspiration may also be a problem in patients with impaired bulbar function (the musculature involved in speech and swallowing).

A multidisciplinary approach, in particular physiotherapy and SALT input, is essential in managing these patients.

Non-intubated patient

- Monitor gas exchange for hypoxia and CO_2 retention – aim for S_pO_2 > 95% on room air. Hypoxia may worsen agitation or mask confusional state. An inability to maintain gas exchange may precede deterioration in neurological condition.
- Ensure gag is adequate (diminished gag in isolation may not necessarily be an indication for intubation however must be monitored due to risk of airway compromise).
- In neuromuscular respiratory failure (GBS and MG) hypoxaemia, decreased tidal volume, dyspnoea and abnormal blood gases are all late findings and are poor indicators of need for ventilatory support. More sensitive indicator of progressive respiratory failure is forced vital capacity (FVC). As FVC falls, spontaneous coughing weakens and there is greater difficulty clearing secretions. Tracheal intubation generally performed if FVC drops below 15ml/kg, but may be undertaken at higher FVC if patient also has bulbar weakness.
- Facial CPAP and nasopharyngeal airway contraindicated in TBI patient with facial or base of skull fracture.
- Risk of sputum retention if cough ineffective.
- Position to maximize gas exchange – side lying, sitting up, early mobilization.

Intubated patient

- Minimum F_iO_2 to maintain parameters.
- PEEP up to 12cmH$_2$O will not increase ICP.
- Ensure ET tapes not impeding jugular venous drainage.
- Head elevation (unless contraindicated).

Chest physiotherapy and suctioning

- In TBI and SAH patients consider increasing sedation or administering bolus prior to chest physiotherapy or suctioning to prevent vigorous coughing or biting on tube.
- For routine chest management pre-oxygenate with 100% O_2 prior to suctioning, if possible limit to 3 catheters to clear secretions, allow short rest between sessions to avoid hypoxia and hypercarbia.
- Manual hyperinflation can be used with caution if PEEP and CO_2 allow (hypocapnoea can increase the risk of cerebral ischaemia).

Neurogenic pulmonary oedema

- Recognized complication in severe TBI and poor grade SAH. Observe for dyspnoea, cyanosis, pallor, sweating, weak rapid pulse, and production of pink frothy sputum. Treat by manipulation of ventilation (increasing F_iO_2, control of CO_2, increasing PEEP) and reducing ICP.
- Consider frusemide if not responsive to above measures.

Early tracheostomy

- Consider in patients with persistent poor neurology or significant bulbar problems.
- In conditions where there is progressive respiratory muscle failure (as in GBS or MG) early tracheostomy will be required due to need for prolonged ventilatory support.
- Double lumen tracheostomy recommended.

Cardiovascular

Cardiovascular instability can occur in neuroscience patients as a result of increased sympathetic activity, increased catecholamine release, autonomic dysfunction, or injury to the brainstem.

Heart rate and rhythm

- ECG changes are common, especially in TBI, SAH, and GBS. Life threatening arrhythmias require prompt treatment. However, most ECG abnormalities in acute CNS disorders do not require therapeutic intervention.
- Continuous ECG monitoring essential.
- Acute MI and cardiac causes must be excluded in all cases.

Blood pressure

Close monitoring is required to detect and treat hypotension and hypertension promptly (see specific conditions for parameters).

Temperature

- Maintain normal temperature at 35.5–37°C (elevations in temperature worsen outcome in brain injury, and pyrexia should be investigated and treated).
- Treat pyrexia with paracetamol and cool if necessary. Do not induce hypothermia (no proven benefits at this time as treatment for raised ICP).
- Persistent hyperpyrexia resistant to treatment may be result of damage to hypothalamus (usually high temperature sustained without peaks and troughs), but microbiological causes must be excluded.

Sedation, analgesia, and NMBAs

- Use with caution in GBS and MG.
- Sedation has a 2-fold purpose in TBI and SAH – it acts as a cerebral protective agent for the management of ICP and it facilitates controlled airway management.
- Sedation and analgesia should always be administered via continuous infusion to maintain effective levels.
- Propofol and fentanyl are commonly used and are given concurrently. Dose will depend on the reason for use and patient requirement. Monitor effect of sedation levels on ICP and adjust accordingly to reduce risks associated with high drug doses.
- NMBAs have no direct effect on ICP, but may facilitate ventilation.

For management of raised ICP

- Propofol and fentanyl infusions titrated to reduce ICP.
- Consider adding midazolam and reducing propofol if hypotension problematic or if sedation to be continued for >48h (however, some level of propofol should be maintained due to cerebroprotective properties).
- In cases where ICP remains unacceptably high and unresponsive to maximal doses of sedation consider thiopentone bolus, followed by infusion if ICP responsive to bolus dose (reduce other sedative agents once thiopentone infusion commenced).
- Consider using morphine instead of fentanyl if long term analgesia required

For management of airway and to aid ventilation

Propofol and fentanyl in lowest dose to manage patient in the short term. Consider using midazolam and fentanyl or morphine if prolonged therapy required.

Fluids and electrolytes

Fluid regulation can be affected by direct injury to hypothalamus or pituitary gland, or compression from surrounding oedema. Adequate circulating blood volume reduces risk of cerebral ischaemia secondary to hypovolaemia. Depleted volume states require close monitoring and prompt treatment.

Several factors should be considered in fluid management of patients with neurological conditions – clinical and laboratory assessment of volume status, effects of different fluids on CPP and cerebral oedema, osmotic therapy, and water and electrolyte disturbances.

Fluid therapy

- Normal saline or colloid to restore or maintain normovolaemia.
- CVP 5–10mmHg.
- Avoid glucose containing solutions unless blood glucose <5mmol/l (increase in glucose levels in ischaemic brain allows anaerobic glycolysis and accumulation of lactic acid).
- Maintain Hb >7 (unless higher level clinically indicated).
- Do not fluid restrict unless clinical condition demands (i.e. cardiac history or clinically overloaded), or to manage sodium and water disturbance (see Algorithm 4, Fig. 13.4).
- In SAH minimum intake 3l in 24h.

Electrolytes

- Normal parameters (unless specific indications for higher level, e.g. ↑ K^+ if cardiac history).
- Risk of Na^+ abnormalities especially in TBI and SAH (Na^+ levels of <125mmol/l can cause nausea, anorexia, emesis, confusion, obtundation, seizures). Hyponatraemia (serum Na^+ <135mmol/l has associated morbidity and mortality if left untreated.
- Blood glucose 5.5–9mmol/l (tight glycaemic control used only in patients with associated sepsis as risk of critically low brain glucose levels if systemic glucose is low).
- Maintain magnesium ~1mmol/l (may help reduce seizure activity and maintain cell function).
- Maintain phosphates ~1mmol/l (low phosphates may contribute to respiratory muscle weakness and can delay weaning from mechanical ventilation).

Sodium and water balance: hypernatraemia

MAY BE DUE TO **DEHYDRATION** (secondary to use of osmotic agents for ICP control),
DIABETES INSIPIDUS (seen in severe TBI or major cerebral insult due to gross generalised
brain swelling), **PITUITARY DYSFUNCTION** (trans-sphenoidal surgery/craniopharyngioma - these
patients usually require input from endocrinology team)
OR MAY BE SEEN IN PATIENTS WHO ARE **BRAIN STEM DEAD**

DIABETES INSIPIDUS LEADS TO RAPID FLUID & ELECTROLYTE DEPLETION
AND SHOULD BE TREATED PROMPTLY ONCE DIAGNOSIS IS ESTABLISHED ON
CLINICAL FINDINGS AND **CONFIRMED BY LABORATORY RESULTS**

CONSIDER TREATING SERUM SODIUM >150–155mmol/l

DIABETES INSIPIDUS (DI)	**DEHYDRATION**
Signs	**Signs**
☑ LOW CVP (<5mmHg) ☑ HIGH URINE OUTPUT (>1000ml in 4h) ☑ LOW SPECIFIC GRAVITY (≤1.005) ☑ NORMAL URINARY SODIUM (20– 60mmol/l) ☑ HIGH SERUM OSMOLARITY (>305mmol/kg) ☑ LOW URINE OSMOLARITY (<350mmol/kg) *Occurs acutely over hours and is not related to the administration of fluids or osmotic agents*	☑ LOW CVP (<5mmHg) ☑ LOW URINE OUTPUT (<0.5ml/kg/hr) ☑ HIGH SPECIFIC GRAVITY (≥1.020) ☑ TACHYCARDIA AND HYPOTENSION ☑ 'DRY'ON CLINICAL ASSESSMENT *High urinary output associated with osmotic agents is not sustained*
Treatment	**Treatment**
AIM TO CONSERVE FLUID VOLUME AND ELECTROLYTES BY REDUCING URINE OUTPUT GIVE 0.4mcg desmopressin iv *Repeat after 30 min if urine output remains high* CONSIDER 5% DEXTROSE WHEN SERUM SODIUM ≥**155mmol/l** • *Consider risks of increased brain swelling in TBI due to water load* • *Keep blood glucose 5.5–9mmol /l* CONSIDER **WATER VIA NG/OG TUBE**	**AIM TO ESTABLISH NORMAL URINE OUTPUT BY NORMALIZING FLUID VOLUME AND ELECTROLYTES** USE **ISOTONIC FLUIDS** TO RESTORE NORMOVOLAEMIA *Increase fluid intake if indicated with careful assessment of patient's needs* *(Consult with dietician if risk of refeeding syndrome)*
Monitor	**Monitor**
CARDIOVASCULAR STATUS *(Risk of instability due to intravascular volume depletion and loss of electrolytes)* **FLUID BALANCE** **URINE AND SERUM OSMOLARITY** *(may need to be repeated several times in 24h period as DI may return once desmopressin wears off)*	**CARDIOVASCULAR STATUS** *(Risk of instability due to intravascular volume depletion and loss of electrolytes)* **FLUID BALANCE** **SERUM SODIUM** **RENAL FUNCTION**

Fig. 13.2 Algorithm 2a. Sodium and water balance: hypernatraemia.

Sodium and water balance: hyponatraemia

2 MAIN CAUSES:
SYNDROME OF INAPPROPRIATE ANTIDIURETIC SYNDROME HORMONE (SIADH)
AND CEREBRAL SALT WASTING (CWS)
(Na+ levels of <120–125mmol can cause nausea, anorexia, emesis, confusion, obtundation, and seizures)

ACCURATE **DIAGNOSIS** BASED ON **CLINICAL FINDINGS** *(IMPORTANTLY VOLUME STATUS)* AND
LABORATORY RESULTS ESSENTIAL AS TREATMENT MARKEDLY DIFFERENT

MANAGEMENT DEPENDENT ON PATIENT CONDITION, RATE AT WHICH
SODIUM FALLS AND BY HOW MUCH

CONSIDER TREATING SERUM SODIUM ≤ 130mmol/l

SIADH
Dilution of Na+ due to water retention

Signs

☑ HIGH CVP – no evidence of dehydration
☑ LOW SERUM SODIUM (<135mmol/l)
☑ LOW URINE OUTPUT (<0.5ml/kg/h)
☑ NORMAL SPECIFIC GRAVITY
☑ LOW SERUM OSMOLARITY (<280mmol/kg)
☑ URINE OSMOLARITY>SERUM OSMOLARITY
☑ NORMAL URINARY SODIUM (>18mmol/l)
☑ ABSENCE OF PERIPHERAL OEDEMA
☑ NORMAL THYROID, ADRENAL, RENAL
FUNCTION

Treatment
AIM TO RESTRICT INTAKE OF WATER

FLUID RESTRICTION

*Dependent on individual patient requirements
-consider risks in patients with SAH*

*(In SAH patient with low Na+ assume CSW until
sure of diagnosis of SIADH because of
consequences of fluid restriction)*

*Hypertonic saline may be required in severe cases
but seek senior advice*

CSW
Fluid and Na+ depletion

Signs

☑ LOW CVP
☑ HIGH URINE OUTPUT
☑ NORMAL SPECIFIC GRAVITY
☑ HIGH/NORMAL SERUM OSMOLARITY
☑ VARIABLE URINE OSMOLARITY
☑ HIGH URINARY SODIUM (>60mmol/l)

Treatment
AIM TO REPLACE SODIUM AND WATER WITH SODIUM
CONTAINING ISOTONIC FLUIDS

In severe cases consider
HYPERTONIC SALINE *(1.8%)* for **24–48 h**
*via central venous line to increase sodium concentration by
maximum 8–10mmol in 24 h*
(1.8% saline can be given peripherally but not if treatment >24h)

*The rate of infusion should be prescribed for each patient
individually and daily target rise in Na+ set*

Hypertonic saline usually started at around 30–40ml/h

Once daily target achieved hypertonic saline should be stopped

(Rapid increase or decrease can cause myelinolysis)

Monitor

CARDIOVASCULAR STATUS
FLUID BALANCE
URINE AND SERUM SODIUM AND OSMOLARITY
(BD urine /serum Na+ osmolarity if patient receiving hypertonic saline)
GLASGOW COMA SCALE

Fig. 13.2 Cont'd—Algorithm 2b. Sodium and water balance: hyponatraemia.

Nutrition

TBI patients in particular have an induced hypermetabolic and hypercatabolic state resulting in increased energy and protein requirements.

Early enteral feeding can reduce nitrogen loss, and is associated with improved clinical outcome and fewer infections.

- Commence nutritional support as soon as possible: normal diet and fluids if patient is able otherwise enteral feeding should be considered and commenced as soon as possible.
- If there is any doubt about adequacy of bulbar function a SALT assessment must be made prior to eating and drinking in all neuroscience patients.
- Early referral to dietician for individualized feeding regime is essential.
- Delayed gastric emptying is not uncommon and prokinetics are often required to assist with gastric emptying in patients with large aspirates.
- Gut protection other than feeding is not usually necessary unless indicated by patient history or prolonged poor absorption.
- If patient is prescribed phenytoin feed must be stopped for 2h before and after administration (feed will reduce absorption of phenytoin, making it difficult to achieve therapeutic blood levels).
- Sliding scale insulin may be required (be aware of risks of hypo- and hyperglycaemia).
- There is an increased risk of paralytic ileus in TBI with associated spinal injury and in GBS.

Elimination

Cerebral injuries can lead to disorders of fluid regulation, and abnormalities must be detected early and treated promptly.

Constipation occurs as a result of immobility and reduced gastric motility, especially in spinal injury and GBS, and when high levels of opiates have been used.

Renal

- Monitor fluid balance and urinary chemistry (may be an increase in urinary loss of various electrolytes).
- Observe for DI – treat promptly once diagnosis made (see Algorithm 2a, Fig. 13.2). Accurate diagnosis is essential – exclude mannitol administration as contributing factor.

Bowels

- Early activation of local bowel management protocol to prevent constipation (see 📖 Aneurysmal subarachnoid hemorrhage, p. 310).
- Early prescribing of aperients.
- Severe constipation or obstruction can lead to diaphragmatic splinting and compromise ventilation.
- Straining to pass a stool can contribute to high ICP by increasing intra-abdominal and intra-thoracic pressure, and decreasing venous return.
- Increased risk of paralytic ileus in spinal injury and GBS.
- Commence spinal bowel regime for patients with spinal cord injury on admission.

Positioning and mobility

Patients with neurological dysfunction are at risk of developing structural deformity, and early intervention will help maintain limb function and facilitate rehabilitation. Management requires a multidisciplinary approach.

- TBI patients require clinical and radiological examination to detect associated spinal injury and should be managed as per local policy.
- Elevate head of bed 15–30° once normovolaemia established (and after spinal clearance in TBI patients).
- Maintain neutral body alignment: avoid head rotation, neck flexion or hyperextension, extreme hip flexion.
- Turning and repositioning can be associated with transient rises in ICP, but is important for chest management and pressure relief. Consider bolus of sedation prior to turning (rises in ICP may be avoided if head and neck are kept in alignment).
- Early assessment and treatment by physiotherapist. Limbs may require splinting (risk of loss of range of movement, muscle stiffness, contractures, foot drop, shoulder subluxation, and ulnar nerve damage).
- Careful positioning of limbs in patients with loss of sensation (keep in neutral mid-position, supported with pillows).
- Forced bed rest in SAH prior to definitive treatment of aneurysm.
- DVT prophylaxis: graduated elastic stockings and mechanical calf compression device (see 📖 Anticoagulation therapy, p. 456).
- Anticoagulants contraindicated in early phase of some conditions.

Oral and eye care

- Risk of corneal damage in patients with cranial nerve dysfunction. Requires meticulous eye care and low threshold for ophthalmic consultation. Consider lubricating eye ointment to prevent corneal abrasions.
- Oral care as per local policy.
- Prioritize care to limit unnecessary interventions and avoid clustering of activities to minimize sensory stimulation.

Sleep deprivation

- For awake patients (GBS and MG) who have prolonged ITU admission this can be a particular problem. Sleep patterns should be established early and night sedation considered.
- Patients recovering from TBI and SAH can safely have night sedation once fluctuations in neurology are no longer of concern.

Communication

- Patients without cognitive deficits will require communication aids as soon as sedative agents stopped. Early intervention from SALT will identify most appropriate aids for individual patients (alphabet board or picture cards in early stages may be helpful). Patients with cognitive, memory and language problems will require expert assessment and retraining.
- If prolonged intubation anticipated early tracheostomy will aid lip reading.

Traumatic brain injury (TBI)

The two main causes of secondary brain injury correlating with increased mortality and morbidity are: failure to correct systemic hypoxaemia and hypotension, and delay in appropriate surgical management.

Extradural haematoma (EDH)

- Blood in extradural space (between skull and dura).
- 90% associated with skull fracture and rupture of middle meningeal artery.
- Mortality ~20% if poor GCS at time of surgery.
- Requires prompt diagnosis and evacuation of clot.

Subdural haematoma (SDH)

- Blood between dura and arachnoid layers due to tearing of cortical veins and may have underlying brain injury.
- Prognostically worse than EDH.
- Poor outcome more likely if SDH is bilateral, accumulates rapidly, or >4h delay in removal of clot.
- Chronic subdural can occur weeks after injury.

Traumatic subarachnoid haemorrhage

Seen in association with other brain injury and presence implies severe brain injury, therefore higher mortality and morbidity.

Intracerebral haematoma

- Usually affects white matter or basal ganglia.
- Can cause delayed neurological deterioration.

Contusions and lacerations

- Superficial areas of haemorrhage usually affecting frontal and temporal lobes sustained as brain hits bony protruberances of skull at site of impact (coup injury) and opposite side during deceleration (contrecoup injury).
- Contusions usually increase in size 24–72h after injury and patient can deteriorate rapidly.

Diffuse axonal injury (DAI)

- Commonest cause of coma, vegetative state, subsequent disability, and is attributed to tearing of nerve fibres at junction between grey and white matter.
- Severe DAI patient often in deep coma (may have normal CT and initially normal ICP).

Skull fracture

- Evidence of major impact – most involve vault.
- High incidence of associated intracranial haematoma.
- Base of skull fracture more difficult to exclude radiologically – observe for clinical indicators (most leaks close spontaneously):
  - peri-orbital bruising (panda eyes);
  - retro-auricular bruising (Battle's sign);
  - CSF leak from nose (rhinorrhoea) or ears (otorrhoea).

Care of the patient with traumatic brain injury

Management aimed at prevention of secondary brain injury (optimization of gas exchange, correction of hypovolaemia and timely neurosurgical intervention). Hypotension (SBP <90mmHg) and hypoxia (P_aO_2 < 8kPa) are the most predominant factors in secondary brain injury, and have high correlation with morbidity and mortality.

- Full neurological assessment according to NICE guidelines for patients with GCS $\geq$ 9. These patients are at risk of deteriorating from secondary complications. In addition to GCS, limb and pupil triggers, observe for changes that require closer observation and immediate review by supervising doctor (such as development of agitation, severe or increasing headache, persistent vomiting – all possible signs of raised ICP). Aim for S_pO_2 > 95% on room air (observe for hypoxia and CO_2 retention, which may indicate deteriorating neurology).
- Patients with GCS $\leq$ 8 require sedation, intubation, and ventilation, therefore, clinical assessment no longer possible, but continue pupil checks at least hourly. Consider follow-up CT scan in 24h or earlier if clinically indicated, especially if not ICP monitored (seek advice from neurosurgeon). Aim for P_aO_2 > 13kPa and P_aCO_2 4.5–5kPa (remember PEEP up to 12cmH$_2$O will not increase ICP). Intubated patients should be ventilated with adequate sedation and analgesia (important not only to facilitate ventilation but also for management of ICP) and also NMBAs if needed.
- Consider sedation, intubation, and ventilation in patient with significantly deteriorating conscious level, even if not in coma, or to manage extremely agitated patient.
- SBP > 120mmHg or MAP > 90mmHg (vasopressor, usually noradrenaline, may be required to counteract hypotensive effects of sedation in ventilated patients). If ICP monitored target BP to maintain CPP = 60mmHg (CPP = MAP – ICP).

- ECG changes most commonly seen are peaked P waves, prolonged QT interval, heightened T waves, ST segment elevation or depression. Bradycardia associated with hypertension and widening pulse pressure is indicative of severe swelling and brainstem herniation.
- Aim for normal temperature (35.5–37°C) – in acute phase hyperthermia should be treated since it will exacerbate cerebral ischaemia and adversely affect outcome.
- Headache and nausea: paracetamol, morphine, codeine (remember persistent headache can be sign of raised ICP). Pain may increase confusional state or agitation.
- Aim for normovolaemia using normal saline or colloid (avoid glucose containing solutions unless blood glucose <5mmol/l).
- Commence enteral nutrition (see Figure 13.3).
- Blood glucose 5.5–9mmol/l (risk of critically low brain glucose levels if systemic glucose is low).
- Monitor urine output: observe for DI in acute phase; later SIADH or CSW (see 📖 Fluids and electrolytes, p. 298).

Specific ICP directed therapy
Further active treatment of ICP is only indicated if evidence of neurological deterioration due to intracranial causes, e.g. pupillary dilatation, deteriorating motor function (see Figure 13.3).
- Hyperventilation P_aCO_2 4.0–4.5kPa.
- Mannitol given as bolus dose 0.25–1g/kg over 20min. (Powerful osmotic diuretic therefore adequate fluid resuscitation essential. Repetitive doses can increase ICP especially when given as continuous infusion. Chronic therapy not associated with improved outcome).
- Head elevation 15–30° (when thoracolumbar fracture excluded and patient adequately volume resuscitated).

Precautions and contraindications
- Anticoagulant therapy is contraindicated in acute phase. Only given on advice from neurosurgeon.
- Base of skull fracture (BOS) – observe for clinical indicators. Oral route for all tubes until fracture excluded. If fracture confirmed orogastric tube for 10–14 days then consider change to nasogastric. Prophylactic antibiotics not usually prescribed but consult with neurosurgeon.

ICP Directed Therapy

Therapy and parameters on admission

➢ Sedate with **propofol** and **fentanyl**
➢ Arterial blood gas – $P_aO_2 > 13$kPa, P_aCO_2 4.5–5.0kPa
➢ **MAP** $\geq$ 90mmHg or SBP > 120mmHg
➢ Blood glucose **5.5–9mmol/l** and temperature **35.5–37°C**
➢ **Hourly pupil** checks
➢ Commence **spine** clearance algorithm (see Fig 13.4) head of bed 15–30° once thoracolumbar spine cleared

Therapeutic goals once ICP monitoring commenced

ICP < 25mmHg
CPP = 60mmHg
To attain CPP ensure adequate fluid resuscitation before starting vasopressors
Insert oesophageal Doppler if indicated

ICP < 20mmHg
Continue current therapy and parameters
Neurosurgeons may consider waking patient to assess neurology
Consider spine clearance and requirements for further imaging prior to wake up

---

ICP 20 – 25mmHg

Check
☑ Pupils – equal and reacting?
☑ ET tapes – not tight and impeding venous drainage?
☑ Patient – head and neck in neutral alignment? Return to supine position
☑ Arterial blood gases – P_aCO_2 within parameters, adequate P_aO_2?
☑ Infusions, lines and connections – patent, no leaks or cracks in taps or tubing?

Ensure
⇨ Adequate sedation   ⇨ give bolus and observe effect

Consider
⇨ Increasing rate of sedation, adding midazolam and bolus of muscle relaxant followed by infusion

---

ICP > 25mmHg

Repeat checks as before and

- Manipulate ventilation - P_aCO_2 4–4.5kPa

- Commence active cooling - **35–36°C**

- Consider **thiopental** bolus and infusion

- Consider insertion of $S_{vj}O_2$ catheter to allow further manipulation of P_aCO_2

☎ **Neurosurgeon for further management plan**
CSF drainage or decompressive craniectomy may be considered

Fig. 13.3 Algorithm 3. ICP-directed therapy.

Aneurysmal subarachnoid haemorrhage (SAH)

Around 60% of SAH (bleeding into subarachnoid space and CSF) results from rupture of saccular aneurysm (dilatation in wall of artery). Other causes include arteriovenous malformation, hypertension, tumour, bleeding diathesis, anticoagulation, and idiopathic.

Clinical status (GCS) on admission (after initial resuscitation and stabilization) is the single most important independent predictor of outcome. The World Federation of Neurological Surgeons (WFNS) Subarachnoid Haemorrhage Grading Scale (which grades the severity of the bleed) is used to guide treatment, and predict morbidity and mortality (Table 13.2).

Table 13.2 World Federation of Neurological Surgeons Subarachnoid Haemorrhage Grading Scale

WFNS grade	GCS	Motor deficit
I	15	Absent/present
II	14–13	Absent
III	14–13	Present
IV	12–7	Present or absent
V	6–3	Present or absent

Complications of subarachnoid haemorrhage

- **Rebleeding** (initial bleed self-limiting as clotting cascade activated):-
  Untreated aneurysms are at risk of rebleeding and is the commonest cause of early death with a mortality rate of 80% (can occur at any time – most frequently from 3rd to 11th day with peak incidence ~ 7th day).
- **Cerebral vasospasm** (narrowing of cerebral artery): leading cause of death and disability, and present in 20–30%, with blood products around large arteries at base of brain most likely cause – occurs 3–5 days post-ictus or delayed up to 21 days with highest risk at days 3–14.
- **Hydrocephalus** (dilation of ventricles): occurs when blood impairs re-absorption or intraventricular flow of CSF either acutely (first few days) or chronically (second week). Can cause acute deterioration in conscious level and requires insertion of an external ventricular drain.
- **Seizures:** can occur at any stage especially if cortical damage has occurred.

Diagnosis

- **Computerized tomography:** first line investigation, will also show associated problems, such as hydrocephalus, intracerebral haematoma, and may help identify site of aneurysm.

- **Lumbar puncture:** only carried out when CT imaging negative, but history suggestive of SAH.
- **Digital subtraction angiography:** definitive investigation for diagnosing aneurysms and for treatment planning (15–20% of patients will have normal angiogram and aetiology is unclear, but may be venous haemorrhage).
- **Cerebral angiography:** ideally performed within 24h.

Treatment

Definitive treatment is to secure the aneurysm to prevent rebleeding. Early treatment eliminates the risk of rerupture and enables intensive management of vasospasm.

Endovascular: coiling

- Approach via femoral artery – aneurysmal sac obliterated by filament coils, which cause thrombosis by inducing flow stagnation.
- Can follow on from diagnostic angiography in one procedure.

Surgical: clipping

Metal clip placed across neck of aneurysm to prevent re-rupture.

Drug therapy

Regardless of whether patients are coiled or clipped, nimodipine is commenced as soon as diagnosis of SAH confirmed (nimodipine significantly lowers the incidence of death as a result of delayed cerebral ischaemia and the occurrence of cerebral infarcts).

- Dose – 60mg 4-hourly for 21 days (can cause hypotension – if BP affected give 30mg 2-hourly).
- Usually absorbed well in patients fed via nasogastric tube, but if absorption a problem give intravenously (must be given via central line and run concurrently with normal saline 40ml/h via dedicated lumen).

Care of the patient with aneurysmal subarachnoid haemorrhage

Management is aimed at stabilizing and optimizing patient for aneurysm obliteration, and preventing secondary cerebral insults. Initial priorities include adequate ventilation and oxygenation, haemodynamic stability, and control of raised ICP. Extremes of blood pressure should be avoided – high BP is more likely to cause rebleed and low BP to exacerbate hypoxic or ischaemic cerebral damage from vasospasm.

- Full neurological assessment if GCS ≥. Record observations 1-hourly for first 24th, thereafter consider reducing to 2-hourly dependent on patient condition.
- Patients with GCS ≤8 require intubation and sedation (propofol and fentanyl) for airway management and ventilation, therefore clinical assessment no longer possible, but continue 1-hourly pupil checks. Sedation should be adequate to prevent coughing on ET tube if aneurysm untreated (can induce hypertension and increase ICP). Clinical assessment will determine future management, therefore, short-acting sedative agents preferred.

- $S_pO_2 > 95\%$ on room air or $P_aO_2 > 13$kPa and normal P_aCO_2 in ventilated patients. Do not hyperventilate due to added risk of ischaemia from vasospasm.
- Poor grade SAH patients in particular at risk of neurogenic pulmonary oedema.
- Maintain normal BP for patient – hypotension (SBP < 120mmHg) treated initially with fluids, use vasopressors only if unable to maintain circulation or urine output. Treat sustained hypertension (SBP > 160mmHg) with short-acting agent preferably iv to allow careful titration, e.g. labetalol. (Be aware of hypotensive effects of sedative agents in ventilated patients.)
- ECG changes commonly associated with SAH are ST segment depression, bundle branch block, sinus arrhythmias. MI must be excluded, however, in acute phase pharmacological management of ECG abnormalities should be implemented with care.
- Headache and nausea common can be severe and can persist for many days (resulting hypertension can increase risk of rebleeding). Give regular analgesia – paracetamol, dihydrocodeine, morphine (PCA for suitable patients) and anti-emetics (cyclizine) prescribed on admission. NSAIDs not recommended prior to treatment of aneurysm (see ⌨ Precautions and contraindications).
- Minimum intake 3l in 24h – normal saline/colloid (avoid glucose containing solutions unless blood glucose <5mmol/l).
- Patient is at risk of water and electrolyte imbalance – CSW and SIADH most commonly seen (see Fig. 13.2).

Precautions and contraindications

- NSAIDs not recommended in patient with untreated aneurysm (antiplatelet effects can increase risk of rebleeding), but may be considered once aneurysm has been treated.
- Anticoagulant therapy contraindicated due to risk of rebleeding in untreated aneurysm.
- Bowel management from admission with aperients prescribed regularly (straining at stool increases risk of aneurysm rebleed) – do not give suppositories or enemas in untreated aneurysm (valsalva manoeuvre).
- Do not mobilize until aneurysm treated – forced bed rest with head of bed elevation up to 15° with side to side lying for comfort and meals (if treatment decision for conservative management seek advice from neurosurgeon on timing of mobilization).

Management of cervical spine

ON ADMISSION

- TREAT AS UNSTABLE – APPLY MIAMI J COLLAR
- CONSIDER HISTORY AND CLINICALLY EXAMINE SPINE
- 5 PERSON LOG ROLL - WHEN THORACIC AND LUMBAR INJURY EXCLUDED
  3 PERSON LOG ROLL

C-spine can only be cleared on x-ray when patient is GCS 15

Once intubated CT scan is required

↓

IMAGING

CT SPINE (**OCCIPUT-T2**) and **LATERAL C-SPINE X-RAY** WITHIN 24 HOURS IF PATIENT STABLE

IF **NO** FRACTURE OR DISLOCATION SEEN	FRACTURE OR DISLOCATION PRESENT
Collar for potential ligament damage *but* only required when turning if patient sedated	Straight bed tilt to aid ICP management When thoracic/lumbar # excluded nurse 15–30° head up 3 person log roll is sufficient
Patient can be nursed 15–30° head up No need for log roll or straight bed tilt ▼	**STABLE CERVICAL #** If fully sedated/paralysed collar can be removed to aid ICP management when patient is supine Collar applied for turning and side lying If only lightly sedated collar must be applied at all times
Apply collar for 'waking' When awake test neck for tenderness or pain Consider dynamic flexion/extension X-rays if patient co-operative to check for instability For confused patients with no limb deficits remove collar and mobilise If unexplained limb deficit, MRI spine as soon as clinically possible	**UNSTABLE CERVICAL #** Collar must be applied at all times Management is dictated by precise nature of injury and its stability Await instructions from spinal team

Fig. 13.4 Algorithm 4. Management of cervical spine.

Guillain-Barre syndrome (GBS)

GBS is an acute inflammatory neuropathy affecting the peripheral nervous system (usually demyelination with secondary axonal degeneration). Complications include respiratory failure, respiratory or cardiac arrest, sepsis, pulmonary embolism, or general medical complications of intensive care.

Signs and symptoms

Patient experiences weakness, usually maximal 3 weeks after onset, and mild sensory symptoms, typically glove and stocking paraesthesia from the feet up, gradually involving rest of body depending on severity. Patients may describe infectious illness in 4 weeks prior to onset of symptoms suggesting immune basis for inflammatory process with both bacterial and viral agents implicated. Recovery usually begins 2–4 weeks after progression of weakness stops, but may be delayed for months depending on severity.

- Cranial nerves commonly affected (especially facial/bulbar).
- Areflexia (loss of tendon jerks) an early sign.
- Respiratory muscle weakness.
- Autonomic dysfunction common (usually persistent tachycardia and hypertension, but severe parasympathetic manifestations can occur).

Diagnosis

- History of presenting symptoms (progressive weakness of more than one limb with duration of progression less than 4 weeks).
- Clinical assessment (areflexia).
- Laboratory studies of CSF and blood.
- Nerve conduction studies (EMG).

Treatment

Supportive measures
- Good general medical and nursing care.
- Intensive care management.
- Rehabilitation.

Specific therapy
Both plasma exchange (PX) and intravenous immunoglobulin (IVIg) therapy effective in promoting recovery, particularly if given within 1 week of onset of symptoms or when there has been rapid deterioration in limb power. Due to ease of administration IVIg is now treatment of choice

Care of the patient with GBS

- If possible assess motor and sensory function 4-hourly, and cranial nerve function, in particular III, V, VI, VII, IX, X, XII.
- Early tracheal intubation indicated if respiratory muscle weakness occurs (i.e. if vital capacity falls to between 15 and 20ml/kg) or bulbar function compromised. Intubation often difficult due to autonomic instability. Early tracheostomy if prolonged period of artificial ventilation anticipated. Sedation for ventilation normally only in first 24–48h. When recovering FVC reaches 20ml/kg respiratory weaning usually commenced.

- Autonomic dysfunction is usually benign and specific therapeutic intervention is not required, but monitor closely to detect life-threatening instability.
- Persistent tachycardia (>120bpm) ± paroxysmal hypertension. Severe blood pressure swings treated symptomatically – colloid for hypotension. Pressor drugs with caution, antihypertensive therapy used only for prolonged hypertension – use short-acting agents. Postural hypotension can occur with increased incidence of cardiac arrhythmias, in particular bradycardia induced by vagal stimulation.
- Cardiac arrhythmias can be induced by vagal stimulation during suctioning.
- Pain common problem arising from immobility, inflamed nerves, and denervated muscles. Can be refractory to simple analgesics (often severe, usually neurogenic and worse with remyelination). Types of pain – paraesthesia (tingling, stinging, pins and needles), dysaesthesia (burning), backache and sciatica, meningism (meningeal irritation from swollen nerve roots), joint pain, and occasionally visceral pain (related to autonomic dysfunction). Simple analgesics and NSAIDs effective in relieving musculoskeletal symptoms (paracetamol and NSAIDs should be prescribed routinely). Anticonvulsant agents, such as gabapentin effective for paraesthesia and dysaesthesia. Tricyclic antidepressants such as amitriptyline effective for neurogenic pain. Prescribe opioids (e.g. meptazinol) if pain persists. Night sedation to promote sleep and facilitate rehabilitation.

Precautions and contraindications

- Urinary retention and constipation common. Paralytic ileus can develop as result of autonomic dysfunction.
- Potential risk of autonomic instability – gradually sit up to 70° in bed to assess blood pressure. Tilt table patient when BP stable to ensure patient can tolerate postural changes, use semi-reclining wheelchair.
- Autonomic instability causes fluctuating pulse and blood pressure, and extreme sensitivity to effects of drugs, in particular sedatives, analgesics, inotropes.

Myasthenia gravis (MG)

Myasthenia gravis (MG) is an autoimmune disease affecting the neuromuscular junction, specifically the acetylcholine (ACh) receptor sites, characterized by relapses and spontaneous remissions. Without treatment, 20–30% of myasthenics will die from the disease, 39–50% improve spontaneously, and the remainder continue to worsen or remain symptomatic. Its cause is unknown, but thymus gland may play some role in autoimmune process, since 80% of MG patients have thymic hyperplasia and 15% have thymic tumours.

Signs and symptoms

Characterized by weakness and fatigability of voluntary muscles, typically of eye, face, and mouth – classic signs and symptoms include:

- Ocular problems of ptosis and diplopia.
- Facial or bulbar weakness (difficulty swallowing, managing saliva).
- Dysarthria (voice nasal, weak, fades when talking).
- Weakness and fatigability of skeletal muscle exacerbated by exercise and worsening as day goes on (usually relieved by rest).
- Loss of strength in limbs – arms more affected than legs and proximal muscles more affected than distal muscles.
- Neck muscle weakness with head falling forward.
- Respiratory muscle weakness (not usually affected in isolation).

Diagnosis

- History and physical examination.
- Electromyography (EMG) – may include diaphragmatic EMG.
- Laboratory testing (should include anticholinesterase drug testing – Tensilon test – and detection of anti-ACh receptor antibodies).
- MRI/CT scan to determine if thymus gland is enlarged.

Treatment

No single therapy that works best for all patients; therefore, treatment based on individual's response to specific therapies.

Symptomatic therapy with anticholinesterase agents

- Pyridostigmine.
- Neostigmine (rarely used).

Disease modifying approaches

- **Prednisolone:** given until sustained improvement seen (initially within 3–4 weeks), then given on alternate days, and gradually reduced over months to lowest level necessary to maintain improvement. Worsening of symptoms occurs in 50% of patients after commencing, and may result in severe bulbar and respiratory muscle weakness, sometimes requiring tracheal intubation and ventilation.
- **Azathioprine:** produces improvement in most patients after 4 months, but may not show significantly until up to 12 months. Improvement persists while drug is given, but weakness may return 2–3 months after drug stopped or dose reduced.

- **Thymectomy:** thymus gland thought to be responsible for production of auto-antibodies in MG. Thymectomy produces best results in young patients with a short history of MG and in the absence of thymoma. As treatment for MG thymectomy should always be an elective procedure, with patient's MG well stabilized prior to surgery. Response to thymectomy may take up to 2 years to show improvement with the ultimate aim of maintaining the patient on lower doses of immunosuppressive medication.
- **Plasma exchange (PX) and intravenous immunoglobulin (IVIg):** PX and IVIg therapy used to produce rapid, but short-term improvement of severe symptoms. Almost all patients will improve after PX (improvement may begin after first exchange and seen within 48h in most patients, continuing for weeks or months after course of PX).

Care of the patient with myasthenia gravis

- ICU management will vary depending on whether admission is as a result of acute deterioration in patient with known MG or of new onset in previously undiagnosed MG patient.
- In severely ill patients the first priority is to maintain adequate ventilation and protection of airway. Respiratory insufficiency is due to respiratory muscle weakness and may be complicated by aspiration pneumonia secondary to bulbar weakness.
- Hypoxaemia, decreased tidal volume, dyspnoea, and abnormal arterial blood gases are all late findings in neuromuscular respiratory failure and are poor indicators of need for ventilatory support. More sensitive indicator of progressive respiratory failure is forced vital capacity (FVC). As FVC falls spontaneous coughing weakens and there is greater difficulty clearing secretions. Tracheal intubation generally performed if FVC drops below 15ml/kg but may be undertaken at higher FVC if patient also has bulbar weakness.
- Acute deterioration in known myasthenic patient – important to distinguish between myasthenic and cholinergic crisis. (see Algorithm 5, Fig. 13.5).

Precautions and contraindications

- A number of drugs (including some aminoglycoside antibiotics) exacerbate blockade at neuromuscular junction and use of all drugs must be carefully considered.
- Some drugs, such as antispasmodics, carry warning against their use in MG.
- Decision to extubate patient with MG after an anaesthetic should be taken with caution.

Myasthenic or cholinergic crisis

FVC < 15ml/kg
Stop ChE inhibitors
Both are **medical emergencies** that require prompt tracheal intubation
and assisted ventilation

↓

Establish whether **Myasthenic** or **Cholinergic** crisis

Tensilon test

Edrophonium chloride *(short-acting cholinesterase inhibitor)* given as diagnostic test
and produces rapid, but brief return of muscular power
Used to distinguish between myasthenic crisis (ACh deficiency) and cholinergic crisis
(excess of ACh due to overdose with anticholinesterase drugs)

This **test may not be appropriate in crisis** if patient unable to co-operate as delay in
intubation while test carried out may prove life-threatening

Tensilon test should be carried out by skilled personnel in environment that can
facilitate emergency respiratory and cardiovascular management

Atropine, the antidote to the muscarinic side effects of edrophonium, should be
available during testing

Myasthenic crisis	**Cholinergic crisis**
Usual cause is infection and signs and symptoms are that of myasthenia	Over-medication with anticholinesterase drugs. Symptoms include abdominal cramping and diarrhoea (muscarinic effects), profound generalised weakness, excessive pulmonary secretions and impaired respiratory function (nicotinic effects)
↓	
Give ChE inhibitor	
↓	↓
ChE inhibitors should be resumed at dose lower than before crisis and gradually increased	**Give atropine**
Any underlying cause such as infection or electrolyte abnormalities, in particular hypokalaemia, hypocalcaemia and hypermagnesemia, should be treated	↓
Consider steroid therapy Immunosuppression	Re-introduce ChE inhibitors gradually ChE inhibitors should be resumed at dose lower than before crisis and gradually increased
Plasma exchange	

Weaning from ventilation based on improved **FVC** and **MG**

Fig. 13.5 Algorithm 5. Myasthenic or cholinergic crisis.

Infection and inflammation of central nervous system

CNS infection can have potentially devastating consequences and requires immediate medical attention. Patients often need urgent airway protection, mechanical ventilation, and control of raised ICP. They may also require management for seizure control or because agitation makes them difficult to manage, necessitating sedation and respiratory monitoring.

Infection can be:
• **Regional:** meningitis (meninges, usually arachnoid and pia, and intervening subarachnoid space).
• **Diffuse:** encephalitis (brain tissue ± inflammation of meninges).
• **Focal:** brain abscess (intracerebral or subdural – empyema).

Signs and symptoms

Clinical presentation depends on part of CNS affected.

Meningitis
Certain features are common to all types of meningitis, but the speed at which they develop and their intensity varies depending on causative organism. Even with modern treatment, mortality is significant and many of those who survive will have complications of hydrocephalus, blindness, deafness, or cognitive deficits or epilepsy.
• The majority of viral causes self-limiting, resolve spontaneously with only supportive treatment and patient makes full recovery.
• Other forms, in particular bacterial meningitis, constitute serious, life-threatening illness.
• Fever, headache, neck stiffness, non-blanching haemorrhagic rash (meningococcal meningitis).

Encephalitis
Altered mental status.

Brain abscess
Focal neurology.

Diagnosis
• History and examination.
• Blood culture and CSF analysis.
• Lumbar puncture is essential to establish diagnosis, but patients in a coma, with focal neurological signs or papilloedema, must first undergo CT scan to exclude mass lesion.
• If CT scanning is not immediately available, commence antibiotics after taking blood samples for culture, rather than risk significant and perhaps fatal delay in initiating treatment.
• CSF results may show moderate increase in pressure, raised white cell count, raised protein, and normal or low glucose level.

Investigations and treatment

See Algorithms 6 and 7 (Figs 13.6 and 13.7)

Investigations and tests for CNS infection

SUSPECTED CNS INFECTION

PRIORITIES OF MANAGEMENT
BLOOD CULTURES
COMMENCE BROAD SPECTRUM
ANTIBIOTICS AND ANITVIRAL THERAPY
FULL SUPPORTIVE THERAPY FOR THE ITU PATIENT
CONSIDER LIKELY CAUSES FROM PATIENT HISTORY

CONSIDER CEREBRAL MALARIA
⇨ *TREATMENT IV QUININE*

STANDARD TESTS
M C & S
Inflammatory markers
Paired CSF and plasma glucose
Oligoclonal bands and paired serum

INVESTIGATIONS

✓ CT scan - if scan shows brain abscess surgical management essential

✓ Lumbar puncture (safe if patient not in coma and has no focal
   neurological signs or papilloedema)

✓ CSF analysis

✓ Look for meningococcal rash

✓ EEG in any patient with unexplained alteration in consciousness

✓ If TB meningitis suspected
   ⇨ look for BCG scar
   ⇨ do mantoux test
   ⇨ look for signs of primary TB on chest X-ray

✓ Consult with microbiologist/virologist

✓ Continue broad spectrum antibiotic and antiviral therapy until causative
   organism identified

✓ EDTA and serum sample stored for PCR/antibody studies

✓ Possible brain biopsy

Fig. 13.6 Algorithm 6. Investigations and tests for CNS infection.

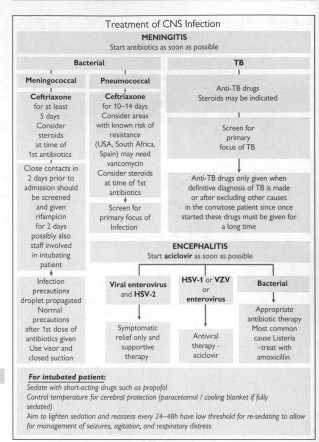

Fig. 13.7 Algorithm 7. Treatment of CNS infection.

Generalized convulsive status epilepticus

Status epilepticus (SE) is a clinical term referring to a series of generalized seizures without recovery of consciousness between attacks lasting for at least 30 min.

Diagnosis

- Diagnosed by observation – seizures characterized by loss of consciousness, tonic (ongoing) and/or clonic (rhythmic) muscle activity, tongue biting, and urinary incontinence.
- As duration of seizures increases, convulsive activity may become less obvious as depleted cerebral oxygen supplies are unable to meet demand (electromechanical dissociation), with perhaps only subtle twitching remaining as outward sign that seizures persist.

Causes

- Metabolic abnormalities.
- CNS infection.
- Traumatic or vascular brain injury.
- Cerebral tumours/space occupying lesions.
- Cerebral anoxic/hypoxic damage.
- Pre-existing epilepsy.
- Non-compliance/withdrawal anticonvulsant drug therapy.
- Drug toxicity.
- Chronic alcoholism.

Care of the patient with status epilepticus

SE carries high risk of mortality and morbidity. Management is aimed at terminating seizure, preventing occurrence once status controlled, investigating and managing precipitating causes and managing potentially serious and cumulative complications

- Many patients will respond to 1st line treatment with benzodiazepines.
- All anti-epileptic medication has sedative effect.
- Nurse in recovery position.
- Give oxygen therapy.
- Continuous ECG, BP, and pulse oximetry monitoring.
- Reduce risk of injury during seizures by removing unnecessary equipment from immediate vicinity.
- Consider anti-epileptic drugs in treatment algorithm (see Fig. 13.8).
- During prolonged status (60–90min) outward signs of motor activity diminish despite presence of continued electrographic seizures, and the patient will require sedation with general anaesthetic agents necessitating intubation and ventilation.
- Management aimed at suppressing activity by titrating agents to neurophysiological monitoring (portable EEG) until burst suppression of such activity achieved.
- Supportive treatment of intubated patient until seizures stop and patient regains consciousness.

Treatment

See Algorithm 8 (Fig. 13.8).

Algorithm for treatment of Status Epilepticus

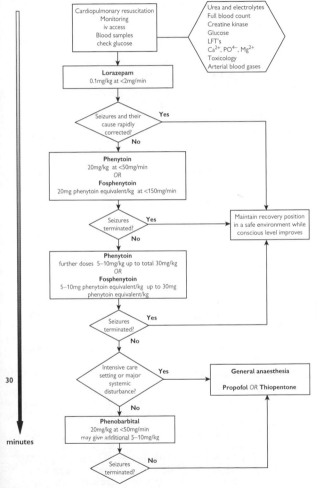

Fig. 13.8 Algorithm 8. Algorithm for the treatment of status epilepticus.

Brainstem testing and organ donation

Brainstem death (BSD)

BSD is defined as 'irreversible loss of the capacity for consciousness, combined with irreversible loss of the capacity to breathe'. In the UK there are three stages in diagnosis of brain death – preconditions, exclusions, and clinical tests.

Preconditions

- Diagnosis compatible with BSD.
- Evidence of irreversible structural brain damage.
- Apnoeic coma dependent on mechanical ventilation.

Exclusions

- Causes of reversible coma and factors causing central depression excluded.
- Absence of effects of sedative, hypnotic, analgesic and muscle relaxant drugs confirmed.
- Primary hypothermia excluded.
- Metabolic disorders considered with particular emphasis on correction of abnormal sodium, glucose and pH levels.

Clinical tests

Tests to confirm absence of brainstem reflexes and presence of persistent apnoea.

Test procedure

- 2 doctors make diagnosis of BSD (senior clinicians registered for >5 years – one a consultant, the other a consultant or senior registrar).
- Preconditions and exclusions must have been satisfied before tests carried out.
- In adults, no formal requirement for specified time interval between two sets of tests.

Care of the patient for BSD tests

Brainstem death can lead to a potentially very unstable patient due to loss of autoregulatory and brainstem function – cardiovascular instability and water and electrolyte imbalance can occur and must be treated promptly to meet criteria for testing.

- Early involvement of donor liaison nurse recommended to support staff and family.
- Central line and arterial line mandatory for management. Keep MABP ≥ 60mmHg – vasopressors as required to maintain organ perfusion (usually noradrenaline), but subject to patient requirements. May require pitressin in severe hypotension and where levels of vasopressor support are very high.

- Continuous ECG and arterial monitoring (be aware of possible cardiac arrhythmias and treat life-threatening arrhythmias if continuing to testing).
- Maintain temperature > 35°C for testing (damage to hypothalamus may cause loss of temperature regulation).
- Continue feeding and hydration. Maintain glucose within normal limits. Monitor electrolytes – be aware that Na^+ can rise rapidly and K^+ can be quickly lost in presence of DI (if Na^+ high give water via NGT or 5% glucose, and use sliding scale insulin to keep BM < 10mmol/l).
- Monitor fluid balance especially urine output and observe for diabetes insipidus (DI), and treat promptly (see Fig. 13.2).
- Continue chest physiotherapy to optimize oxygenation.

Equipment required for testing

- Ophthalmoscope.
- Ice and shallow container.
- 50ml lueur lock syringe and quill.
- Gauze.
- Narrow gauge suction catheter connected to oxygen tubing with suction hole occluded.
- Blood gas syringes.

Brainstem function tests

Optic (II), oculomotor (III) (midbrain)
Fixed diameter pupil, unreactive (directly or consensually) to light.

Trigeminal (V), facial (VII) (midbrain)
Absent corneal reflex.

Acoustic (VIII), abducens (VI) (pons)
Absent vestibulo-ocular reflex.

Facial (VII), accessory (XI) (midbrain and medulla)
- No motor response within cranial nerve distribution and no limb response to supra-orb/supra-orbital nerve pressure.
- Absent grimacing to pain.
- No head movement.

Glossopharyngeal (IX), vagus (X) (medulla)
- No gag reflex in response to suction catheter into trachea.
- No slowing of heart rate.
- No respiratory movement when disconnected from ventilator.

Testing for apnoea
- Reduce rate to allow P_aCO_2/O_2 o rise to 5.0kPa pre-testing.
- Pre-oxygenate with 100% oxygen for 10 min.
- Disconnect from ventilator.
- Insufflate oxygen at 6l/min via suction catheter placed in ET tube to maintain adequate oxygenation during testing.
- Allow $P_aCO_2O_2$ to rise to 6.65kPa.
- Confirm no spontaneous respiration.
- Reconnect to ventilator.

Limb and trunk movements
Reflex movements of limbs and trunk may occur in brainstem dead patients due to spinal reflexes. Their significance should be explained to staff and relatives to enable them to understand that movements do not involve conscious voluntary movement, i.e. do not originate in cerebral cortex.

Documentation
Documented time of death is the time of the 1st set of brainstem death tests when diagnosis of brain death confirmed, and not when mechanical ventilation discontinued (Legally, time of death recognized when 1st set of tests indicates brainstem death, but death cannot be pronounced and certified until after completion of second set of tests).

Approaching the family of a potential organ donor
- Collaborative approach (intensive care team involved in care of patient and Donor Liaison Nurse), ideally in interval between two sets of brainstem tests.
- If proceeding to organ donation continue invasive monitoring and intensive care procedures according to UKT/ICS guidelines. If not, give appropriate time to relatives and then discontinue all infusions and ventilation.

Renal disorders

Acute renal failure

Terms associated with acute renal failure

- **Acute renal failure**: an inability of the kidneys to remove the waste products of metabolism after correction of haemodynamic and mechanical causes.
- **Oliguria**: urine output <0.5ml/kg/h in an adult. Usually due to a sudden and sustained fall in renal perfusion causing the glomerular filtration rate to fall, thus resulting in a decrease in urine output.
- **Non-oliguric ARF**: adequate volumes of urine are produced, but levels of urea and creatinine remain high.
- **Pre-renal ARF**: renal tubules remain intact, and conserve salt and water during renal hypoperfusion, but urine output is decreased. When normal perfusion/pressure is restored, urine output returns to normal. If ischaemia continues, acute tubular necrosis may develop.
- **Acute tubular necrosis (ATN)**: necrosis of tubular cells caused by ischaemia or exposure to toxic molecules/drugs. This is actually an uncommon histological finding. In most cases of ARF (except for specific conditions such as glomerulonephritis), kidney histology looks normal.

Causes of acute renal failure

Many cases occur in patients with pre-existing disease (e.g. diabetes, hypertension, etc.), but can occur *de novo*.

Pre-renal
- **Hypovolaemia:** e.g. haemorrhage, burns, gastrointestinal losses, excessive diuresis, loss to extracellular spaces (ascites, sepsis, pancreatitis).
- **Hypotension:** myocardial dysfunction, arrhythmias, valvular dysfunction.
- **Obstructive hypotension:** pulmonary embolus, pericardial tamponade.

Renal (intrinsic)
- **Renal 'shutdown':** no gross abnormality seen. Causes include sepsis, other shock states, persisting hypoperfusion, hepatorenal syndrome.
- **Tubular damage:** haemorrhage, burns, shock states, nephrotoxins (e.g. radiographic contrast, aminoglycosides), eclampsia, pancreatitis, haemoglobin/myoglobin (e.g. rhabdomyolysis), multiple myeloma.
- **Cortical necrosis:** nephrotic syndrome, renal artery occlusion/thrombosis, glomerulonephritis, polyartertis nodosa, post-streptococcal infection, Goodpasture's syndrome, Wegener's granulomatosis, Henoch–Schönlein purpura.
- **Acute interstitial nephritis:** drugs including penicillins, NSAIDs.
- **Vascular:** emboli (NB. Infective endocarditis).

Post-renal
- **Raised intra-abdominal pressure** (impedes renal venous drainage).
- **Intra-ureteral:** bilateral calculi, papillary necrosis, crystals (e.g. uric acid), tumour, blood clot.
- **Extra-ureteral:** retroperitoneal fibrosis, tumour, aneurysm.
- **Bladder obstruction:** prostatic hypertrophy, bladder tumour, blood clot, calculi, functional neuropathy.
- **Urethral obstruction:** e.g. stricture, phimosis, blocked urinary catheter.

Investigations and diagnosis of acute renal failure

Investigations
The focus of the investigations is identification of the cause of the renal dysfunction so that appropriate corrective action may be taken.

Urine
- Urinalysis.
- Microscopy, culture, and sensitivities.
- Electrolytes, osmolality, urea, and creatinine.
- Creatinine clearance (marker of glomerular filtration rate).
- Urine:plasma ratios of urea, sodium, and osmolality.
- Myoglobinuria.
- Examination for stones ± measurement of urate, oxalate, etc.

Blood
- FBC.
- Co-agulation screen.
- U&Es, creatinine, calcium, phosphate, magnesium, glucose.
- Urate.
- Arterial blood gases.
- Liver function tests.
- Creatinine kinase (rhabdomyolysis).
- Autoantibodies (e.g. ANCA for Wegener's granulomatosis).

Radiology
- **Abdominal X-ray:** identifies renal calculi.
- **Renal ultrasound:** determines renal size, detects obstruction.
- **Urography** (X-ray with contrast): determines renal size, presence of obstruction, and suspected trauma.
- **Isotope renography:** determines renal function, size, vasculature, and outflow.
- **CT scan.**

Other
- 12-lead ECG.
- **Renal biopsy:** if renal failure is unexplained and a histological diagnosis is required. Not recommended if only single kidney or uncorrected coagulation abnormalities.

Diagnostic results
Urine
- Microscopy:
  - acute nephritis – white blood cells and casts;
  - acute tubular necrosis – tubular epithelial cells and casts;
  - glomerulonephritis – granular and red cell casts.
- Urinary indices (see Table 14.1).

Table 14.1 Diagnostic urinary indices for pre-renal and renal oliguria

Test	Pre-renal	Renal
Specific gravity	>1020	1010
Osmolality (mOsmol/kg)	>500	250–300
Sodium (mmol/l)	<15	>40
Urea (mmol/l)	>250	<160
Urine:plasma osmolality ratio	>1.3:1	<1.1:1
Urine:plasma urea ratio	>10:1	<4:1
Urine:plasma creatinine ratio	>40:1	<20:1

Blood investigations
- See Table 14.2.
- **Blood gas analysis:** usually shows a metabolic acidosis with a low bicarbonate, a significant base deficit and a low pH.

Table 14.2 Blood investigations in acute renal failure

Test	Normal value	Value in acute renal failure
Full blood count	Haemoglobin (Hb): 12—18 g/dl	Hb normal or low with anaemia or dilutional effect
	White blood cells (WBC): $(4-11) \times 10^9$/litre	WBC normal or raised if accompanying infection/ inflammation
Platelet count	$(150-400) \times 10^9$/litre	Normal (but function may be decreased or low, e.g. in systemic lupus erythematosus)
Sodium	132–144 mmol/l	Normal, high, or low
Potassium	3.3–4.7 mmol/l	Normal, high, or low
Urea	2.5–6.6 mmol/l	Raised
Creatinine	55–120 µmol/l	Raised
Phosphate	0.8–1.4 mmol/l	Usually raised
Glucose	Fasting <5.5 mmol/l	Normal
Osmolality	285–295 mOsm/l	Usually raised
Magnesium	0.75–1.0 mmol/l	Variable
Calcium	2.12–2.62 mmol/l	Normal or low

Reproduced with permission from *Critical Care Nursing*, Adam and Osborne (2005), Oxford University Press.

Further information

Adam SK, Osborne S. (2005) *Critical Care Nursing*. Oxford: Oxford University Press.

Management of acute renal failure (ARF)

Airway and breathing

- Monitor respiratory rate, pattern, and airway maintenance. Kussmaul breathing (rapid, deep respirations) may develop secondary to acidosis. continuous pulse oximetry.
- Monitor arterial blood gases and administer oxygen therapy as required.
- Respiratory failure, necessitating endotracheal intubation and ventilation, may develop secondary to:
  - deterioration in conscious level (secondary to uraemia);
  - pulmonary oedema due to fluid overload;
  - pre-existing respiratory failure.
- Note type and colour of secretions (e.g. oedema, frank blood).

Circulation

- Continuous monitoring, including ECG, CVP ± cardiac output.
- Maintain adequate circulating volume, BP, and cardiac output.
- Treat arrhythmias (NB. Peak T waves may indicate hyperkalaemia).
- Monitor K^+ level: treat hyperkalaemia promptly as this can lead to ventricular arrhythmias and asystole. For immediate treatment give 10ml of 10% calcium chloride to stabilize the myocardium followed by 50ml of 50% glucose containing 10–20 units of soluble insulin infused over 30–60min, and repeated as necessary.

Fluid balance

- Monitor all fluid intake and output hourly. Excess fluid overload should be avoided.
- Suspect catheter blockage if sudden oligoanuria develops, and exclude by bladder irrigation and/or replacement of catheter. In patients with nephrostomies, stents, or urostomies, rule out possibility of obstruction. If post-surgery or trauma, consider the possibility of blood clots causing obstruction, an anastomotic leak, or ureteric rupture.
- If obstruction has been excluded and the patient remains oliguric, optimize circulating volume by giving aliquots of 200ml colloid. Record CVP (or stroke volume) prior to and after each fluid bolus. If there is a sustained rise ≥3mmHg (or ≥10% in stroke volume), adequate filling has probably been achieved. If not, then give a further fluid bolus.
- Diuretics (e.g. furosemide, mannitol) can be tried if oliguria persists despite adequate filling and BP. They do not improve renal function, but may convert oliguric to polyuric renal failure, and thus assist with fluid balance (see Table 14.3).
- If circulating fluid volume has been optimized and the patient remains oliguric, fluid intake should be restricted to replace urine output and insensible losses only; renal replacement therapy should be considered.

Nutrition

The patient in ARF is often extremely catabolic and nutrition should be commenced as soon as possible. Enteral nutrition is preferable, has fewer complications (e.g. line-related sepsis) and maintains gut integrity. Renal failure patients should not be treated differently to other patients, but consideration should be given to the fact that:

- Total body water and sodium overload is usually present so volumes may need to be restricted (using higher concentration feeds).
- Amino acid losses occur with haemofiltration.
- B group vitamins are water soluble and can be removed during renal replacement therapy.

Electrolyte and trace elements should be administered either routinely (e.g. weekly basis) and/or according to blood levels.

Other

- Drug dosages or timings may need to be adjusted if they are renally excreted. Examples include penicillins, aminoglycosides, digoxin. A pharmacist should be consulted and blood levels taken, if appropriate.
- If the patient is anuric, remove the urethral catheter to reduce the risk of infection.

Table 14.3 Actions of furosemide and mannitol

Drug	Action	Dosage in renal failure
Furosemide (loop diuretic)	May increase intratubular flow, preventing obstruction	20–100mg bolus, followed by an infusion of 5–10mg/h
	May cause vasodilation of glomerular capillaries	
	May inhibit tubuloglomerular feedback, increasing GFR	
	May decrease oxygen consumption	
Mannitol (osmotic diuretic)	May reduce cell swelling and decrease tubular cell injury	500mg/kg (i.e. 5ml/kg of 10% solution or 2.5ml/kg of 20% solution)
	May increase extracellular volume and therefore cardiac output	
	Increase in extracellular fluid volume may cause pulmonary oedema	
	May decrease blood viscosity and systemic oncotic pressure causing increase in GFR	
	May increase intratubular flow, preventing obstruction	
	May cause vasodilation of glomerular capillaries	

Renal replacement therapy: basic principles

Indications for replacement therapy
- Metabolic acidosis (e.g. pH <7.3 and falling).
- Hyperkalaemia (e.g >6 mmol/l and rising).
- Fluid overload or to create space for nutrition and other inputs.
- Severe uraemic symptoms (confusion, pericarditis, vomiting etc.).
- Elevated and rising urea (e.g.>30mmol/l) and creatinine (e.g. >300μmol/l).
- Clearance of nephrotoxins or other toxins.

Aims of replacement therapy
- To relieve fluid overload and restore and maintain fluid balance.
- To remove waste products of metabolism (i.e. urea and creatinine).
- To correct and maintain an acceptable electrolyte balance.

Types of renal replacement therapy
- Continuous venovenous haemofiltration (CVVH).
- Continuous venovenous haemodialysis (CVVHD).
- Continuous venovenous haemodiafiltration (CVVHDF).
- Intermittent haemodialysis (IHD).
- Slow continuous ultrafiltration (SCUF).
- Continuous arteriovenous haemofiltration (CAVH).
- Peritoneal dialysis (PD) is now rarely used in critical care.

Vascular access
- Extracorporeal circuits that do not use a pump (CAVH) require an arterial vascular access to supply sufficient pressure to drive blood around the circuit and provide adequate filtration pressure.
- If a blood pump is used in the circuit, blood flow is not dependent on arterial pressure and so access can be gained from a vein.
- A 'double-lumen' cannula inserted in a large vein (e.g. internal jugular, femoral, or subclavian) is routinely used for pump-driven circuits. One lumen draws blood from the patient, while blood is simultaneously pumped back through the other. This lumen enters the vein more proximally to prevent recirculation (see Fig. 14.1, p. 341).

Basic physiological principles
Diffusion
- This is movement of solutes across a semi-permeable membrane from an area of high concentration to one of lower concentration.
- A concentration gradient is necessary for diffusion to occur.
- Molecules with smaller molecular weights (MW) move across the semi-permeable membrane more easily than those with larger MW.
- A semi-permeable membrane has a defined pore size and any molecules exceeding this will not pass through.

- Diffusion is affected by the resistance offered by the membrane; this is related to its thickness, and the size and shape of the pores.
- Diffusion is utilized in haemodialysis and haemodiafiltration.

Ultrafiltration
- This is bulk movement of water plus permeable solutes through a semi-permeable membrane.
- Water molecules are small and pass through any semi-permeable membrane.
- The driving force of ultrafiltration can be either an osmotic gradient or hydrostatic pressure.
- In osmotic ultrafiltration, water is drawn across a semi-permeable membrane from a hypotonic solution into a hypertonic solution. It is utilized in peritoneal dialysis.
- In hydrostatic ultrafiltration, water is forced across a semi-permeable membrane by a hydrostatic pressure exerted across the membrane. It is utilized in haemofiltration and haemodialysis.

Buffers
- To treat the metabolic acidosis a buffer must be provided in either the dialysate fluid or the replacement fluid (for haemofiltration).
- Lactate is commonly used as the buffer for haemofiltration and is metabolized to bicarbonate in the liver. In liver failure, the lactate will not be metabolized and blood levels will rise.
- Bicarbonate itself can be used as a buffer for renal replacement therapy, but cannot be given with calcium because of the risk of chalk formation.
- Acetate is often used as a buffer in short-term dialysis. It is not generally used for continuous renal replacement therapy as it is metabolized by muscle, and this may be affected by hypoperfusion. It is also associated with increased haemodynamic instability, making it unsuitable for critically ill patients.
- Excess lactate buffer can cause a metabolic alkalosis; in this case, replacement fluid with a lower lactate content can be substituted.

Types of renal replacement therapy

Continuous venovenous haemofiltration (CVVH)

A pumped method using a double-lumen cannula (see 🕮 Renal replacement therapy: basic principles; Vascular access, p. 338) sited in a large vein (or two separate venous cannulae) for blood outflow and return. Alarms and monitoring devices are incorporated, and high filtration rates can be maintained. There are potential dangers in removing and replacing large volumes of fluid and solutes, and there is a considerable nursing workload involved.

Continuous venovenous haemodiafiltration (CVVHD)

Requires a dialysate solution running through the filter in a direction that is counter-current to the blood, and on the opposite side of the membrane. Filtration still occurs because a pressure gradient exists, but diffusion can be utilized to facilitate the removal of solutes without the need to remove such large volumes of fluid. The flow rate of the dialysate can be up to 2l/h. The same nursing issues as CVVH apply.

High (or ultra-high) volume haemofiltration

The removal of high volumes (up to 6l/h for limited periods) of filtrate during continuous haemofiltration. These high rates have been associated with improved removal of inflammatory mediators, but is time-consuming, labour-intensive, and expensive. Clinical benefits are uncertain.

Assisted haemo(dia)filtration techniques

A range of machines are available with varying modes of operation. They must be set up and used by adequately trained staff as there is a risk of user error and patient complications:

- Some machines operate on specific time cycles over a number of hours, others operate on an hourly basis.
- All fluid intake (nutrition, drugs, infusions, buffered replacement fluid) must be balanced against losses, including the filtrate.
- A target fluid balance (positive or negative) is determined on the basis of clinical assessment of body and intravascular volume status.
- Most machines incorporate pumps for replacement fluid, dialysate fluid, blood, and filtrate fluid.
- Alarms to indicate abnormal pressures within the circuit are also an essential part of the system.
- If haemodiafiltration is used, the volume of dialysate infused must be subtracted from the total filtrate volume to obtain the actual filtrate volume (more advanced systems will do this automatically).
- Fluid balance recordings must be documented carefully to avoid confusion and prevent accidental hypo- or hypervolaemia.
- Blood flow through the circuit should be between 100 and 200ml/min in order to reduce clotting risk without damaging the filter with extreme pressures.
- Filters are usually hollow fibre membranes made from biocompatible products, such as polyacrilonitrile.

Continuous arteriovenous haemofiltration (CAVH)

Blood flows through the extracorporeal circuit (driven by the patient's own arterial BP) from an arterial cannula and returns via a venous cannula. A pump can also be inserted into the circuit. This method is rarely used because the lack of pressure alarms and dependence on arterial pressure makes it unsafe and inefficient.

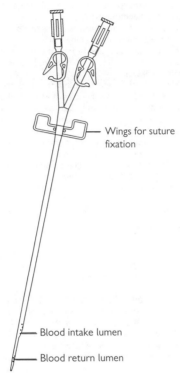

Wings for suture fixation

Blood intake lumen

Blood return lumen

Fig. 14.1 Double-lumen vascular cannula for venovenous haemo(dia)filtration. Reproduced with permission from *Critical Care Nursing*, Adam and Osborne (2005), Oxford University Press.

Further reading

Adam SK, Osborne S. (2005) *Critical Care Nursing*. Oxford: Oxford University Press.

Haemofiltration

General principles

- This is a hydrostatic ultrafiltration process with mass movement of plasma water and solutes across a semi-permeable membrane.
- Blood on one side of the membrane exerts a hydrostatic pressure causing water and solutes to move from the plasma across the membrane to become the 'haemofiltrate'.
- Constant draining of the filtrate ensures a negative pressure on the other side of the membrane, maintaining a pressure gradient.
- Protein and cellular contents of the blood do not cross the membrane due to their large molecular size. In general, molecules >35kDa are not filtered (albumin is 64kDa).
- This process is not selective; removal of waste products is achieved only by removal of an accompanying load of water and other solutes.
- The volume of filtrate removed can greatly exceed 2l/h ('ultra-high haemofiltration); to maintain haemodynamic stability, similar volumes must be replaced concurrently to the desired fluid balance.
- The replacement fluid should be isotonic and replace solutes lost in the filtrate.
- Continuous anticoagulation of the circuit is usually necessary unless the patient is significantly auto-anticoagulated.
- Haemofiltration allows continuous control of uraemia and fluid balance, but its efficiency is low, it restricts patients mobility and necessitates constant patient-centred activity that can disrupt rest and sleep.

Nursing interventions

Monitoring

- Haemodynamic monitoring should be continuous to detect hypovolaemia, hypotension and arrhythmias.
- Monitor plasma potassium at least 4-hourly, unless patient is very stable.
- Monitor core temperature and maintain >36°C. Heat loss from blood in the extracorporeal circuit and infusion of large volumes of room temperature replacement fluid can reduce body temperature. Replacement fluid can be warmed prior to infusion, and circuit tubing wrapped in aluminium foil to reduce heat losses.
- Monitor circuit pressures and blood coagulation laboratory profiles.

Rest and sleep

Ensure the patient is allowed adequate rest and sleep. Position circuit tubing to prevent kinking and obstruction of blood flow, and thus avoid setting off machine alarms and the risk of filter/circuit clotting.

Psychological care

The sight of large volumes of blood in the extracorporeal circuit can be frightening for patients and relatives. To reduce anxiety, discussion regarding renal replacement therapy as a treatment should be introduced before its commencement. A constant and reassuring nursing presence will also support the patient and their family.

Safety

- Vascular access should be in view or inspected regularly (particularly after position change or patient movement).
- Circuit tubing should be supported or clamped in position, and checked for kinking or undue tension.
- Haemofiltration machines should be positioned so that urgent access to the patient is still possible.
- Circuits should incorporate clamps to ensure that inadvertent disconnection does not result in severe blood loss.

Intermittent haemodialysis

- Blood is pumped into an extracorporeal circuit, where it is anticoagulated prior to passage through an artificial kidney (dialyser).
- The kidney contains multiple hollow fibres or sheets, which form the semi-permeable membranes.
- Dialysate fluid is pumped on the opposite side of the semi-permeable membrane to the blood and in a counter-current direction.
- Waste products move by diffusion from the blood, across the membrane and into the dialysate solution.
- Blood flows of up to 600ml/min can be achieved.
- The clearance of small molecules depends on the concentration gradient across the membrane. Clearance can be improved by increasing the counter-current dialysate flow rate (usually set at 500ml/min).
- Water is removed by ultrafiltration achieved by the exertion of a pressure across the membrane (the transmembrane pressure, TMP).
- The dialysate fluid is usually supplied in concentrated form and needs to be diluted with water. Proportionators mix the correct volume of water and dialysate solution, and are either incorporated in the machine or are situated centrally.
- Large quantities of water are used (approx 120l per session); these must be sterile and specially treated (either by reverse osmosis or ion exchange resins).
- The patient can be weighed pre- and post-dialysis to calculate fluid loss.
- Plasma urea and electrolytes and a coagulation screen should be taken before and after each 2–4h dialysis session.
- Numerous monitoring and alarm systems are incorporated, which must be observed, recorded, and acted upon.

Advantages

- The most effective method of clearing waste products.
- Intermittent – only requires anticoagulation during the procedure and makes fewer demands on nursing time.
- The patient can be mobile between sessions.
- Closed circuit poses less infection risk to staff (e.g. hepatitis B, HIV).

Disadvantages

- Specially trained staff required.
- Adequate fluid must be removed during the session (usually 2–4h) to allow nutrition and other infusions to be given for the following 24–72h.
- A negative balance may be required at the end of the session causing rapid fluid shifts and leading to potential haemodynamic instability.
- Provides only episodic control of uraemia.
- Hypoxaemia, hypotension and complement activation are associated with cheaper types of membrane.
- Equipment and water supply can be expensive.
- The first session should be brief because of the risk of disequilibrium syndrome (see 📖 p. 345).

Complications

Cardiovascular

Continuous cardiovascular monitoring, pulse oximetry, and regular blood gas monitoring are essential.

- **Hypotension:** secondary to hypovolaemia and the use of acetate buffer solutions.
- **Arrhythmias:** due to hyper- or hypokalaemia, and/or hypovolaemia.
- **Hypoxaemia:** caused by cuprophane membranes, which are thought to cause cytokine activation, oxygen removal, and shunting.

Muscle cramps, nausea, and vomiting

Experienced by many patients. Common predisposing factors are hypotension, excess fluid removal, and low plasma sodium.

Disequilibrium syndrome

Caused by the rapid removal of urea, which results in a decreased concentration in the plasma compared to the cerebrospinal fluid (CSF). The resulting osmotic gradient causes water to move into the CSF and brain tissue. The patient presents with headache, vomiting, restlessness, convulsions, and even coma. A severely uraemic patient should not experience an initial reduction in plasma urea >30% during dialysis.

Acute haemolysis

Can be caused by overheated, hypotonic, or contaminated dialysate fluid. The patient complains of chest tightness, back pain, and dyspnoea. Hyperkalaemia can result from the release of potassium from the haemolysed red cells.

Anticoagulation therapy for extracorporeal circuits

Anticoagulation

- Necessary to prevent platelet and coagulation system activation in response to contact with a foreign surface (circuit and filter).
- Ineffective anticoagulation causes clotting in the filter; this is time-consuming to replace, expensive, and bad for the patient as it decreases efficiency and wastes blood (a circuit contains 150–200ml blood).
- Too much anticoagulant can cause bleeding from cannula sites or spontaneously into skin or brain, or from bowel or lung.
- Heparin is the most commonly used anticoagulant (usually mixed molecular weight 'unfractionated' heparin). Low molecular weight heparin is harder to monitor because it requires an anti-Factor Xa assay and is therefore rarely used.
- 5–20 IU/kg/h heparin is usually infused proximal to the filter. The dose required during haemofiltration is less than haemodialysis.
- A pre-filtration heparin bolus of 2000–5000IU may also be given if there are difficulties with filter clotting.
- If the patient develops heparin-induced thrombocytopenia syndrome (HITS), all heparin must be stopped.
- If the patient has an adverse reaction to heparin (e.g. thrombo-cytopenia) or is at risk of bleeding (e.g. post-surgery), epoprostenol (PG1$_2$) or alprostadil (PGE$_1$) can be given instead at 2.5–10ng/kg/min.
- Refer to 📖 Chapter 19, pp. 445–470, for further information, other anticoagulation alternatives, and adverse effects.

Troubleshooting frequent filter clotting

- Ensure adequate pre-filter use priming has been undertaken.
- Maintain blood flows at >150ml/min.
- Check for kinking or obstruction of double-lumen cannula (femoral placement is a particular problem).
- If arterial (outflow) circuit pressures are high, check vascular access for signs of obstruction.
- If filter pressures are high check filter for signs of clotting and if necessary reduce blood flow rate if above 150ml/min.
- Consider swopping access on the double lumen cannula as an interim measure if this is unsuccessful.
- Consider cannula change if pressures remain high and filter clot is likely.
- If repeated filter clotting occurs with full anticoagulation, consider pre-dilution using replacement fluid added prior to the filter to reduce viscosity (this will reduce filter efficiency, however).

Tests to assess anticoagulation during renal replacement therapy

All measure the anticoagulation effect of heparin.

Activated clotting time (ACT)

- Blood is added to a tube containing siliceous earth, which accelerates the clotting process.
- The tube is placed in a machine (e.g. Haemochron), which automatically tilts/rotates it and measures the time taken (in seconds) until clot formation is detected.
- ACT is normally maintained at 200–250s for haemodialysis and 150–220s for haemofiltration.

Whole blood partial thromboplastin time (WBPTT)

- 0.2ml of actin FS reagent (Thrombofax) is added to 0.4ml blood to accelerate the clotting process.
- This is set in a heating block at 37°C for 30s and tilted every 5s until a clot forms.
- During haemodialysis the WBPTT would be maintained at the baseline value plus 40–80% (approximately 120–140s) and during haemofiltration a baseline value plus 50%.

Activated partial thromboplastin time (APTT)

- Blood is added to a tube containing oxalate or citrate (to stop coagulation by calcium binding).
- Phospholipid (an activator) and calcium (to reverse the effect of the oxalate or citrate) are mixed with the sample and the time measured until a clot forms.
- APTT should be checked 4–6h after starting a heparin infusion.
- Aim for 1.5–2.5 times the control value.

Specific disorders associated with acute renal failure

Acute glomerulonephritis

This refers to a specific set of renal diseases in which an immunological mechanism triggers inflammation and proliferation of glomerular tissue. This can result in damage to the basement membrane or capillary endothelium. Sudden onset haematuria, oliguria, and proteinuria accompanies renal dysfunction. Granular red cell casts are present in urine. Clinically, it is associated with hypertension and peripheral oedema.

Causes of acute glomerulonephritis

Systemic causes

- **Wegener's granulomatosis:** necrotizing vasculitis affecting small- and medium-sized vessels in kidneys, lungs and nasal cartilages.
- **Collagen vascular diseases** (e.g. systemic lupus erythematosus): causes renal deposition of immune complexes.
- **Hypersensitivity vasculitis:** often associated with eosinophilia.
- **Polyarteritis nodosa:** causes vasculitis of the renal arteries.
- **Henoch–Schönlein purpura:** causes generalized vasculitis.
- **Goodpasture's syndrome:** antibodies to type IV collagen may rapidly result in oliguric renal failure and haemoptysis.
- **Drug-induced** (e.g. gold, penicillamine).
- **Cryoglobulinaemia:** abnormal quantities of plasma cryoglobulin.

Post-infectious causes

- **Group A streptococcal infection** (e.g. sore throat, upper respiratory tract): usually occurs a week or more after the acute infection.
- **Other specific agents:** including other bacteria, fungi, viruses, parasites, e.g. malaria, filariasis), atypicals (e.g. Legionnaire's disease).

Renal diseases

- **Berger's disease:** immunoglobulin-related nephropathy due to deposition of IgA and IgG.
- **Membranoproliferative glomerulonephritis**: deposition of complement causes expansion and proliferation of mesangial cells.
- **Idiopathic rapidly progressive glomerulonephritis.**

Hepatorenal syndrome

Development of ARF in patients with chronic liver disease with ascites and portal hypertension. It may be caused by alterations in splanchnic circulatory tone and renal blood supply. The renin-angiotensin-aldosterone and sympathetic nervous systems are activated with profound renal vasoconstriction. It is associated with a high mortality. Liver transplantation is the definitive treatment with normalization of renal function occurring soon after the transplant. Risk factors include:

- Infection: particularly spontaneous bacterial peritonitis.
- Acute alcoholic hepatitis.
- Large volume paracentesis without albumin replacement.
- Gastrointestinal and variceal bleeding.

Rhabdomyolysis

The breakdown of striated muscle releasing myoglobin, which causes a combination of pre-renal, nephrotoxic, and obstructive acute renal failure.

Causes
- Direct trauma, crush injury, burns.
- Muscle compression from prolonged immobility (surgery, coma).
- Metabolic illness (diabetic metabolic decompensation).
- Myositis.
- Temperature extremes.
- Toxins – alcohol, solvents, drug abuse.
- Muscular dystrophies.
- Excessive muscle activity.

Substances released by damaged muscle
- Potassium, leading to hyperkalaemia; this may be resistant to glucose and insulin therapy and require urgent or haemodialysis or haemo-diafiltration (dialysis is more effect than filtration alone).
- Hydrogen ions, leading to a metabolic acidosis.
- Phosphate, leading to hyperphosphataemia.
- Creatine, leading to an elevated creatinine kinase (usually >5000IU/l).
- Myoglobin leading to myoglobinuria; myoglobin is oxidized by hydroperoxides in the kidney generating potent oxidizing ferryl-myoglobin. This is nephrotoxic, especially with co-existing acidosis and volume depletion. It can obstruct renal tubules.

Management
- Maintain good circulating volume to ensure high urine output.
- Forced alkaline diuresis (6–10L fluid/day including 1.24% sodium bicarbonate for 3–5 days) to maintain urine pH>6 using 1.24% sodium bicarbonate. Alkalinization stabilizes the oxidizing form of myoglobin.
- Treat hyperkalaemia.
- Renal replacement therapy may be needed if renal failure is established.
- Compartment syndrome may require treatment (referral to surgeons) with decompression fasciotomies.
- Avoid NSAIDs and use opiate analgesia.
- Treat the underlying cause.

Gastrointestinal dysfunction and nutrition

Overview of physiology I

Functions of GIT

The major functions of the GIT are:
- Breakdown of complex nutrients.
- Absorption of predigested molecules.
- Movement of foodstuff though the digestive tract.
- Elimination of waste matter.
- Recycling of materials used in digestion.
- Protection of vulnerable internal organs from ingested organisms.

Control of functions

Most of the functions are under the control of the autonomic nervous system (sympathetic and parasympathetic). Voluntary control occurs at the upper oesophagus, external anal sphincter, and oropharyngeal cavity controlling intake and allowing excretion to occur at convenient times.

Sympathetic stimulation decreases gut motility, increases sphincter tone and decreases exocrine (via a duct, e.g. bile) and salivary secretions. This occurs with increased catecholamine release. Parasympathetic stimulation increases motility, decreases sphincter tone, and increases exocrine secretions. Thus, secretion, absorption, and motility are controlled by the interaction between the sympathetic and parasympathetic stimuli. GI secretions and their functions are listed in Table 15.1.

Movement of food, chyme (semi-digested food and gastric enzymes), and faecal material is by peristalsis (contraction of smooth muscle in waves).

Oropharyngeal cavity and oesophagus

Food is broken down in the mouth mechanically and by enzymes, such as salivary amylase and lingual lipase. A food bolus is produced, which is swallowed and propelled down the oesophagus by peristalsis.

Saliva and mucus production occur in the mouth and mucus produced in the oesophagus helps food to slide down.

Saliva is an important component of protection and digestion.

Stomach

The function of the stomach is primarily digestive, but the highly acidic environment also protects against foreign organisms. Gastric acid secretion is regulated by gastrin and has a diurnal rhythm, which is higher in the evening and lower in the morning. Distension of the stomach and the presence of digested protein in the intestine will stimulate further gastric acid release. Between 1 and 2l of gastric juice are produced each day and this can be increased by the presence of a nasogastric tube.

Table 15.1 Important gastrointestinal secretions

	Contents	Function
Saliva	Salivary amylase	Starch-digesting enzyme
	Mucus	Lubricates and binds food with enzymes
	Lingual lipase	Lipid-hydrolysing enzyme
	Lysozyme	Cell wall breakdown enzyme, which protects against bacteria
	Lactoferrin	Iron-chelating agent, which protects against bacteria
	Secretory IgA	Immunoglobulin, which is active against viruses and bacteria
Gastric juice	Pepsin	Protein-digesting enzyme, which functions in an acidic environment
	Hydrogen ions	Maintains low pH for protection and pepsin activity
	Intrinsic factor	Facilitates absorption of vitamin B_{12} by small intestine
	Gastrin	Promotes growth/repair of mucosa and secretion of HCl and pepsinogen
Pancreatic juice	Trypsin, chymotrypsin, elastase, carboxypeptidase	Protein digestion – trypsin is activated in the duodenum by enterokinase and then activates other enzymes
	Lipase and esterase	Fat digestion – catalysis of hydrolysis
	Amylase	Carbohydrate digestion
	Nuclease	Nucleic acid digestion
Small intestine	Bicarbonate	Neutralizes post-gastric acid
	Enterokinase	Converts trypsinogen to trypsin (active form)
	Secretin and CCK	Stimulate pancreatic secretion
	Maltase, lactase, sucrase	Conversion of carbohydrates to simple sugars

Overview of physiology II

Pancreas and gall bladder

Both exocrine and endocrine secretion occurs in the pancreas. Cholecystokinin (CCK) stimulates enzyme secretion by pancreatic cells in response to the presence of amino acids, peptides, and fatty acids in the small intestine. Endocrine secretions include insulin and glucagon, and exocrine secretions include bicarbonate, water, and a variety of protein, starch, and fat digesting enzymes.

The gall bladder holds and concentrates bile, which emulsifies fat, ionizes fat-soluble vitamins, and suspends cholesterol, triglycerides, and lipoproteins in the blood.

Small intestine

This is a vital area of the GI tract as absorption of food takes place primarily in the duodenum and jejunum. In addition, other highly complex mechanisms are associated with this part of the GI tract.

Secretion of water and bicarbonate by Brunner's glands allow the chyme (semi-digested food and enzymes) to be diluted and the acidity neutralized.

Secretion of a range of digestive enzymes allows conversion of carbohydrates to simple sugars, fats to fatty acids/monoglycerides and protein to dipeptides/amino acids that are absorbed.

Approximately 7–10l/24h of water enter the small intestine and all but approximately 600ml is reabsorbed.

Colon and rectum

Further water (around 500ml) is re-absorbed in the colon, together with sodium, potassium, chloride, and bicarbonate. The colon secretes mucus to lubricate the faecal material and protect the mucosa. Folic acid and ammonia are also absorbed in the colon.

The rectum fills intermittently with faecal matter, which would initiate relaxation of the internal sphincter if not voluntarily overridden. If appropriate, relaxation of the internal and external sphincters allows faeces to move into the anal canal and from there to be expelled.

Liver function

The liver hepatocytes perform a large number of essential metabolic functions. The liver has the ability to regenerate itself, and has both an arterial (hepatic artery) and a venous (portal vein) blood supply, as well as venous drainage. The portal vein comes from the mesenteric circulation, and contains nutrients for storage and synthesis, as well as debris for filtration and phagocytosis. It supplies approximately three-quarters of the blood flowing through the liver.

Hepatocyte functions

Hepatocytes are the main liver cells and perform multiple functions.

Glucose homeostasis

In order to maintain a constant level of glucose available for energy, the liver is able to store, release, and manufacture glucose. Glucose is stored as glycogen.

Degradation of drugs for excretion

- Fat-soluble drugs are metabolized by hepatic enzymes in a specialized part of the hepatic cell into water-soluble substances, which can be excreted in bile or urine.
- Synthetic (the drug is conjugated with substances, such as glucuronic acid) and non-synthetic breakdown (the drug is altered by oxidation, reduction, or hydrolysis) occurs in the hepatocyte.
- Conjugation usually causes loss of drug activity (e.g. paracetamol or morphine), but when 2 drugs are both metabolized by the same microsomal enzymes there may be prolongation of drug effect.
- Decreased hepatic function may lead to impaired excretion and prolonged drug effect.

Protein metabolism

Hepatocytes synthesize plasma proteins, such as albumin, globulins, transferrin, and caeruloplasmin (a protein binding copper in the plasma). Protein is also deaminated, and ammonia is converted to urea and transaminated (amino acids moved from one protein to another).

Synthesis of coagulation factors

These vital components of haemostasis include fibrinogen, prothrombin and factors I, II, V, VII, IX, and X.

Elimination of bilirubin

Haem, a product of the breakdown of haemoglobin, is not water-soluble and must be conjugated with glucuronic acid by hepatocytes and actively transported into bile to be excreted via the stool.

Production of bile

The liver synthesizes cholesterol from which the primary bile acids (cholic and chenodeoxycholic acid) are produced. Bile is secreted and then bile acids are re-absorbed into the portal blood in specific ileal sites.

Fat metabolism

Hepatocytes synthesize lipoproteins from a combination of fats (e.g. cholesterol) and apoprotein. They also assist in the conversion of carbohydrate and protein into fat (lipogenesis).

Mineral storage

Hepatocytes store up to 60% of excess iron and vitamins including A, D, K, B12, and folate.

Hormone catabolism

Hormones catabolized by the liver include steroids, insulin, oestrogens, and contraceptive drugs.

Glycogen storage

Glycogen is a polysaccharide of glucose, and acts as a short-term form of energy storage found mainly in the liver and muscle.

Gluconeogenesis

Glucose is formed from lactate, pyruvate, amino acids, or glycerol by enzymes in the liver cell.

Glycogenolysis and glucose release

If blood glucose levels fall, glycogen is broken down by enzymes in the hepatocytes into glucose, which is then released into the circulation.

Immune function and the gastrointestinal tract

Due to the direct exposure to potentially harmful organisms associated with ingestion, and due to the large number of commensal bacteria living in the gut, the GI tract has a highly sophisticated immune defence system. This consists of both mechanical and cellular forms of protection.

Mechanical protection

- Gastric pH is highly acidic and kills most organisms.
- Gut mucosa acts as a physical barrier.
- Secreted mucus prevents bacterial adherence.

Immunological protection

- Secretory immunoglobulin A (IgA) is secreted by Peyer's patches and prevents bacterial adherence to and, thus, penetration of mucosal cells.
- High numbers of lymphocytes and macrophages in the intestinal wall trap, and phagocytose bacteria which do penetrate the intestinal wall.
- Mesenteric regional lymph nodes provide fast antigen-specific responses.
- Fixed organ-specific macrophages, such as Kupffer cells in the liver and spleen trap, and phagocytose bacteria, which have entered the portal circulation.

In the healthy person, this protection is highly effective, but as soon as critical illness develops components of the defence become compromised.

Effect of critical illness on the gastrointestinal tract immunity

- Decreased ability to maintain acidic gastric pH.
- Altered permeability of the mucosal wall due to:
  - sepsis;
  - hypovolaemia and decreased intestinal perfusion;
  - ischaemia;
  - endotoxaemia
- Increased bacterial numbers in the intestine due to overgrowth, stasis, or loss of commensal bacteria due to antibiotic use.
- Immunocompromise due to sepsis and SIRS, drugs such as steroids, stress.

The patient is then more vulnerable to secondary infection, which may rapidly become overwhelming.

Maintenance of mucosal integrity is thought to be supported by early enteral nutrition, which supports the fast replicating enterocytes and lymphocytes by providing direct sources of nutrients.

Gastrointestinal dysfunction: diarrhoea

This symptom of gastrointestinal dysfunction is common amongst critically ill patients with a reported incidence of 15–52%.

A number of factors have been implicated (see Table 15.2), which can be divided into infective and non-infective causes.

A clear definition of diarrhoea has not been determined being variously:
- >3 stools per day.
- Loose or fluid consistency.
- Stool weight >300g/day.

Prevention

The increase in *Clostridium difficile* (*C.difficile*)-related diarrhoea is caused by use of broad spectrum antibiotics, which kill commensal gut organisms allowing *C.difficile* to proliferate. Good antibiotic practice should include:
- A clear, specific antibiotic policy minimizing the use of broad spectrum antibiotics.
- Antibiotics should be prescribed with a stop date.
- Antibiotic requirement should be reviewed on a daily basis.

Other important preventive measures are hand hygiene, wearing gloves and aprons for close contact, chlorine-based disinfectants, source isolation of patients.

Maintenance of the integrity of the gut mucosa is also useful in reducing diarrhoea and early enteral nutrition will assist with this.

Management of diarrhoea (general)
- Rectal examination to rule out faecal impaction with overflow.
- Send stool specimens (usually 3) for culture and sensitivity and *C.difficile* toxin.
- Review Drug Chart for diarrhoea-inducing drugs and discontinue any that are not essential. (NB. Also ensure any laxatives are discontinued!)
- Consider use of alternative enteral feed, e.g. fibre-containing, pre- and probiotic additives.
- Protect skin from excoriation (see Table 15.3).
- High level of monitoring and management of electrolytes (K^+, Na^+, Mg^{2+}), and fluid balance.

Infective causes
- Appropriate antibiotic treatment after culture and isolation of the organism involved.
- Metronidazole or vancomycin for *C.difficile* infection.

Non-infective causes
- Abdominal X-ray if ischaemic or inflammatory bowel disease is suspected (or there is bloody diarrhoea).
- Administer anti-motility agents, such as loperamide or diphenoxylate.
- If malabsorption is likely to be the cause, consider semi-elemental feeds.

Table 15.2 Causes of diarrhoea

Infective causes	Non-infective causes
Clostridium difficile	Drugs – containing sorbitol, laxatives(!), ACE inhibitors, broad-spectrum antibiotics, etc.
Enterococcus coli	Malabsorption, e.g. in hypoalbuminaemia
Salmonella	Intolerance of solutes, e.g. lactase deficiency
	Increased secretion of chloride ions related to toxins or neoplasms
Other tropical diseases, such as amoebic dysentery, *Shigella* cholera, giardia, etc.	Overflow with faecal impaction
	Inflammatory bowel disease, diverticulitis

Table 15.3 Prevention of skin excoriation from faecal contact

Unbroken skin	Broken skin
Careful washing with every episode of diarrhoea	Careful washing
Application of barrier cream after each episode of diarrhoea	Use of spray-on barrier film
	Consider use of bowel management system (flexible rectal catheter with balloon seal and collection bag)

Gastrointestinal dysfunction: constipation

The incidence of constipation in the critically ill patient is more common than is generally supposed, occurring in 15% of all critically ill patients and up to 80% of ventilated patients. The definition of constipation is subjective, but is usually taken as >3 days without a bowel movement. However, in patients who are fed parenterally, there may be minimal gastrointestinal content and waste for excretion, and expected bowel movements may be less frequent.

Recent studies show an association between length of time to bowel movement and length of stay in intensive care. It seems that severity of illness is associated with degree of gastrointestinal dysfunction.

Critically ill patients are prone to constipation due to:
- Immobility.
- Effects of sepsis and shock on GI tract motility.
- Opiate reduction of GI tract motility.
- Loss of stimulus of food passing through the oesophagus.
- Muscle wasting, which may include the muscles of defaecation (diaphragm, abdominals, levator ani).

Managing constipation in the critically ill
- Maintaining an accurate record of bowel movements ensures that constipation is picked up and managed appropriately.
- Careful monitoring and maintenance of the patient's hydration.
- If there is no evidence of bowel movement after 3 days, a per rectum examination should be carried out, to confirm the presence of stool in the rectum.
- If there is stool in the rectum, a stimulant (usually a glycerin suppository) can be administered.
- If there is no stool in the rectum an osmotic laxative should be commenced.
- If the patient is enterally fed, it may be worth switching to a fibre-containing feed.
- If there is no response after a further 3 days, switch to an alternative laxative (such as a stimulant) or an enema (Micralax®) should be carried out (see Table 15.4).
- Neostigmine infusion has been used with some success if there is still no response to maximum therapy.
- There is a risk of stercoral perforation (perforation of the gut by hardened faeces or a foreign body).
- Care should be taken if there is any suspicion of obstruction. or pseudo-obstruction. or the patient has recently had abdominal surgery.

Table 15.4 Laxatives

Type	Effect	Examples
Bulking or hydrophilic agents	Soluble fibres draw water into the gut and provide bulk to the stool	Psyllium, bran, methylcellulose
Osmotic agents	Draw water into the colon and increase the volume and water content of the stool	Lactulose, polyethylene glycol, sorbitol
Lubricants	Ease the passage of the stool by altering consistency	Liquid paraffin, seed oils
Stimulants	Act by irritating and increasing the motility of the gut	Senna, castor oil, cascara
Others	Serotonin (5-HT$_4$) agonist increases secretions and motility	Tegaserod

Further information

van der Spoel JI, Oudemans-van Straaten HM, Kuiper MA, et al. (2007) Laxation of critically ill patients with lactulose or polyethylene glycol: a two-centre randomized, double blind, placebo-controlled trial. *Crit Care Med* **35**, 2726–31.

Gastrointestinal dysfunction: gastric hypomotility and vomiting

Vomiting in the critically ill, although rare, is high risk as the patient may aspirate gastric contents, leading to significant complications, such as pneumonia. High gastric residual volumes can be an early indicator of hypomotility and need to be managed pro-actively.

Even patients with cuffed tracheal tubes are not completely protected from the risk of aspiration as it is still possible for gastric contents to be aspirated past the cuff.

Gastro-intestinal hypomotility

Multiple factors contribute to gastrointestinal hypomotility in the critically ill, many of these are difficult to manage, coming as a consequence of both critical illness itself and interventions needed to manage it (such as catecholamine infusions). The stomach itself is most sensitive to these factors and other parts of the GI tract, such as the small intestine may continue to function.

Management of gastrointestinal hypomotility
- Monitoring and early recognition (checking gastric residual volumes 2–4-hourly during instability).
- Continue low volume enteral feeding.
- Commence prokinetic agents (e.g. metoclopromide and erythromycin).
- Semi-recumbent positioning (head-up 35–45°).
- Post-pyloric feeding.

Vomiting

This is a high risk event that should be responded to immediately. Causes of vomiting are multiple, including ileus, bowel obstruction, drugs, chemical irritants, neurological events, e.g. ↑ intracranial pressure, enteritis, pancreatitis.

Management of vomiting
- Turn off enteral feed.
- If intubated, carry out endotracheal suction.
- If ↓ level of consciousness, or poor cough or gag reflex, carry out suctioning of mouth and pharynx.
- Administer anti-emetics as prescribed.
- Clean linen and wash as required.

If the patient is awake and aware, they will need privacy, support, and reassurance from the nurse, as well as the obvious receptacle and tissues. Mouthwash or water should be offered afterwards. Review the enteral feeding regime with medical staff.

Factors contributing to gastrointestinal hypomotility in the critically ill

- Cellular cytokines and kinases released locally during reperfusion injury.
- Cytokine actions on the enteric nervous system.
- Increased intracranial pressure.
- Release of endotoxin or corticotropin (a stress response agent).
- Effects of ischemia on motor function.
- Concomitant drug therapy, e.g. opiates, catecholamines.

Factors increasing the risk of aspiration of gastric contents

- ↓ level of consciousness.
- Diminished or absent cough or gag reflexes.
- Incompetent oesophageal sphincters.
- Delayed gastric emptying.
- Paralytic ileus.
- Displacement of enteral feeding tube (can be associated with vigorous coughing or retching).
- Presence of an enteral feeding tube.

Acute gastrointestinal haemorrhage

Clinically important gastrointestinal bleeding occurs in 2.8% of mechanically ventilated patients. The risk of bleeding is increased with renal failure and reduced by enteral nutrition. Causes vary from ulceration (30–50%) to inflammation (5–15%), varices (5–10%), Mallory-Weiss tears (15%) and tumours (1%).

Acute gastrointestinal bleeding manifestations

- **Haematemesis:** usually if the bleeding point is above the duodenojejunal junction.
- **Melaena:** ranging from virtually unaltered blood to black and tarry, depending on site, volume, and rate of bleeding, and thus time spent in the GI tract.

Management of gastrointestinal haemorrhage

GI bleeding may be the cause of the patient's admission to critical care or may occur while the patient is critically ill.

Initial assessment

- Ensure the airway is uncompromised/protected – if not, this must be dealt with first.
- Visual inspection of skin colour/mucosa, patient responsiveness, evidence of sympathetic activation such as sweating.
- Assess peripheral circulation using capillary refill time, level of limb cooling, etc.
- Assess haemodynamic status – heart rate, rhythm, blood pressure, CVP, cardiac output or index, stroke volume, etc.
- Assess oxygenation status – respiratory rate, peripheral oxygen saturation, ABGs.
- Assess metabolic status – pH, base deficit, lactate levels, degree of respiratory compensation (pCO_2).

Priorities of management

Fluid resuscitation: replacement and stabilization of blood loss. Volume replacement is essential and can maintain circulation even when haemoglobin (Hb) is reduced to levels of less than 5g/dl. Artificial colloids, e.g. gelatin or starch based colloids, should commence immediately with the addition of blood products when available and as needed to maintain Hb. between 7 and 10g/dl, and support coagulation.

- If Hb. is <5g/dl. with ongoing bleeding and no cross-matched blood is available, consider use of O negative blood.
- Inspired oxygen should be increased to >F_iO_2 0.6 until ABG results show pO_2 levels and then adjusted to maintain pO_2 > 12kPa.
- The patient will require enormous support and reassurance, as well as information about what is happening.
- Determine the cause of bleeding - endoscopic examination will be necessary to determine and, in some cases, treat the cause of bleeding.
- Commence a proton pump inhibitor intravenously.
- If bleeding continues surgery may be required.

Acute liver failure

Severe liver dysfunction occurs up to 3 months after an initial precipitating cause. The patient exhibits jaundice, encephalopathy, coagulopathy, and hypoglycaemia.

Classification of acute liver failure
- **Hyper acute liver failure:** encephalopathy seen within 7 days of onset of jaundice.
- **Acute liver failure:** encephalopathy seen within 8–28 days of onset of jaundice.
- **Sub-acute liver failure:** encephalopathy seen 29–84 days from onset of jaundice.
- Prognosis is very poor in all groups without liver transplantation.

Management of acute liver failure

Most treatment is supportive in nature, until the acute insult can resolve. Specialist liver transplant centres should be consulted when managing these patients.

Encephalopathy (see Table 15.5)
Thought to be due to breakdown products from ammonia produced by intestinal bacteria acting on dietary proteins. Management is aimed at limiting their absorption by the gut.
- Low protein (<40g/day) intake.
- Oral lactulose and magnesium sulphate enemas.
- Avoid sedation agents such as benzodiazepines.
- Monitor patient's mental state and reduce sensory overload by maintaining a quiet environment with minimal handling, quiet speech, and reassurance.
- Grade III and IV encephalopathy may require intubation, ventilation, and ICP monitoring.

Coagulopathy
Hepatic synthesis of fibrinogen, factor V, VII, IX and X is impaired resulting in prolonged prothrombin time and poor clotting. Management constitutes monitoring coagulation and preventing or avoiding bleeding risks.
- Avoid prolonged/excessive suctioning, intramuscular injections, vigorous mouth care.
- Maintain high level of awareness of bleeding risk.
- Prophylactic H_2 antagonists or PPIs.
- Vitamin K (10mg once daily for 2–3 days).
- Give fresh frozen plasma, whole blood, and platelets if spontaneous bleeding occurs or prior to invasive procedures to normalize clotting and maintain Hb.

Renal failure and hepato-renal syndrome

Hepato-renal syndrome is the development of renal dysfunction in patients with acute or chronic, severe liver disease in the absence of any other identifiable causes of renal pathology. It is thought to be related to decreased renal blood flow. It has a poor prognosis and prevention is best.

- Correct any precipitating cause (e.g. hypovolaemia).
- Avoid nephrotoxic drugs and high dose furosemide.
- If anuric renal failure occurs, the treatment of choice is continuous haemodiafiltration, rather than dialysis due to the impact the fluid shifts in dialysis can have on cerebral perfusion.

Precipitating causes of acute liver failure

- Alcohol.
- Drug overdose (commonly paracetamol).
- Viral hepatitis (A, B, C, E).
- Idiosyncratic drug reactions.
- Ingestion of toxins.

Table 15.5 Grades of encephalopathy

0	Normal awareness
I	Mood change, slow mentation, disturbed sleep, usually alert, and lucid
II	Drowsiness, inappropriate behaviour, arousable, and conversant
III	Marked confusion and disorientation, agitation, stuporose, but rousable
IV	Unrousable to minimal stimuli or no response to noxious stimuli; decerebrate or decorticate

Cerebral oedema is common in Grade III and IV encephalopathy. ICP monitoring facilitates prompt recognition and treatment.

Prognosis is worse as the grade of encephalopathy increases.

Pancreatitis I

This is an acute condition, which is mild and self-limiting in 80% of cases, but can result in multiple organ dysfunction and death in 20%. This is the group that will require critical care. It occurs in 1 in 10 000 people commonly associated with alcohol abuse or gallbladder disease (75% of cases). Pancreatitis occurs as a result of activation of pancreatic enzymes within the pancreas, rather than in the duodenum (see 📖 Overview of physiology II, p. 354). This causes autodigestion of tissue and an acute inflammatory response. Irritant factors and obstruction of the ductules that trap enzymes within the pancreas are thought to be the mechanism of pathology.

Diagnosis can be difficult, involving a combination of investigations, CT scans, and exclusion of other causes of the signs and symptoms.

Complications, such as pseudocysts (walled-off collection of pancreatic enzymes) and biliary obstruction from the swollen head of pancreas can occur.

The patient suffers severe pain, nausea, and vomiting, and will require careful pain management, and psychological support as in severe cases symptoms continue for prolonged periods, and there is no definitive treatment.

Management

Compromised respiratory function

- Respiratory complications occur in 30–50% of patients and up to 70% are hypoxaemic. ARDS, pleural effusions, and atelectasis may all contribute. Patients should be given oxygen therapy, CPAP, and IPPV to maintain oxygenation as required.

Correction of hypovoloemia and fluid volume imbalances

Auto-digestion releases vasoactive substances resulting in loss of fluid into the extravascular and particularly the peritoneal space. Splanchnic vascular constriction will further damage the pancreas by reducing perfusion:

- Maintain intravascular volume with colloid or crystalloid.
- Volume load against CVP or stroke volume with the aim of preserving organ perfusion and renal function with a urine output > 0.5ml/kg/h.

Haemodynamic disturbances

Hypotension and arrhythmias occur related to the acute inflammatory process, as well as hypovolaemia, hypocalcaemia, hypokalaemia, and possible myocardial depressant factors.

- Continuous monitoring of BP and ECG.
- Inotropes or vasoconstrictors may be needed.

Signs and symptoms of acute pancreatitis

- Acute epigastric and peri-umbilical pain.
- Nausea and vomiting.
- Abdominal distension associated with a small bowel ileus or pseudo-cyst in severe disease.
- Low grade pyrexia, occasionally hypothermia.
- Shock: ↑pulse, ↓ BP, etc.
- Retroperitoneal haemorrhage showing as either:
  - Grey–Turner sign – grey discoloration (bruising) over the flanks; or
  - Cullen's sign – bruising in and round the umbilicus.

Associated abnormal laboratory data (not always present)

- Serum amylase is high (usually > 1000IU/l).
- Serum lipase is high in 75% of cases.
- Total calcium levels are decreased (this may be due to hypoalbuminaemia or extravascular precipitation).
- Ionized calcium levels may also decrease due to intraperitoneal combination with free fatty acids.
- Hyperglycaemia is common (this is related to either hyperglucagonaemia or, more commonly, insulin deficiency).
- Hyperbilirubinaemia.
- Raised transaminase and alkaline phosphatase levels.
- Hypoalbuminaemia.

Signs of hypocalcaemia

- **Chvostek's sign:** twitching of the lip and cheek in response to tapping of the side of the face over the facial nerve in the parotid gland.
- **Trouseau's sign:** carpopedal spasm with wrist and metacarpophalangeal joints flexed, and interphalangeal joints extended when a blood pressure cuff. Placed on the same arm is inflated to just above systolic pressure (the response should occur within 2 min).

Pancreatitis II

Pain

This is caused by extravasation of inflammatory exudate and enzymes into the retroperitoneum and distension of the pancreatic ducts.

- Analgesia is essential – pethidine is first choice and morphine should be avoided (increased sphincter of Oddi spasm).
- Other methods of pain relief, such as warmth, positioning, and relaxation, may also help.
- Continuous nasogastric aspiration and nil by mouth will limit pancreatic stimulus to release enzymes.

Correction of electrolyte imbalances

Imbalance in calcium, magnesium, phosphate, and potassium occur due to GI fluid losses (interstitial space, nasogastric drainage, vomiting, diarrhoea). Intraperitoneal saponification can also reduce calcium levels. Levels should be monitored and corrected as required.

Hyperglycaemia

This can occur secondary to hyperglucagonaemia and insulin deficiency.

- Requires frequent monitoring of blood glucose.
- Insulin infusion titrated to blood glucose levels should be used.

Nutrition

Food in the stomach will have a stimulant effect on enzyme production in the pancreas. However, jejunal feeding is now successfully used and has been shown to be beneficial even in severe pancreatitis. Elemental feeds may also be less stimulant. If jejunal feeding tube placement in unsuccessful, then parenteral nutrition can be instituted. Give jejunal feeding with standard or semi-elemental feed

Secondary infection

Can occur with an increased risk of mortality. No benefit has been shown for use of prophylactic antibiotics and preventive measures, such as those to reduce VAP, are essential.

Drainage of abscesses/necrosis/pseudocysts

Radiologically-guided drainage of abscesses or pseudocysts may be necessary, and very occasionally surgery may be indicated, although this remains controversial.

Nutrition: assessment

Malnutrition leads to increased morbidity and mortality in the critically ill patient. Increased susceptibility to infection, poor wound healing, and delayed recovery are associated with poor nutrition in the critically ill. Early delivery of enteral nutrition has benefits in trauma, head injury, and surgical patients.

Assessment of malnutrition

Many of the usual methods of assessing nutritional state are not applicable to the critically ill patient (see Table 15.6). Use of baseline weights can be a starting point, but ongoing assessment of nutritional status is complex and often difficult. Widespread oedema will disguise loss of muscle mass, which will only become evident once improvement occurs and the fluid is re-distributed.

Assessment of the correct mode of nutrition should start with assessment of ability to take oral diet, gut function, and impact on disease state.

Modes of nutritional delivery

- Oral diet should be the first choice if the patient can swallow adequately, has a functioning gut and can consume sufficient nutrition to meet their needs.
- Enteral nutrition should be used if the gut is functioning, but the patient is unable to swallow.
- Parenteral nutrition should be used if the gut is not functioning.

Assessment of gut function

Bowel sounds

Absence of bowel sounds is not an absolute indicator of dysfunction unless associated with other markers, such as pain, distension, and vomiting. Listen for up to 2min to confirm absence of bowel sounds.

High volumes of nasogastric aspirate (gastric residual volume)

There is no definitive level to indicate dysfunction, but repeated aspirates of >200ml after a 4h period should limit enteral feed increases in delivery volume and trigger the use of prokinetics (drugs that increase gastric motility and emptying). Ongoing high levels of aspirate following these measures or association with other markers may indicate the need for parenteral nutrition.

Vomiting/regurgitation of feed

- Risk of aspiration is high and endotracheal intubation is not totally protective, despite a fully inflated tube cuff. The patient should be nursed 30–45° to the horizontal to reduce the risk of regurgitation. Enteral feeding should be stopped and the patient assessed for other signs of intolerance.
- If there is no evidence of an abdominal disorder (pain, abdominal distension) then prokinetics, such as metoclopramide, may be given and feed re-started cautiously at a low rate.

Diarrhoea

Persistent diarrhoea may be a marker of ongoing gut dysfunction and should be managed as described in 📖 Gastrointestinal dysfunction: diarrhoea, p. 360.

Table 15.6 Assessment of malnutrition

Method of assessment	Applicable in critical care
Daily weight	Affected by fluid retention and oedema, no indication of components of weight gain/loss
Mid-arm muscle circumference	Affected by oedema, slow to change
Triceps skin-fold thickness	Affected by oedema, slow to change
Hand-grip dynamometry	Affected by patient compliance/awareness
Nitrogen balance	Affected by renal dysfunction, large body pool of nitrogen
Albumin levels	Commonly low in the critically ill due to: (i) Fluid shifts producing comparative dilution (ii) Movement of proteins into extravascular spaces through leaky capillary membranes (iii) Dilution by infusion of artificial colloids (iv) Decreased liver production due to liver dysfunction associated with the disease state
Serum transferrin	Raised in iron deficiency and frequently under-estimates nutritional status in the critically ill
Indirect calorimetry	Allows day-to-day assessment of energy requirements, but does not give a full view of nutritional state

Nutrition: enteral

In the acute phase of critical illness, nutrition should provide sufficient calories and protein to maintain body weight and reduce nitrogen loss. The level of catabolism associated with the stressed state of critical illness does not allow the replenishment of body stores until the recovery phase.

Care of the enterally fed patient

Safe delivery of enteral feed requires monitoring of tube placement and integrity, checking for tolerance of feed, and ensuring the required volumes are delivered.

Monitoring tube placement

Enteral feeding tubes can migrate into the oesophagus, pharynx, and trachea/bronchi. Any misplacement will result in the delivery of feed into the lungs. The most effective bedside method of checking tube placement is to test the pH of fluid aspirated from the tube. Gastric contents should have a pH of <4, although this is affected by proton pump inhibitors (e.g. omeprazole) and H_2 antagonist drugs (e.g. ranitidine). If there is any doubt about the position of the tube a CXR should be carried out. Checks of tube placement should be carried out routinely (during checking of feed tolerance), following any vigorous retching or coughing, and if feed is found in the mouth or bronchial secretions.

Preventing tube obstruction

Internal diameters in fine bore feeding tubes are very small and easily occluded. Administration of crushed tablets down the tube should be avoided. Soluble or linctus forms of the drug should be requested instead. Flushing with 20ml of water following any drug delivery (solutions and linctus) or following aspiration of feed will reduce encrusting.

Checking for tolerance of feed

Gastric residual volumes should be checked 4-hourly when feeding is first commenced and then 8-hourly once the feed has been running without large amounts of residual volumes. This may differ according to unit protocols.

Feed should be stopped briefly (the length of time depends on local protocol) and then gastric contents aspirated using a 50ml syringe. There is no evidence to suggest contents should be discarded or returned, and this will depend on unit protocol.

Gastric residuals of less than 200ml are acceptable and feeding should continue. Feeding rates should be adjusted to cover for any stoppage time prior to aspiration.

Repeated (>2) residual volumes of > 200ml, or if accompanied by abdominal distension or pain indicate a problem with tolerance of feed. Feed should be stopped/reduced and use of prokinetic drugs considered if there are no acute signs of abdominal dysfunction. Jejunal feeding should be considered if this continues in spite of prokinetics.

Advantages of enteral nutrition

- Nearer normal physiologically, using GI route for absorption and stimulating normal enzyme/hormone involvement.
- Preservation of gut mucosal integrity.
- Cheaper than parenteral nutrition.
- No central venous access thus reducing risks of insertion, infection, etc.
- May modify the immune response to stress if administered in the early stages following trauma.

Disadvantages of enteral nutrition

- May be associated with increased volumes of diarrhoea.
- Difficulty ensuring patients receive/tolerate the volume of feed they require to meet energy and other needs.
- Requires GI tract function.
- May be associated with increased VAP risk.

Table 15.7 Prokinetic agents

Prokinetic agents	Dose	Action
Metoclopromide (dopamine$_2$ receptor antagonist)	10mg NG or IV TDS	Acts centrally to increase GI motility
Erythromycin (motilin receptor agonist)	80–250mg IV or NG QDS	Acts locally to increase gastric migratory complexes and motility

Nutrition: enteral feeding complications

Many of the complications associated with enteral feeding can be avoided by using the correct formula (see 📖 Nutrition: feeds and daily requirements, p. 382) and being meticulous in management of the tube itself.

Mechanical (tube-related)

- **Knotting of the tube** can occur with increased curling in stomach. Endoscopic or even surgical removal may be necessary.
- **Clogging or blockage** can occur due to fragments of inadequately crushed tablets, adherence of feed residue, and incompatibilities between feed and medication given (e.g. phenytoin). Attempts should be made to flush the tube with 20ml water, some authorities advocate coca-cola, but there is no evidence for this. A solution of sodium bicarbonate may help for alkaline drugs, such as ranitidine. Prevention is the best approach.
- **Incorrect placement** (usually in the bronchial tree). See 📖 Nutrition: enteral, p. 376.
- **Nasopharyngeal erosions and discomfort:** the patient's nostrils should be checked for signs of pressure externally. The tube should not be left in for longer than the recommended time.
- **Sinusitis and otitis:** the tube should be changed at recommended intervals (see 📖 Nutrition: enteral feeding tube types, p. 380). Aseptic technique should be used for insertion.
- **Oesophageal reflux and oesophagitis:** tube placement should be checked regularly and the patient nursed at 45°
- **Tracheo-oesophageal fistula:** the tube should be changed at recommended intervals (see 📖 Nutrition: enteral feeding tube types, p. 380). Never use force in placing the tube. Consideration should be given to placing a PEG if the tube is likely to remain in for longer than 12 weeks.

Nausea and vomiting

This can be caused by gastric intolerance, high infusion rates, fat or lactose intolerance, hyperosmolality. Stop the feed and aspirate the stomach. Commence prokinetic agents if there are no other signs of abdominal dysfunction.

Aspiration

See 📖 Nutrition: enteral, p. 376.

Diarrhoea

See 📖 Gastrointestinal dysfunction: diarrhoea, p. 360.

Abdominal distension/delayed gastric emptying

This can be due to critical illness itself (see 📖 Immune function and the gastrointestinal tract, p. 358), and also feed formula (associated with high density, high lipid content), medication (e.g. opiates), ileus, gastric atony, medical conditions, such as pancreatitis, diabetes, malnutrition, or post-vagotomy. Stop the feed and review/treat potential causes.

Cramping
High fat content formulae and malnutrition-related malabsorption have been associated with cramping. Reducing the feed rate may help. Occasionally buscopan can be given for cramping.

Constipation
This is more common than previously thought and can be caused by opiate infusions, previous laxative abuse, long-term feeding regimens (particularly low-fibre formulae). See 📖 Gastrointestinal dysfunction: constipation p. 362.

Hyperglycaemia
This is associated with sepsis, age, renal insufficiency, diabetes, steroid therapy, and high caloric density formulae. Regular blood glucose monitoring is essential when commencing feed.

Hypercapnia
Higher than required levels of carbohydrate in feeds can produce large amounts of CO_2 that require increased minute volumes and respiratory rate in order to be excreted. This may precipitate ventilatory failure in the patient with compromised respiratory function or in the weaning patient. Accurate calculation of the patients nutritional requirements are essential

Electrolyte and trace element abnormality
Sodium, potassium, phosphate and magnesium abnormalities can be associated with enteral feeding. Monitoring of blood levels on a daily basis should be carried out when commencing enteral nutrition.

Nutrition: enteral feeding tube types

Nasogastric feeding is indicated when swallowing is compromised or there is upper GI obstruction. Gastric function is required.

Nasojejunal feeding is indicated when gastric function is compromised.

Wide-bore nasogastric tubes

Made from polyvinyl chloride (PVC) size 12–16 Fr. Length 90–110cm. Suitable for short-term use only, they should be replaced with a fine-bore feeding tube and not left in place for more than 7–10 days. PVC will degrade with continued contact with gastric acid.

Fine-bore nasogastric tube

- Available in a range of materials and sizes 8–10 Fr. PVC tubes should not be used for longer than 14 days.
- Polyurethane tubes can be left in place for up to 6 weeks and are the material of choice for enteral feeding.

Nasojejunal tube

Available in a range of materials and sizes 6–12 Fr. Length should be 130 cm or more.

Percutaneous gastrostomy tube (PEG)

Placed either surgically or percutaneously via endoscopy. Size 14–18 Fr. They are suitable for long-term feeding. Materials are either polyurethane or silicone.

Percutaneous jejunostomy tube (PEJ)

Placed either surgically or endoscopically. It is usually placed in the proximal jejunum so that elemental feeds are unnecessary.

Placement of all enteral tubes should be documented with time, date, and length of insertion. Length of insertion should be re-checked for nasogastric and nasojejunal tubes every time aspiration occurs, and a high level of awareness of potential displacement should be maintained.

Nutrition: feeds and daily requirements

Enteral feeding

- Enteral feed is an iso-osmolar solution containing whole protein, carbohydrate, and a combination of triglycerides. Standard feed delivers 1 cal/ml, although special formulations are available which deliver 1.5 cal/ml.
- Most feeds no longer contain lactose.
- Feeds are designed to deliver the correct nutritional requirements within a suitable overall volume over a 24h period.
- For example, 1800ml of standard enteral feed will deliver 1800kcal, 72g protein, and 72g fat per day. In addition, daily multivitamin, trace element and electrolyte requirements will also be met.
- Special feeds are available such as high fibre, low sodium, 50:50 fat to carbohydrate, low protein, and immune-enhanced (containing omega 3 fatty acids, nucleotides, arginine, and/or glutamine).

Parenteral feeding

Parenteral feeding solution is provided as pre-mixed bags prepared in sterile conditions. Separate component delivery is no longer considered good practice. Constituents are either a standard formula or can be tailored to individual need. Volume of the bags are usually 2000–2400ml over 24hr. Occasionally, higher volume regimens, up to 3000ml, are used. There are specific multivitamin, trace element, and electrolyte daily requirements.

Re-feeding syndrome

Is seen when nutrition is first started following a prolonged period of semi-starvation. There is rapid uptake of glucose, potassium, phosphate, and magnesium into cells and the serum concentration falls dramatically. This is particularly evident in phosphate due to poor prior intake of phosphate, increased glucose phosphorylation and augmented intracellular transport of phosphates once feeding is restarted. Plasma phosphate levels below 0.3–0.5mmol/l can cause haemolysis, rhabdomyolysis, respiratory failure, and hamper weaning attempts. This may persist for several days after adequate replacement. Other effects include arrhythmias, decreased myocardial contractility, 2,3-DPG deficiency, seizures, diminished tissue sensitivity to insulin, abnormal calcium and magnesium metabolism, decreased sensitivity to vasoactive drugs, generalized tissue hypoxia, and ATP deficiency.

Feeding should be started slowly in this case and serum electrolytes monitored on a daily basis (Table 15.9).

Table 15.8 Daily nutrient requirements

Nutrient	Amount per day	Influencing factors
Protein (nitrogen)	0.7–1.0g/kg/day (0.15–0.3g/kg/day)	Hypermetabolism can increase protein requirements to 1.5–2.0g/kg/day
Carbohydrate	Need will depend on the patient's energy requirements, two-thirds of which are usually provided by carbohydrate, and one-third by fat A useful quick estimate of requirements is: Male – 25–30kcal/kg/day Female – 20–25kcal/kg/day	Patients with respiratory insufficiency or weaning after long-term ventilation may not handle the amount of carbon dioxide produced when intake outstrips requirement. Ratios of fat to carbohydrate should change to 50:50
Fat	Only necessary in very small amounts to prevent fatty acid deficiency. Usually, amount delivered contributes to providing energy (see above) It forms between one-third and one-half of total calories required A useful quick estimate of requirements is 0.8–1.0g/kg/day	Tolerance of intravenous fat can be limited (see parenteral nutrition complications) and the amount delivered may need to be adjusted if this is the case.

This table represents a guide and each patient should be assessed individually.

Table 15.9 Daily electrolyte requirements

Typical daily requirement	Additional factors
Sodium 70–100 mmol/day	More may be needed with loop diuretic therapy or increased gastro-intestinal losses such as diarrhoea or fistulae, etc.
	Less may be needed in oedema and hypernatraemia
Potassium 70–100mmol/day	More may be needed during early repletion, post-obstructive diuresis, loop diuretic therapy and increased GI losses
	Less may be required in renal failure
Magnesium 7.5–10mmol/day	As above
Calcium 5–10mmol/day	
Phosphate 20–30mmol/day	More may be needed in early nutritional repletion when there may be dramatic falls in serum phosphate (see re-feeding syndrome)
	Less may be required in renal failure

Table 15.10 Recommended daily requirement

	Recommended daily requirement		Effects of deficiency
	Enteral (μmol/l)	Parenteral (μmol/l)	
Zinc	110–145	145	Impaired cellular immunity, poor wound healing, diarrhoea
Chromium	0.5–1.0	0.2-0.4	Insulin-resistant glucose intolerance, elevated serum lipids
Copper	16–20	20	Hypochromic microcytic anaemia, neutropenia
Iodine	1–1.2	1.0	
Selenium	0.8–0.9	0.25-0.5	Cardiomyopathy
Molybdenum	0.5–4.0	0.2–1.2	
Manganese	30–60	5–10	CNS dysfunction
Fluoride	95–150	50	

Table 15.11 Daily vitamin requirements

Vitamin	Recommended daily requirements	
	Enteral nutrition	Parenteral nutrition
A (retinol) 5000 (µg)	600–1200	800–2500
B1 (thiamine) (mg)	0.8–1.1	3–20
B2 (riboflavin) (mg)	1.1–1.3	3–8
Niacin (mg)	2–18	40
B6 (pyridoxine) (mg)	1.2–2.0	4.0–6.0
B12 (cyanocobalamine) (µg)	1.5–3.0	5–15
C (ascorbic acid) (mg)	40–60	100
D (cholecalciferol) (µg)	5	5
E (δ and α tocopherol) (mg)	10	10
Folic acid (µg)	200–400	200–400
K (phytomenadione) (µg/kg)	1	0.03–1.5
Pantothenic acid (mg)	3–7	10–20
Biotin (µg)	10–200	60

Parenteral nutrition: care of the patient

- Parenteral nutrition in the critically ill generally requires central venous access although some solutions (<800 osmol) can be delivered via peripheral venous routes.
- Triple or quadruple lumen central venous catheters can be used for parenteral nutrition delivery providing that one lumen is dedicated solely to this. Care of the catheter must be meticulous due to the increased risk of infection.
- Problems with parenteral nutrition can be associated with catheter insertion, the catheter itself or metabolic disturbance.
- Many of the potentially serious complications associated with parenteral feeding can be avoided or controlled by rigorous monitoring and observation of the patient. A high index of suspicion for complications should also be maintained.

Insertion of central venous catheter

Pneumothorax

This is a recognized complication, occurring in 1.5% of cases, but more likely with inexperienced operators, left-sided insertion, obesity, chest deformity, CPAP, and IPPV. Use of ultrasound-guided insertion has reduced this.

Arterial puncture

Accidental puncture of the carotid artery often only requires digital pressure to control it. Subclavian artery puncture can cause significant bleeding especially in patients with coagulation abnormalities, including platelet dysfunction. Accidental injury to the thoracic duct may produce chylothorax and, although rare, can occur with a left-sided approach.

Catheter misplacement

Usually misdirection into the neck from the subclavian approach, more common with right-sided approaches due to the anatomy. Can also pass down the subclavian vein from a jugular approach, perforate a vessel and place the catheter into the neck tissue, mediastinum, or pericardium. This may result in a large haematoma, upper airway obstruction, hydro- or haemopneumothorax, or pericardial tamponade.

The presence of a central venous catheter

Infection

Bacterial and fungal infections occur in between 3 and 7% of patients. The infecting organism is commonly *Staphylococcus aureus* (a skin commensal). Most infections are thought to be due to poor insertion technique or failure to observe infection control protocols (see ☐ Preventing complications: hospital acquired infection, p. 80).

Metabolic

Hyperglycaemia

Causes include persistent gluconeogenesis, blunted insulin response, decreased sensitivity to insulin, impaired peripheral utilization of glucose or phosphate, and chromium deficiency. Late development in a stable patient may signal a new infection or complication.

Hypoglycaemia

Sudden discontinuation of feed may induce hypoglycaemia, particularly if the patient is receiving insulin concurrently. Insulin should be discontinued or reduced prior to stopping the feed and, if this is not possible, 10–20% glucose may be commenced. Blood glucose should be frequently monitored.

Hyperlipidaemia

Lipid clearance can be impaired in liver disease. Rapid infusion of lipid may also result in transient hyperlipidaemia.

Hepatic dysfunction

Abnormal liver function tests (LFTs) and fatty infiltration of the liver can develop in carbohydrate-based parenteral nutrition. It is treated by reducing the amount of calories or increasing the proportion of fat.

Acid-base disturbances

Hyperchloraemia can develop from amino acid metabolism, but the resulting acidosis is usually mild and most amino acid preparations contain acetate as a buffer. Metabolic alkalosis can be seen with diuretic use, continuous nasogastric drainage or corticosteroid therapy if concomitant replacement of sodium, potassium, and/or chloride ions is inadequate.

Electrolyte imbalance

Generally, sodium, potassium, chloride, and bicarbonate are monitored and corrected before problems occur. However, significant body deficiencies may not be reflected by plasma levels due to the effect of pH and serum albumin levels, or hormonal influences, such as aldosterone or ADH, which are often altered in the critically ill. Occasionally, magnesium, calcium, and phosphate may become imbalanced.

Other complications associated with parenteral feeding are rare, but include:

- Precipitation of respiratory failure and failure of weaning due to excessive carbohydrate administration (see earlier).
- Hyperosmolar states with an excessive osmotic diuresis.
- Abnormal platelet function and hypercoagulability states.
- Anaemia after prolonged use of iv lipids.

Systemic inflammatory response syndrome, sepsis, and multiple organ dysfunction

Introduction and definitions

In spite of a huge amount of research aimed at understanding the pathogenesis of SIRS and sepsis, and translating this into improved clinical management, mortality remains high, with up to 50% of patients still dying from severe sepsis and septic shock.

The systematic inflammatory response syndrome (SIRS) is a non-specific generalized inflammatory response of the body to an extrinsic insult, of which infection is one of many possible triggers.

The lack of clinically-specific definitions of the condition, the varying causes and the numerous co-morbidities (e.g. cancer, immunosuppression, COPD) has made early identification and management difficult.

International guidelines have been produced by a consensus conference based on best evidence and these will be outlined.

Definitions

- **Infection:** inflammatory response to the presence of micro-organisms or the invasion of normally sterile host tissue by those organisms.
- **Bacteraemia:** the presence of viable bacteria in the blood.
- **Sepsis:** systemic inflammatory response with an infective cause.
- **Severe sepsis:** sepsis complicated by organ dysfunction or hypoperfusion.
- **Septic shock**: sepsis-induced hypotension (BP < 90mmHg or reduced by 40mmHg from baseline without another cause), which is unresponsive to fluid resuscitation with manifestations of hypoperfusion, such as oliguria, altered mental state, etc.
- **Multi-organ dysfunction syndrome**: presence of altered organ function in an acutely ill patient, such that homeostasis cannot be maintained without intervention.
- **Apoptosis:** genetically programmed cell death.
- **Anergy:** a general loss of immune responsiveness indicating deficient T cell function.
- **Septicaemia:** an imprecise term used in a number of different ways to describe:
  - the presence of micro-organisms or their toxins in the blood;
  - sepsis syndrome.

Systemic inflammatory response syndrome (SIRS)

The systemic inflammatory response to a variety of severe clinical insults is manifested by two or more of the following conditions:
- Temperature >38° or <36°C.
- Heart rate >90beats/min.
- Respiratory rate >20breaths/min or hyperventilation with a P_aCO_2 <4.3kPa (32mmHg).
- WBC >12 000 or <4000cells/mm^3, or >10% immature forms.

Triggers of SIRS

- Infection.
- Trauma.
- Pancreatitis.
- Major burns.
- Major surgery without adequate organ perfusion.
- Haemorrhage/major blood-transfusion.
- Ischaemic tissue.
- Periods of inadequate perfusion followed by reperfusion.
- Miscellaneous, e.g. drug-related, near-drowning, pulmonary embolus etc.

Overview of physiology

Although the prevailing view of the physiology of SIRS is of an overwhelming and inappropriately exaggerated immune response to a trigger, more recent research has shown that there may be a variety of immunological responses. These range from anti-inflammatory to hyper-inflammatory. When immunosuppression occurs as an anti-inflammatory response, there may be increased susceptibility to further infection. Stimulation of the inflammatory response will cause release and activation of a complex range of inflammatory mediators from white cells, concomitant activation of inflammatory pathways, and endothelial damage. These result in major alterations to fluid and blood flow redistribution, vasodilatation, microvascular obstruction, altered mitochondrial function, and increased/altered metabolic demand. The consequences of this may be organ dysfunction, varying from 'mild' to severe, and affecting one or more organs.

White cell activation (macrophages, neutrophils, monocytes, lymphocytes)

The primary function of white cells is surveillance and phagocytosis of pathogens. Macrophage-presented pathogens stimulate lymphocytes to form sensitized cells and pathogen-specific antibodies. Phagocytosis by release of proteases and oxygen-derived free radicals (highly reactive oxygen-based molecules that are highly destructive) occurs causing local tissue damage.

Effects of inflammatory pathway activation

- **Complement pathways:** complement is an initiating and enhancing pathway activated by antigen/antibody complexes or specific micro-organisms. If regulated and localized, it is protective, but if systemic activation occurs there will be overwhelming vasodilatation, increased capillary permeability and phagocytic activation.
- **Coagulation and fibrinolysis:** systemic disruption of the haemostatic balance between coagulation and fibrinolysis will lead to coagulopathy, and ultimately disseminated intravascular coagulation (DIC). This can cause vascular obstruction, with potential for tissue ischaemia, and organ damage and bleeding from depletion of clotting factors and platelets
- **Kallikrein/kinin:** kallikrein/kinin cascades are initiated at the same time as the coagulation cascade in SIRS and sepsis through factor XII. This appears to enhance the inflammatory response and the fibrinolytic cascade. Bradykinin is a potent mediator produced by the cascade that causes vasodilatation and increased capillary permeability, as well as potentiating the complement pathway.

Effects of endothelial damage

Widespread endothelial damage causes release of vasoactive and pro-coagulant substances (e.g. thromboxanes, nitric-oxide, and prostaglandins). Platelets are activated, and stick to each other and the exposed sub-endothelial surface. This potentiates coagulation and increases capillary permeability with the resulting reduction in intravascular fluid volume. This is sometimes known as 'third-spacing' of fluid.

Non-specific physiological alterations in sepsis and SIRS

- **Cellular**: inhibition of mitochondrial processing of oxygen.
- **Vascular**: systemic vasodilation, increased microvascular permeability, endothelial damage, microvascular obstruction, selective vaso-constriction, and shunting (blood flow past poorly ventilated alveoli reducing oxygenation).
- **Systemic**: hypermetabolism, hyperglycaemia and insulin resistance, protein catabolism and gluconeogenesis, fatty acid mobilization and increased oxidation, increased lactate production.

Disseminated intravascular coagulation (DIC)

DIC is a systemic activation of clotting cascades, producing widespread microvascular clots that rapidly utilize available clotting factors, depleting essential components in the clotting cascade, such as platelets, preventing necessary clotting, and preventing limitation of haemorrhage from any exposed skin surface or micro-trauma.

Further information

Hotchkiss RS, Karl IE. (2003) Medical progress: the pathophysiology and treatment of sepsis. *N Engl J Med* **348**, 138–50.
Levy B, Fink M, Marshall J, et al. for the International Sepsis Definitions Conference (2003) SCCM/ESICM/ACCP/ATS/SIS International Sepsis Definitions Conference. *Crit Care Med* **31**, 1250–6.

Organ manifestations of SIRS/sepsis I

Respiratory: acute lung injury/acute respiratory distress syndrome

Acute lung Injury (ALI)

- Diffuse acute pulmonary infiltrates seen on CXR associated with decreased pulmonary compliance.
- P_aO_2:F_iO_2 ratio <300mmHg (40KPa).
- PAOP of <18mmHg (i.e. non-cardiogenic origin for pulmonary changes).
- Precipitating factor.

Acute respiratory distress syndrome (ARDS)

ARDS is defined as all of the above, but P_aO_2:F_iO_2 ratio is <200mmHg (26.7kPa). There is usually evidence of respiratory failure.

Pathogenesis of ARDS

Three phases have been identified:
- Inflammatory or exudative.
- Proliferative.
- Fibrotic.

However, these phases are not distinct and commonly overlap (see Table 16.1).

Patient assessment

The patient is commonly agitated and distressed, pale and sweaty with increased work of breathing, altered mental state (confusion/drowsiness), dyspnoeic, and tachypnoeic.

Lung fields

Auscultation of the chest may detect either isolated or generalized crackles or wheezes, or may have no added sounds.

Chest X-ray

The typical early picture is non-specific with clear lungs or scant infiltrates. There may be unilateral lobar consolidation or diffuse lung involvement, depending on precipitating factors. Later in the disease process, interstitial oedema will be evident, and the picture is one of diffuse lung infiltrates, sometimes called 'white-out'.

Pulse oximetry

Hypoxaemia is common from early stages of the disease with S_pO_2 of <90% on air. Initially, this will improve with additional inspired oxygen, but requirements may continue to rise making CPAP and/or IPPV necessary.

Pulmonary secretions

These are initially minimal, loose, and white. As the disease progresses, they become thicker and more profuse, often due to secondary infection. Specimens should be sent for microbiological culture.

Arterial blood gases
In the early stages, a low P_aO_2 is seen with a normal or low (from hyperventilation) P_aCO_2 and a normal or moderately raised pH.

As the patient tires, P_aCO_2 may rise, and pH may fall due to a mixed respiratory and metabolic acidosis.

Pulmonary function
Pulmonary compliance is reduced, resulting in increased airway pressures, so volume and pressure should be controlled in the ventilated patient. The ARDS-net study suggests tidal volumes of 6–8ml/kg and plateau pressure <30cmH$_2$O should be achieved to avoid barotraumas.

Table 16.1 Pathogenesis of ARDS and its effect on the patient

Phases of pathogenesis of ARDS	Pathophysiology	Dysfunction	Patient effect
Inflammatory phase	Disruption of alveolar epithelium and endothelial damage, mediator release. Increased capillary permeability, neutrophil and platelet aggregation, pulmonary vasoconstriction	Altered microcirculatory flow and V/Q mismatch. Movement of fluid into the interstitium (space between cells). Atelectasis and decreased lung compliance	Hypoxaemia, dyspnoea, tachypnoea, tachycardia and agitation
Proliferative phase	Damage to the parenchyma from mediators and macrophage action	Fibrotic tissue reduces alveolar elasticity decreasing lung compliance. Progressive alveolar collapse and further shunting result in increasing hypoxaemia	Increased work of breathing, decreased tidal volumes, and carbon dioxide retention
Fibrotic phase	Increasing fibrotic tissue replace alveolar epithelial tissue and deranged vasculature	Alveolar obliteration, and interstitial thickening decrease gas exchange. Fibrosis and scarring further reduce lung compliance	Poor gas exchange contributes to hypoxaemia. Recovery of lung function takes up to 12 months and in some cases poor function will persist

Organ manifestations of SIRS/sepsis II

Cardiovascular

Cardiovascular dysfunction in MODS is related to the loss of peripheral vaso-autoregulation and hypoxaemia. This is often confounded by a myocardial depressant effect.

Reduced arterial and venous tone results in reduced pre- and afterload. This is related to high levels of nitric oxide (NO) produced from increased expression of the inducible form of NO synthase. Nitric oxide is a potent vasodilating mediator resulting in relaxation of arterial and venous tone and profound vasodilatation. Tissue hypoxia increases cardiac output by increasing heart rate and contractility, and a reduced afterload increases the capacity of the heart to respond. This results in the classic 'hyperdynamic' circulation with warm peripheries, low blood pressure, and a bounding pulse or dynamic arterial waveform.

Depression of myocardial function can occur even after correction of hypoxia, acidosis, and electrolyte disturbance suggesting that components of the inflammatory response itself may have a depressant effect on myocardial contractility. This is seen as a reduced ventricular ejection fraction and biventricular dilatation.

Gastrointestinal and hepatic

- **Splanchnic vasoconstriction:** in response to decreased blood pressure reduces gastrointestinal perfusion.
- **Stomach:** disruption of the mucosal barrier occurs with ischaemia leading to increased risk of ulceration and reduction in normal gastric motility. Poor tolerance of enteral nutrition is also likely. Motor function may also be disrupted leading to ileus.
- **Small intestine and colon:** loss of gut mucosal integrity may lead to bacterial translocation from the intestinal lumen to the portal circulation.
- **Pancreas and gall bladder**: pancreatitis or alcalculous cholecystitis.
- **Hepatic:** the impact manifests later in the disease, although the mechanism is not fully understood. Effects are wide-ranging with prolonged clotting, deranged carbohydrate, protein, and lipid metabolism, impaired detoxification processes, and reduced protein synthesis. Accumulation of drugs metabolized by the liver, such as benzodiazepines, coagulopathy, and bleeding occur.

Renal

Dysfunction is caused by either pre-renal failure from low blood pressure decreasing renal perfusion or as a direct effect of inflammatory mediators. Oliguria with rising blood urea and creatinine, and a reduction in glomerular filtration rate (GFR) are early indicators of dysfunction.

Haematological

Disseminated intravascular coagulopathy occurs to some degree in up to 80% of sepsis patients. In severe cases, it will be seen as bleeding from line sites, and wounds, gums, and mucous membranes with petechiae, purpura and bruising of the skin.

Principles of management of sepsis

Management for the best possible outcomes is based on a combination of the right preventive and supportive actions, as well as the right treatment.

Details of the right treatment interventions are based on the consensus guidelines of the Surviving Sepsis Initiative (2008), which are evidence-based.

- Early goal-directed resuscitation of the septic patient during the first 6h after onset of the condition. This has a mortality reduction of 16%.
- Blood cultures to be taken before antibiotic therapy.
- Prompt imaging studies to confirm potential source of infection.
- Administration of broad-spectrum antibiotic therapy within 1h of diagnosis of septic shock and severe sepsis without shock.
- Re-assessment of antibiotic therapy following availability of microbiology and clinical data to narrow coverage.
- Antibiotic therapy for 7–10 days guided by clinical response.
- Early identification and treatment of identified infection source, e.g. draining of pus, debridement of necrotic tissue.
- Administration of either crystalloid or colloid fluid resuscitation by fluid challenge to restore CVP >8mmHg or S_vO_2 >65%.
- Reduction in rate of fluid administration with rising filling pressures and no improvement in tissue perfusion.
- Use of vasopressors, such as noradrenaline (norepinephrine) or dopamine to maintain an initial target of mean arterial pressure >65mmHg.
- Inotropic therapy (e.g. dobutamine, adrenaline (epinephrine)) when cardiac output remains low despite fluid resuscitation.
- Intravenous hydrocortisone should be given only in septic shock after blood pressure is identified to be poorly responsive to fluid and vasopressor therapy.
- Recombinant activated protein C in patients with severe sepsis and clinical assessment of high risk for death.
- In the absence of tissue hypoperfusion, coronary artery disease, or acute haemorrhage, target haemoglobin of 7–9g/dL.
- Target a low tidal volume and limitation of inspiratory plateau pressure strategy for acute lung injury (ALI)/acute respiratory distress syndrome (ARDS); see detail on 📖 p. 394.
- Apply at least a minimal amount of positive end-expiratory pressure in acute lung injury.
- Head of bed elevation in mechanically ventilated patients unless contraindicated.
- Avoid routine use of pulmonary artery catheters in ALI/ARDS.
- Consider a conservative fluid strategy for patients with established ALI/ARDS who are not in shock.
- Use protocols for weaning and sedation/analgesia; using either intermittent bolus sedation or continuous infusion sedation with daily interruptions or lightening.
- Avoid neuromuscular blockers, if at all possible.
- Institute tight glycaemic control targeting a blood glucose 3.9–8.3mmol/l (70–150mg/dL) after initial stabilization.

- Use of continuous veno-veno haemofiltration or intermittent haemodialysis for renal support if necessary.
- Prophylaxis for deep vein thrombosis.
- Stress ulcer prophylaxis to prevent upper gastrointestinal bleeding using H_2 blockers or proton pump inhibitors.

Further information

Dellinger R, Levy M, Carlet J, et al. (2008) Surviving Sepsis Campaign: international guidelines for management of severe sepsis and septic shock: 2008. *Crit Care Med* **36**, 296–327.

Early goal-directed resuscitation

This includes early recognition of sepsis, and early and effective interventions in order to restore circulating volume and oxygen delivery. In some hospitals this occurs in the Emergency department although, in many others, it will only commence once the patient arrives in critical care. However, it is clear that early initiation of fluid resuscitation, ventilatory support, inotropic therapy and transfusion to achieve a central venous O_2 saturation >65% has resulted in significant reduction in mortality. Thus, resuscitation measures should be initiated as early as possible wherever the patient is situated.

Early initiatives should be evaluated and alternative interventions considered including:
- Use of vasopressors, such as noradrenaline (norepinephrine), or dopamine if the target mean arterial blood pressure remains below 65mmHg.
- Consideration of transfusion of red blood cells if Hb <7mmHg.
- Consider intravenous hydrocortisone for adult septic shock when hypotension responds poorly to adequate fluid resuscitation and vasopressors.
- Consider drotrecogin (recombinant human activated protein C (rhAPC)) in adult patients with sepsis-induced organ dysfunction and clinical assessment of high risk of death (typically APACHE II >25 or multiple organ failure) if there are no contraindications.

Previous treatments no longer used include:
- Low dose dopamine to increase renal perfusion.
- Increasing cardiac output with inotropes to previously determined 'supra-normal' levels.
- Corticosteroids in the absence of shock unless there are endocrine problems or previous corticosteroid dependence.

Early resuscitation in septic patients

Begin resuscitation immediately in patients with hypotension (sys. BP <90mmHg) or elevated serum lactate >4mmol/l – do not delay for ICU admission.

Resuscitation goals should be:
- CVP 8–12mmHg.
- Mean arterial pressure >65mmHg.
- Urine output >0.5ml/kg/h.
- Central venous oxygen saturation >70% or mixed venous >65%.

Potential infective sources

Investigate for infection from:
- Wounds (trauma).
- Wounds (operative).
- Central venous lines.
- Abscesses.
- Necrotic tissue.
- Organ-specific infection/inflammation, e.g. pancreatitis, cholecystitis, meningitis, pneumonia.

These should be identified early and treated.

Further information

Dellinger R, Levy M, Carlet J, et al. (2008) Surviving Sepsis Campaign: international guidelines for management of severe sepsis and septic shock: 2008. *Crit Care Med* **36**, 296–327.

Rivers E, Nguyen B, Havstad S, et al. (2001) Early goal-directed therapy in the treatment of severe sepsis and septic shock. *N Engl J Med* **345**, 1368–77.

Ventilatory management

Ventilatory management for the patient with ALI/ARDS

In order to optimize the level of ventilatory support and minimize the risk of barotrauma:

- IPPV should be set to deliver a tidal volume of 6ml/kg (predicted) body weight with an initial upper limit plateau pressure of ≤30cmH$_2$O.
- P$_a$CO$_2$ should be allowed to increase above normal, rather than increasing the tidal volume and plateau pressure limits. PEEP should be set to avoid extensive lung collapse at end-expiration.
- Prone positioning (see 📖 p. 220) can be used where potentially injurious levels of F$_i$O$_2$ or plateau pressure would otherwise be needed.
- Consider the potential risk to benefit ratio from position changes to prone if cardiovascular instability or other risks are present.
- A conservative fluid strategy should be used in patients with established ALI, but no evidence of tissue hypoperfusion as this is associated with improved outcomes.
- Nurse the patient in a semi-recumbent position, i.e. the head of the bed is raised between 30° and 45°.

Non-invasive ventilation

This can be considered in patients with mild to moderate hypoxaemic respiratory failure, providing they are haemodynamically stable, comfortable, easily rousable, and able to protect/clear their airway.

Weaning

A weaning protocol incorporating a regular spontaneous breathing trial (SBT) should be in place with clear pre-conditions for the SBT. These should include:

- Patients are rousable.
- Patients are haemodynamically stable without needing vasopressors.
- Patients have no new potentially serious conditions.
- Patients have low ventilatory support requirements and low F$_i$O$_2$ levels.

Supportive management

Sedation, analgesia, and neuromuscular blockade in sepsis

Use protocols with a sedation goal for mechanically-ventilated patients. These should include either continuous infusions titrated to a sedation score or daily wakening. Avoid neuromuscular blockers wherever possible, and monitor by daily reduction and assessment of sedation levels.

Tight glucose control

Insulin infusions should be used to keep the blood glucose at 3.9–8.3mmol/l (70–150mg/dL) following a validated protocol for dose adjustment. A glucose calorie source should be provided concurrently. Blood glucose should be monitored initially at 15min intervals until stable at the right level of blood glucose. This can be reduced 1–4-hourly.

Renal support

Maintenance of renal perfusion with adequate fluid resuscitation is essential. If renal dysfunction occurs and indicators for renal support (hyperkalaemia, metabolic acidosis, fluid overload, and rising urea and creatinine), continuous renal replacement should be initiated.

Nutritional support

Early initiation of enteral nutrition where possible is thought to be associated with reduced risk of additional infectious complications.

Maintaining haematological function

Due to the potential for increased harm, red blood cells should only be given when Hb decreases to <7.0g/dL. A higher level may be required in special circumstances (e.g. myocardial ischaemia, severe hypoxemia, acute haemorrhage, cyanotic heart disease, or lactic acidosis). Erythropoetin should not be used to treat sepsis-related anaemia. If there is bleeding or significant coagulopathy, and a planned invasive procedure is needed fresh frozen plasma can be given. Platelets can be given when counts are $10 \times 10^9/l$ regardless of bleeding or $<20 \times 10^9/l$ with a high bleeding risk or for higher platelet counts ($>50 \times 10^9/l$) for surgery or invasive procedures.

Preventive measures

Deep vein thrombosis prophylaxis
Unfractionated or low molecular weight heparin should be used to reduce the risk of DVT in combination with compression stockings or an intermittent compression device where the risk is high.

Stress ulcer prophylaxis
Either H_2 blockers or proton pump inhibitors should be given, although an increased risk for developing ventilator-acquired pneumonia should be considered. Use of enteral feeding may also be protective

Support for the patient and their family
Ensure that both receive regular updates and information on the patient's condition and prognosis. Set realistic expectations and, when appropriate, discuss the need for limitation of treatment measures.

Trauma

Initial management

This can be considered as four distinct phases, beginning at the scene of the trauma until stabilization prior to transfer to the critical care unit.

Primary survey

This takes place at the scene of the trauma by pre-hospital staff and continues in the emergency department. It is concerned with the identification and management of life-threatening injuries, and the following are assessed simultaneously.

Airway maintenance and cervical spine control

- Establish a patent airway by chin-lift or jaw-thrust manoeuvres.
- Remove debris, blood clots and loose fitting false teeth.
- Use of airway adjuncts/suction.
- Give high concentration oxygen therapy.
- Endotracheal intubation, cricothyroidotomy, or tracheostomy may be required.
- Consider cervical spine injuries. Do not hyperextend the neck.

Breathing and ventilation

- Expose the chest to assess respiratory movements.
- Consider the possibility of tension, or open pneumothorax, or flail chest with pulmonary contusions.

Circulation and haemorrhage control

- Assess haemodynamic status (blood pressure, heart rate, capillary refill, skin colour).
- Control external haemorrhage by direct pressure or pneumatic splints.

Dysfunction of the central nervous system

Assess neurological status (level of consciousness, pupillary reaction).

Exposure and examination

Undress the patient for a rapid assessment of injuries to the trunk and limbs.

Resuscitation phase

The management of shock is initiated by replacement of lost intravascular volume, oxygenation re-assessed, and haemorrhage control re-evaluated. If not contra-indicated, a urinary catheter is inserted. Life-threatening conditions identified in the primary survey are constantly re-assessed as management continues.

Secondary survey

This begins after life-threatening conditions have been identified and treated and shock therapy has begun. A thorough head-to-toe assessment is done where each region of the body is examined in detail. Laboratory studies, X-rays, scans, and special investigations, such as peritoneal lavage, are carried out.

Definitive care phase

All injuries are managed comprehensively: fractures are stabilized, the patient is transferred to the operating theatre if immediate surgery is necessary, or stabilized in preparation for transfer to the critical care unit or other specialist area.

Arrival on the critical care unit

Equipment should be prepared and tested prior to the patient's arrival. Depending on the patient's injuries, an appropriate bed or pressure-relieving mattress may be required (e.g. Stryker frame for spinal injuries). Ensure any traction can be affixed to the particular bed used.

Checklist for equipment preparation

- Humidified oxygen mask and delivery system/ventilator.
- Suction.
- Rebreathing bag.
- Volumetric pumps.
- Pressure bags for rapid iv infusion.
- Skin electrodes for ECG monitoring.
- Stethoscope.
- Non-invasive blood pressure measuring device.
- Pulse oximeter and probe.
- Temperature probes.
- Primed transducers for invasive monitoring.
- Trolley for central venous/arterial cannulation.
- Nasogastric tube.
- Blood/body warming devices.
- Chest drain sets.

On arrival, connect the patient to the ECG monitor, and attach to the ventilator or oxygen therapy – check the settings are appropriate. If a central venous cannula is *in situ* connect to the transducer. Check any infusions or drugs in progress are running at the correct rate. Check chest drains are unclamped, patent, and positioned appropriately. Ensure alarm limits are set on monitoring equipment. Make immediate baseline observations of:

- Heart rate and rhythm.
- Blood pressure.
- Central venous pressure.
- Respirations or ventilator settings.
- Temperature.
- Neurological status.
- Drainage volumes (urine, wound, chest).

The correct positioning of the patient will depend upon their injuries. Ensure fractured limbs are carefully positioned and supported, and any traction fitted correctly. If the patient is stable at this point a full nursing assessment should be carried out. If the patient is haemodynamically unstable, ventilatory support inadequate, or the patient is in pain, these aspects must be corrected first.

Nursing assessment

Respiratory assessment

Rate

- Record the respiratory rate if the patient is breathing spontaneously.
- Observe the depth and the presence of stridor and whether the patient is using accessory muscles to aid breathing.
- A rate greater than 20 breaths/min should alert the nurse to the possibility of respiratory compromise.
- Pulse oximetry and blood gas analysis should be used as an adjunct to observation and examination (see 📖 Chapter 6, pp. 117–126).

Chest movements and air entry

- Observe if the chest is moving symmetrically with each respiration and listen for air entry to all regions.
- If chest movement is unilateral or air entry poor in any region consider intraluminal obstruction (e.g. blood clot, tooth), malposition of the endotracheal tube (if intubated), pneumothorax, haemothorax, rupture of a bronchus or pulmonary contusions.
- Bear in mind that the patient may have underlying respiratory disease, such as asthma or COPD.
- If the patient has multiple rib fractures and/or a flail segment this will impair movement of the chest wall, and (if breathing spontaneously) paradoxical chest wall movement may be evident over the flail segment.

Respiratory pattern

- Observe if the pattern of breathing is regular.
- Particular patterns are characteristic of particular head injuries in spontaneously breathing patients. Cheyne-Stokes respiration (periodic, rapid and slow breathing) is seen in bilateral cerebral hemisphere damage, hyperventilation in mid-brain injuries, apneustic (prolonged inspiration) in pontine injuries, and ataxic (random) in medullary injuries.

Skin

- Examine the chest skin for bruising, lacerations, and abrasions, which may indicate underlying injuries (e.g. seat-belt marks).
- Feel for subcutaneous emphysema, which may arise from external injuries (e.g. stab wound) or from internal (e.g. rib fractures lacerating the underlying lung) injuries.
- Observe for cyanosis, which can occur if there is rapid deterioration e.g. due to a tension pneumothorax.

Pain

Determine whether there is pain or tenderness over a particular area of the chest, or on inspiration, which may limit chest movement.

Chest drains

- Check the drains are properly positioned and patent.
- Note the type (blood, haemoserous, air) and amounts of drainage.
- Observe and record if they swing with respiration or are bubbling.

Cardiovascular assessment

- Continuous ECG monitoring should be in progress.
- A 12-lead ECG should be recorded.
- Check central pulses are present.
- The frequency of blood pressure recording will depend on the extent of the injuries.
- Continuous invasive monitoring allows blood pressure changes to be detected immediately, and is essential in multiply injury or shocked patients.
- Changes in blood pressure should not be taken in isolation, but related to changes in other variables, such as heart rate, central venous pressure, pulmonary artery pressures, and stroke volume.
- Consider the effects of drug therapy as a potential cause of blood pressure changes (e.g. sedation, analgesia).

Neurological assessment

- A full neurological assessment must be made to provide a baseline for sequential appraisal and detection of deterioration (see ☞ Neurological observations, p. 288).
- The frequency of recordings will depend upon the patient's injuries, and the actual or potential for head injury.
- The scalp should be examined for lacerations, bruising, and obvious deformity. Bruising behind the ears may indicate bleeding into the mastoid space – a late sign of basal skull fracture. The presence of otorrhea or rhinorrhoea is also suggestive of basal skull fracture.

Renal assessment

- A urethral urinary catheter is usually inserted to monitor urine output.
- In trauma to the urethra, a suprapubic catheter is used.
- Routine urinalysis should be performed and the urine observed for frank haematuria, myoglobinuria (black urine), debris, and clots.
- Examine the genitalia for bruising, lacerations, and oedema.

Gastro-intestinal assessment

- All ventilated patients should have a nasogastric tube inserted unless contraindicated (e.g. nasal or basal skull injuries – in this case an oro-gastric tube is inserted). It should be left to drain freely and aspirated regularly – observe/test for blood.
- Examine the abdomen for bruising and lacerations, rigidity, pain on palpation, and distension.
- Note if there is any rectal bleeding.

Skin and limb assessment

- Note any bruising, lacerations, or swelling.
- Feel the skin and note the colour.
- Check the capillary refill in each limb.
- Check that distal pulses are present, and that pressure dressing, splints, plaster casts, or traction on limbs are not impeding the circulation.
- Record peripheral skin temperature if appropriate to the injuries.
- Ensure pressure is not exerted on healthy skin by plaster casts or traction devices (observe for tissue swelling and breaks in the skin).

Head injuries

Skull fractures alone do not cause neurological disability and severe brain injuries can occur without skull fractures. A patient with a skull fracture, however, is at risk of having or developing intracranial damage. Close observation is necessary to detect early signs of neurological deterioration. Priorities of management in the severely-injured patient are to secure adequate oxygenation, support circulatory resuscitation, and deal with any life-threatening injury before definitive treatment for head injury.

The patient will usually be admitted to the critical care unit after CT scanning has identified the extent of the injury. An unstable neck fracture should be assumed until excluded by appropriate investigation. Any deterioration in conscious level, focal signs (e.g. unilateral pupillary dilatation) or developing neurological deficits should prompt urgent rescanning.

Cardiovascular signs of raised intracranial pressure

- Decreased heart rate.
- Decreased respiratory rate.
- Raised blood pressure.
- Widened pulse pressure.

Consequences of raised intracranial pressure

- Alterations in the level of consciousness.
- Headaches, photophobia, nausea, vomiting.
- Coma.
- Death.

Secondary brain damage

The brain requires continuous perfusion with well-oxygenated blood. A reduction in mean arterial pressure below 60–80mmHg, particularly when intracranial pressure is raised, may cause ischaemic neuronal damage if sustained for more than a few minutes. Damage can be prevented by rapid treatment (see 📖 Neurological observations, p. 288)

Table 17.1 Causes of secondary brain damage

	Cause	Secondary to
Extra cranial	Hypoxia	Brainstem damage causing decreased respiratory drive
		Haemo/pneumothorax
		Pulmonary contusions
		Aspiration pneumonitis/infection
		Fat emboli/pulmonary emboli
		ARDS
	Hypotension	Hypovolaemic shock
Intracranial	Compression from haematomas	Subdural
		Extradural
		Intradural (intracerebral/subarachnoid)
	Venous engorgement leading to cerebral oedema	
	Secondary infection	Meningitis, brain abscess

Reproduced with permission from *Critical Care Nursing*, Adam and Osborne (2005), Oxford University Press.

Management

- Stabilize airway, breathing and circulation to prevent hypoxia and hypovolaemia.
- Maintain normocapnia – a low P_aCO_2 can cause arterial vasoconstriction (and relative cerebral ischaemia) and a high P_aCO_2 vasodilation.
- Avoid high PEEP if possible (increases ICP).
- Osmotherapy – administration of mannitol or hypertonic saline (causes an osmotic diuresis) or furosemide to reduce cerebral oedema.
- Aggressive treatment of seizures (see 📖 Neurological observations, p. 288)
- Adequate nutrition (which needs to be started early).
- Anti-emetics (vomiting increases ICP).
- Active treatment of hyperpyrexia (increases CO_2), maintain nornothermia.
- Nursing procedures: avoid over-stimulation, minimize suction, and physiotherapy, nurse with head-tilt at 30° if possible, neck in neutral position, do not tie endotracheal tube tapes tightly, pre-oxygenate with 100% oxygen prior to and after suctioning to avoid hypoxaemia.

Complications of head injury

- Seizures.
- Coma.
- Diabetes insipidus.
- Infection (from open head wound, CSF leakage, aspiration pneumonia if unconscious at the scene of the accident).
- Gastric dilatation (risk of aspiration).
- Nerve damage.
- Cognitive and language difficulties.
- Sensory problems.
- Personality changes.

Further information

Adam SK, Osborne S. (2005) *Critical Care Nursing*. Oxford: Oxford University Press.

Maxillofacial injuries

Many patients with severe maxillofacial injuries will have other associated injuries and cervical spine trauma must always be suspected. Extreme care is needed when stabilizing the neck when the airway is being secured. Injuries to the face and neck can be life-threatening because they may compromise the airway and cause major haemorrhage.

Specific fractures

- **Mandible:** may cause airway obstruction if bilateral fracture. Often causes haematoma and swelling of the neck and floor of the mouth. Treatment is by internal wiring or plating.
- **Maxilla:** Le Fort I, II, or III. Le Fort II and III are associated with basal skull fractures and may lead to CSF leakage. Nasal intubation must never be performed. Treatment involves internal wiring and plating and intermaxillary fixation. External fixation is often required.
- **Zygoma and orbit: fracture and displacement of the zygoma** can disrupt the lateral wall and floor of the orbit. Subconjunctival ecchymosis and peri-orbital swelling may be present. Unstable fractures require internal or external fixation, stable fractures can be surgically reduced. Fractures of the orbital walls may tear or compress the optic nerve and blindness is immediate and permanent.
- **Nasal:** haemorrhage may be severe and may require nasal packing. Closed reduction and external splinting may be required.
- **Larynx:** may severely compromise the airway and necessitate immediate tracheostomy. Surgical exploration and repair is usually necessary.

Specific management

Airway and breathing

- Soft tissue swelling and oedema can increase insidiously.
- A patient without tracheal intubation is at risk of developing airway problems.
- Ensure oxygen face masks are not tight-fitting if there are facial injuries.
- Never use nasal prongs if there is evidence of rhinorrhoea.
- Observe for increasing difficulty in breathing, stridor, and oedema of the face, neck, and mouth.
- Patients are best nursed upright, if their condition allows, to encourage drainage of blood, saliva, and CSF away from the airway and reduce venous pressure.

Circulation

Significant haemorrhage can occur from closed fractures to the maxilla, nose, and ethmoids and cause profound swelling.

- Wounds.
- Obtain clear guidelines from medical staff regarding specific wound management.
- Check wounds for foreign bodies such as glass.
- Observe for haemorrhage, haematoma and infection.
- Ensure pin sites of external fixation are kept clean and dry.

Mouth

- Mouth care can be difficult, but is essential in patients who have had major oral surgery, and have sutures or skin grafts within the oral cavity, have their jaws wired together or cannot take oral fluids.
- A pair of wire cutters must be available at the bedside if jaws are wired (in order to cut the wires if the patient vomits and the airway is compromised).
- Regular anti-emetics should be given if nauseated as vomiting must be prevented.

Eyes

- Observe for peri-orbital swelling and subconjunctival haemorrhage.
- Pooling of tears may indicate damage to the lacrimal apparatus.
- Proptosis or exophthalmia (bulging eyes) suggest haemorrhage within the orbital walls.
- Foreign bodies (grit or glass) can penetrate the eye and cause pyrogenic infection.

Nose

- Observe for bleeding.
- Rhinorrhoea suggests a cribriform plate fracture. Do not pass a nasogastric tube if present or the cranial cavity may be intubated.

Ears

- Observe for bleeding or otorrhoea.
- Look behind the ears for bruising over the mastoid process (Battle sign), which can indicate a basal skull fracture.

Spinal injuries

These are often associated with other injuries, particularly to the head and chest. Any unconscious, multiply-injured patient must be assumed to have spinal injuries until excluded by expert opinion. The management of the airway, breathing, and circulation must take priority, but precautions must be taken to prevent exacerbation of any neurological damage.

Airway maintenance with cervical spine control

- In high cervical spine injuries, intubation may be required to protect the airway and/or provide a means of ventilatory support. Vertebral fractures above C5 lead to loss of diaphragmatic function and those above C8 to loss of intercostal function. Endotracheal intubation should be carried out by an experienced anaesthetist with an assistant responsible for controlling the head and neck, and minimizing spinal movement.
- A difficult intubation should be anticipated.
- A fibre-optic laryngoscope or bronchoscope should be available.
- Pharyngeal stimulation may provoke a vagal reflex causing severe bradycardia (this can be prevented by administering atropine or glycopyrrolate prior to the procedure).
- The neck must be stabilized at all times using a rigid collar of appropriate size with sand bags on each side of the head.
- Stabilization of the neck must be continued throughout all procedures (e.g. X-rays, CVP line insertion).
- If X rays confirm spinal damage, more definitive stabilization may be considered (skull tongs, halopelvic traction, spinal fusion).

Breathing

- Careful observation is required in a patient with a spinal injury who is breathing spontaneously. Ascending oedema of the traumatized cervical cord may lead to deterioration in respiratory status.
- Equipment for manual ventilation must be at the bedside at all times.
- Blood gas analysis and pulse oximetry should be used to identify hypoxaemia as early as possible.
- Vital capacity should be monitored particularly in patients with fractures above C8. A forced vital capacity <10–15ml/kg body weight may indicate the need for ventilatory support.
- Patients should be nursed on a bed capable of lateral tilting and longitudinal elevation, while keeping the spine straight.
- Patients should be nursed, if possible, with the head tilted up and feet down at 30° to increase functional capacity help prevent atelectasis.
- Regular physiotherapy is essential to help remove chest secretions.
- The use of narcotic drugs (which suppress respiration) should be avoided.

Circulation

- All patients must have vital signs observed and recorded frequently with continuous ECG monitoring.
- Reduced sympathetic outflow between T1 and T12 may cause hypotension and bradycardia (neurogenic or 'spinal' shock).

- Neurogenic shock must be distinguished from hypovolaemic shock (hypotension and tachycardia) as aggressive fluid replacement is detrimental and may precipitate pulmonary oedema.
- Atropine or glycopyrronium bromide (glycopyrrolate) may be needed if the heart rate is <50bpm with associated hypotension (<80mmHg systolic).
- A fluid challenge may be given if the patient is hypotensive and bradycardic, but CVP and/or PCWP measurements must be measured before more fluid replacement is given.
- Hypotension and inadequate tissue perfusion may lead to irreversible neurological damage.
- Abdominal or other occult trauma may not be easily recognized in the tetraplegic patient, since the abdominal wall is anesthetized and flaccid. Signs of visceral perforation and haemorrhage may not be easily apparent.
- Peritoneal lavage, ultrasound and X-ray procedures may be necessary if abdominal trauma is suspected.

Specific nursing management

- A nasogastric tube should be inserted (unless contraindicated) and aspirated regularly. Paralytic ileus and gastric dilatation are common in spinal cord trauma. The patient should have nil by mouth for 48h.
- A urethral catheter should be inserted (unless contraindicated) as urinary retention may develop. Urine output should be monitored regularly.
- Regular urinalysis be performed (and colour observed), body temperature recorded to detect urinary tract infections.
- Regular administration of laxative and enemas as per unit protocol to prevent constipation.
- Prevention of pressure sores and limb deformities with correct positioning of limbs and joints.
- Physiotherapy and passive limb movements to preserve joint motion and stimulate circulation.
- Adequate nutrition to prevent hypoalbuminaemia.

Chest injuries

Nursing priorities
Airway and breathing
- A patent airway must be secured, endotracheal intubation or tracheostomy may be required.
- A chest X-ray will have been taken in the casualty department and any specific chest injuries identified.
- Mechanical ventilation, CPAP, non-invasive ventilation, or oxygen therapy will be instituted according to the patient's condition.
- Any pneumothorax must be identified and drained.
- Continuous pulse oximetry and regular blood gas analysis should be performed in conjunction with respiratory observations to monitor respiratory function.
- The self-ventilating patient requires careful and continuous observation in order to detect respiratory distress, and the need for further intervention.

Circulation
Continuous ECG and monitoring of vital signs is essential.
- Observe for signs of hypovolaemia (tachycardia, hypotension) and frank blood loss via drains and wounds.
- Monitor Hb level.
- Myocardial contusions may give rise to tachyarrhythmias and conduction abnormalities.
- Large blood losses may result from tearing of thoracic vessels and haemothoraces.
- Major cardiac or vascular lacerations may have had haemorrhage arrested by a tamponade effect. Rapid transfusion and the subsequent rise in arterial pressure may result in uncontrollable bleeding.

Specific chest injuries
Pulmonary contusions
Shearing and crushing forces within the thoracic cage cause disruption of the microcirculation. Extravasation of red cells and plasma occurs, and these fluids fill the alveoli. Interstitial haemorrhage and alveolar collapse results, impairing gas exchange. Perfusion is maintained in the unventilated lung segments causing intrapulmonary shunting and hypoxaemia. Management is by treating hypoxia (IPPV, BiPAP, CPAP, oxygen therapy), ensuring adequate pain control and physiotherapy.

Rib fractures
Sharp edges of fractured rib may lacerate the underlying lung or blood vessels. If several ribs are fractured in more than one place, or the broken ribs are combined with fracture dislocation of the costochondrial junctions or sternum, a flail segment can move independently of the rib cage. Management is the same as for pulmonary contusions.

Haemo/pneumothoraces

- **Simple pneumothorax:** air in the pleural cavity caused by damage to lung tissue.
- **Open pneumothorax:** air enters the pleural cavity from a penetrating injury.
- **Tension pneumothorax:** air enters the pleural cavity and increases with each respiration. The affected lung is compressed and collapses, pushing the mediastinal structures to the unaffected side. Cardiovascular collapse will ensue unless immediate decompression is undertaken.
- **Haemothorax:** blood in the pleural cavity.
- **Haemo/pneumothoraces** impair ventilation and may result in hypoxaemia. A chest drain is usually inserted, particularly if mechanical ventilation is necessary, as the likelihood of tension pneumothorax is greatly increased.

Pericardial tamponade

Penetrating or blunt trauma causes the pericardium to fill with blood. Characterized by:
- Tachycardia.
- Raised CVP.
- Decreased blood pressure.
- Decreased cardiac output.

Treatment is by pericardiocentesis.

Myocardial contusions

Caused by blunt trauma to the chest or by deceleration trauma. Characterized by:
- ECG changes (non specific ST segment and T wave changes).
- Dyssrhythmias.
- Elevated cardiac enzymes.

Diaphragmatic rupture

Caused by blunt or penetrating injuries. The abdominal contents may be pushed through the laceration. Surgical repair is usually necessary.

Aortic rupture

Characterized by persistent or recurrent hypovolaemia despite fluid replacement. Frequently fatal.

Major airway injuries

Characterized by:
- Surgical emphysema.
- Stridor.
- Aphonia.
- Haemoptysis.
- Respiratory distress.

Often accompanied by injuries to the oesophagus, carotid artery, and jugular vein, and may be associated with pneumo/haemothoraces.

Abdominal and pelvic injuries

Abdominal injuries

Initial priorities are the maintenance of airway, breathing, and circulation. Specific treatment of abdominal injury should not delay correction of hypoxaemia and tissue hypoperfusion. Urgent laparotomy may be indicated if hypovolaemia persists after adequate fluid replacement and the cause cannot be attributed to other injuries. Observations should include:

- Vital signs.
- The presence of increasing abdominal pain or rigidity.
- Hb.
- Urine output.
- Abdominal pressure (if indicated).

A nasogastric tube should be inserted (unless contraindicated) in order to:

- Decompress the stomach.
- Reduce the risk of pneumonic aspiration.
- Detect the presence of upper gastrointestinal injury (blood in nasogastric aspirate).

Patients with abdominal injuries are particularly at risk of local infection, septicaemia, and multi-organ failure, and must be monitored closely for potential infection (temperature, peritonism, purulent discharge from wounds, or drains) If the spleen has been removed they are at risk of overwhelming bacterial sepsis due to diminished humoral immunity.

Pelvic fractures

These can cause severe and uncontrollable haemorrhage. Continuous recording of vital signs is essential and fluid resuscitation given as necessary. Immobilization and external fixation can help control bleeding, but surgical repair of torn vessels, or angiography and embolization may be required.

Care of pressure areas may pose particular problems and clear instructions must be given by the surgeon as to the degree of mobility the patient is allowed. A pressure relieving mattress is essential as even after external/internal fixation movement remains limited.

Intra-abdominal hypertension

Intra-abdominal hypertension (IAH) occurs when the abdomen distends, abdominal wall compliance decreases, causing a rise in intra-abdominal pressure (IAP). This may result in abdominal compartment syndrome (ACS) and lead to multi-organ failure. IAH is said to be present when the IAP rises to 10–15mmHg. ACS is defined as an IAP > 20mmHg.

Causes of intra-abdominal hypertension
- Trauma.
- Abdominal surgery.
- Gaseous distension (ileus, obstruction, post-laparoscopy).
- Cirrhosis (ascites).
- Bowel ischaemia/infarction.
- Gastrointestinal haemorrhage.
- Pancreatitis.
- Pregnancy.

Effects of intra-abdominal hypertension
Respiratory
- Instigates or aggravates respiratory failure.
- Pushes the diaphragm higher than normal into the chest.
- Reduces functional capacity and compliance.
- High peak airway pressures.
- Reduced tidal volume.
- Atelectasis.
- Hypoxaemia and hypercapnia causing respiratory acidosis.

Cardiovascular
- Decreases preload on left ventricle.
- Increases afterload from left ventricle.
- Reduces cardiac output.
- Elevates SVR.
- CVP and PAWP may rise (even if patient hypovolaemic).

Gastrointestinal
- Visceral perfusion falls when IAP > 10mmHhg.
- Reduces intra-mucosal pH and mesenteric flow if IAP > 15mmHg.
- Severe acidosis in intestinal mucosa and decrease in hepatic and micro-circulatory flow if IAP > 40mmHg.

Renal
- Compression of kidneys and renal veins.
- Decreased glucose re-absorption.
- Fall in GFR.
- Oliguria or anuria.
- Renal failure.

Neurological
- Increases intracranial pressure.
- Decreases cerebral perfusion pressure.
- Increased resistance to cerebral venous drainage.

Management of intra-abdominal hypertension

- Prevention and early detection (delayed wound closure following laparotomy or mesh insertion).
- Supportive measures (pressure controlled ventilation, PEEP, inverse I:E ratios, inotropic and renal support).
- Prokinetic drugs (if secondary to ileus).
- Diuretics and/or haemofiltration (if due to bowel oedema).
- Abdominal decompression.

Patients undergoing surgical decompression are at risk of sudden and severe hypotension, and asystolic cardiac arrest when the abdomen is opened. This may be due to hypovolaemia and reperfusion injury, where mediators and free radicals are released following reperfusion of the splanchnic bed. Volume administration should be given prior to decompression. See 📖 Intra-abdominal pressure measurement, p. 154.

Table 17.2 Burch's grading system for abdominal compartment syndrome

Grade	Bladder pressure (cmH₂O)	Equivalent pressure (mmHg)	Treatment strategy
I	10–15	7–11	Monitor only
II	15–25	11–18	Treatment based on clinical condition
III	25–30	18–26	Most will require compression
IV	>35	>26	All require decompression

Reproduced with permission from *Critical Care Nursing*, Adam and Osborne (2005), Oxford University Press.

Further information

Adam SK, Osborne S. (2005) *Critical Care Nursing*. Oxford: Oxford University Press.

Genitourinary injuries

Upper genitourinary

Renal trauma can be categorized as:
- **Minor:** parenchymal damage, contusions, superficial lacerations.
- **Major:** deep lacerations involving the pelvicalyceal system and/or tears of the capsule.
- **Critical:** renal fragmentation and pedical injuries (renal artery thrombosis, pelviureteric rupture, avulsion of renal vessels). These can cause major blood loss and hypovolaemic shock.

Specific nursing observations
- Vital signs and Hb.
- Urine output.
- Evidence of bruising or swelling over lower thoracic, loin, or upper abdominal areas.
- Pain.
- Rigidity of abdominal wall on affected side.
- Haematuria.
- Ureteric colic if blood clots are passed through the ureter.

The initial management is to stabilize airway, breathing, and circulation before specific investigations are undertaken to diagnose the injury.

Lower genitourinary
Specific nursing observations
- Vital signs and Hb.
- Urine output.
- Inspect urethral meatus for blood.
- Evidence of bruising, particularly of perineum.
- Abdominal pain or rigidity.
- Haematuria.

A urethral catheter must not be inserted in patients with suspected trauma or major pelvic fractures until advised by a urologist.

Musculoskeletal injuries

Management is secondary to resuscitation and control of the airway, breathing, and circulation. Life-threatening conditions include:
- Traumatic amputations.
- Severe crush injuries to the pelvis and abdomen.
- Multiple long bone fractures.
- Vascular injuries.
- Open fractures.
- Haemorrhagic shock (see 📖 Complications following trauma, p. 428) must be identified and treated before definitive treatment of the injury.

Specific observation of limbs
- Colour.
- Temperature.
- Pulses.
- Sensation/pain.
- Local compression (plaster-of-Paris, splints, bandages).

Specific nursing management
Depends on the extent of injuries and degree of immobility.

For the patient in traction
- Frequent and meticulous attention to pressure areas, use of a pressure-relieving mattress.
- Inspect pin sites, keep clean and dry.
- Passive/active limb exercises to non-immobilized joints.
- Traction weights to hang free, knots secure.
- Retain traction when moving the patient, support the weights.

For the patient in a plaster cast
- See 📖 Specific observation of limbs, above.
- Check for constriction due to swelling.
- Check for pain under plaster cast.
- Skin integrity around plaster edge.
- Elevate limb to alleviate swelling.

Potential complications
- **Haemorrhage:** monitor vital signs, Hb, observe wounds, and drains.
- **Compartment syndrome:** see 📖 p. 428.
- **Infection:** monitor temperature, observe wounds, cannulae, and pin sites.
- **Deep vein thrombosis:** inspect calves for swelling and pain, consider anti-embolic stockings/prophylactic anticoagulation.
- **Rhabdomyolysis:** see 📖 p. 349.
- **Fat embolism syndrome:** see 📖 p. 428.

Flaps

Free or pedical flaps are used to correct an anatomical defect. Post-operative survival of the flap depends on good perfusion. Close and frequent observation is essential in order to detect changes as soon as possible. Report changes immediately.

Specific flap observations

- Temperature – core, peripheral, flap.
- Colour.
- Capillary refill.
- Turgidity.
- Pulse.

Specific management

Maintain core-flap temperature difference <1.5°

- Keep warm – body warming device if necessary.
- Keep vessels dilated – iv glyceryl trinitrate.
- Keep Hb <10g/dl to reduce blood viscosity.
- Maintain BP and CVP within set parameters.

Factors detrimental to flap survival

- Hypotension.
- Vasopressors.
- Hypovolaemia.
- Poor positioning.

Complications following trauma

Hypovolaemic shock
Treat urgently to avoid organ failure. Baseline vital signs and sequential monitoring are crucial. Use large-bore cannulae obtain high flow vascular access.

Features
- Tachycardia.
- Hypotension.
- Low CVP.
- Low PAWP.
- Poor peripheral perfusion.
- Oliguria.

Management
Fluid resuscitation may consist of a combination of blood, blood products, colloids, and crystalloids.

Ideally, the response of CVP or stroke volume, and PAWP, should be monitored as boluses of fluid (200ml) are administered. Fluid challenges should be repeated if the response suggests continuing hypovolaemia (see 🕮 Hypotension, p. 250). Normalization of BP, heart rate, cerebration, peripheral circulation, urine output, and improvement in metabolic acidosis are good markers of the adequacy of resuscitation.

Compartment syndrome
Results from swelling, bleeding, or ischaemia within the fascial compartments of the limbs. Interstitial tissue pressure rises as the compartments are unable to expand. When this pressure exceeds that of the capillary bed, local ischaemia of nerve and muscle occurs. Rhabdomyolysis, permanent paralysis or gangrene may result.

Features
- Pain.
- Tense swelling of fascial compartment(s).
- Reduced sensation over the dermatomes supplied by the affected nerves.
- Absence of distal pulses (a late sign – may be irreversible damage).

Management
- Monitor limbs for swelling, abnormal perfusion, temperature differences, pain.
- Remove restrictive dressings.
- Needle manometry (pressures >20mmHg are abnormal).
- Fasciotomy.

Fat embolism syndrome
Fat macroglobules and marrow enter the systemic circulation from bone fractures (usually long bones and pelvis) and cause mechanical obstruction of vessels.

Features
- Hypoxaemia.
- Tachypnoea, tachycardia, pyrexia.
- Hypotension, decreased CO.
- Oliguria.
- Petechiae.
- Confusion, drowsiness, decerebrate signs, convulsions, coma.

Management
- Supportive treatment.
- Supplementary oxygen or mechanical respiratory assistance to correct hypoxaemia.
- Maintain circulatory volume.
- Inotropic support.
- Renal support – CVVHD/dialysis.

Air embolism

Air leaks from the lungs directly into the pulmonary circulation and into the left side of the heart. It can occur in severe lung injury due to a bronchopulmonary vein fistula or from direct penetrating injury to the pulmonary veins. Major cardiovascular collapse follows with associated hypoxaemia. Treatment is to turn the patient on their left side in a head-down, feet-up position, and the air is aspirated from the left ventricle followed by thoracotomy of the injured side.

Burn injuries

Classification
- **Erythema:** redness of the skin, pain, but no blistering.
- **1st degree:** involves only epithelial layer. Skin is red and blisters, blanches on pressure and painful. No residual scarring on healing.
- **2nd degree:** extends to the dermis. Skin is red and blistered. The degree of pain and residual scarring depends on the depth of dermis damaged.
- **3rd degree:** involves full skin thickness. Skin is white with little or no pain. Residual scarring on healing.

Calculation of total percentage of burned skin ('rule of 9')
- Head 9%.
- Arms 9% each.
- Front and back of trunk 18% each.
- Legs 18% each.
- Perineum 1%.

Initial management
- If possible, nurse in protective isolation in an environment with humidity and temperature control.
- Reduce heat and fluid losses by nursing on a heated air fluidized bed, and by early coverage of burnt skin by occlusive dressings and placement of affected limbs in transparent plastic bags.
- Strict asepsis for all procedures and meticulous attention to infection control.
- Continuously monitor vital signs, and fluid input and output.
- Maintain patent airway, humidified supplemental oxygen, or mechanical respiratory assistance.
- Establish intravenous access, and CVP and/or PAWP monitoring.
- Insert arterial line for pressure monitoring and blood sampling.
- Either invasive or non-invasive cardiac output monitoring is needed for accurate titration of fluid.
- Insert nasogastric tube to facilitate enteral feeding and for gastric decompression.
- Insert a urinary catheter.
- Fluid replacement: massive fluid losses can occur. Formulae exist for fluid replacement regimes, but should be used as guidelines and frequent assessment of haemodynamics, urine output, haematocrit, and base deficit should be made. Avoid overzealous fluid infusion to minimize oedema.
- Monitor blood electrolytes and glucose as these can fluctuate widely.
- Ensure adequate analgesia.
- Give tetanus toxoid soon after hospital admission.

- Fluid resuscitation regimen (adapted from Mount Vernon formula):;
  - should be used as a guide only;
  - divide first 36h from the time of the burn into six consecutive periods of 4, 4, 4, 6, 6, and 12h. For each period give 0.5ml 4.5–5% albumin × body wt (kg) × % burn.
- Give blood as necessary to maintain Hb > 10g/dl.
- Commence enteral nutrition as soon as possible.
- Give 1.5–2ml/kg/h 5% glucose.
- Re-assess cardiorespiratory variables and urine output at frequent intervals to determine if fluid replacement is inadequate or excessive. Adjust fluid input as necessary.

Subsequent management

Wound care
- Early application of dressings and silver sulphadiazine cream, which has anti-bacterial properties against Gram negative bacteria.
- Escharotomy to affected limbs or, if circumferential burns, to the neck or chest may be required soon after admission.
- Debridement of necrotic tissue is usually performed within the first few days.
- Early skin grafting usually takes place within 2–3 days in order to provide a protective barrier. Blood loss can be considerable from the grafted area.
- Redress wounds according to unit policy/instructions from surgeons.
- Ensure adequate analgesia prior to/during dressing changes.

Infection
- Monitor body temperature – this may rise to 40°C within 1–2 days and persist for several days, but does not indicate secondary infection.
- Scrupulous attention to infection control procedures.
- Observation of wounds/discharge for signs of infection.
- Appropriate antibiotics given if indicated.

Other considerations
- Aim for early enteral nutrition – calorific intake 20Cal/kg + 50Cal/%burn and 1g/kg + 2g/%burn of protein (also reduces risk of stress ulceration).
- Regular physiotherapy to prevent contractures.
- Avoid suxamethonium from 5 to 150 days post-burn as there is a risk of rapid and severe hyperkalaemia.
- Increased resistance to non-polarizing muscle relaxants may be seen.

Near drowning

Pathophysiology

- **Dry drowning:** laryngospasm caused by the presence of water prevents fluid entry into the lungs.
- **Wet drowning:** inhalation of fluid into the lungs.

Traditionally fresh water drowning was thought to lead to rapid absorption of water into the circulation causing haemolysis, hypo-osmolality, and electrolyte disturbances, whereas inhalation of salt water caused mucosal injury and osmotic pulmonary oedema. In practice, there is little difference as both cause loss of surfactant and severe inflammatory disruption of the alveolar-capillary membrane leading to ARDS. Hypothermia usually accompanies near-drowning and, although protective against organ damage, causes loss of consciousness and haemodynamic alterations.

The major complications of near-drowning are:

- Hypoxia.
- ARDS.
- Multi-organ failure.
- Septicaemia.
- Pneumonia.
- Circulatory failure.
- Electrolyte imbalance.
- Dysrhythmias.
- Renal failure.
- Neurological damage.
- Gastric dilatation.
- Metabolic acidosis.

Management

- Cardiopulmonary resuscitation is often required initially.
- Airway management and oxygenation high concentration O_2 by mask, or intubation and ventilation. Early CPAP/PEEP is useful. High inflation pressures may be required.
- Nebulized β agonists if bronchospasm.
- Haemodynamic monitoring.
- Vasopressors if hypotensive.
- Treatment of dysrhythmias (secondary to hypoxaemia, electrolyte imbalance, acidosis and hypothermia).
- Monitor blood electrolytes and glucose.
- Fluid replacement guided by appropriate monitoring.
- Haemolysis may require blood transfusion.
- Monitor core temperature: rewarm as necessary (see 🕮 Hypothermia, p. 434).
- Monitor urine output: haemolysis may cause haemoglobinuria and consequent acute renal failure.
- Neurological observations: ischaemic cerebral damage and cerebral oedema may occur. Attempts should be made to reduce raised intracranial pressure and maintain cerebral perfusion (see 🕮 Neurological observations, p. 288). Observe for and treat seizures.

- Insert a nasogatric tube for gastric decompression and to avoid aspiration.
- Antibiotic therapy if evidence of aspiration (mud, sand, or particulate matter on suction), otherwise take specimens and treat as indicated.
- Metabolic acidosis may develop following intense peripheral vasoconstriction and hypoxaemia. Lactate levels rise as oxygen delivery to the tissues falls, but should improve as the patient is rewarmed and hypoxia corrected.
- Physiotherapy.

Hypothermia

A sustained core temperature below 35°C (mild, 32–35°C; moderate, 28–32°C; severe, <28°C).

Causes

- Reduced metabolic rate (hypothyroidism, hypopituitarism, malnutrition).
- Immobility (coma, spinal injury, elderly).
- Cold water immersion.
- Exposure/poor living conditions.
- Sepsis.
- Erythroderma (generalized erythema and exfoliation).

Features

- >33°C thermoregulatory mechanisms usually intact, marked shivering.
- <33°C slowness and dysarthria.
- <31°C loss of consciousness, papillary dilatation, hypertonicity, life-threatening cardiovascular dysfunction.
- <28°C rigor mortis-like appearance, impalpable arterial pulse, cessation of respiration.

Management

- Airway management and oxygenation.
- Monitor core temperature.
- Haemodynamic monitoring and detection of dysrhythmias – in the event of cardiac arrest (and no evidence of other fatal disease) full resuscitation should continue until the patient is normothermic. VF is resistant to defibrillation between 28 and 30°C.
- Rewarming (see 📖 p. 435).
- Monitor urine output.
- Fluid replacement.
- Monitor blood glucose.
- Neurological observations.

Complications

- ECG changes: as body temperature decreases sinus bradycardia is followed by atrial flutter and fibrillation. The PR interval, QRS, and QT interval are prolonged. Atrial activity then ceases, ventricular fibrillation is common at <30°C leading to asystole at <28°C.
- Decreased CO and BP.
- Hypoxaemia due to hypoventilation and ventilation-perfusion mismatch.
- Respiratory acidosis due to increased CO_2 levels.
- Polyuria and electrolyte imbalance due to impaired tubular function and reduced responsiveness to ADH (anti-diuretic hormone).
- Cerebral depression due to decreased cerebral blood flow.
- Metabolic acidosis due to increased lactate and other metabolites.
- Hyperglycaemia due to decreased insulin release, glucose metabolized from liver glycogen, pancreatitis may develop.

Rewarming

Passive

Suitable for mild hypothermia.
- Rewarm slowly (0.5–1°C/h).
- Warm environment.
- Reflective space blanket/warm air blanket.
- Extra blankets.
- Cover exposed skin (e.g. scalp).
- Remove wet clothes.

Active

Used in moderate hypothermia.
- Heated humidified respiratory gases.
- Warmed intravenous fluids.
- Electrically heated mattress or pads.

Core warming

Rapid rewarming for severe hypothermia.(1–5°C/h).
- Peritoneal/haemodialysis.
- Extracorporeal circuits (heart bypass).
- Gastric and bladder lavage with warmed fluids.

The major incident and critical care

Setting up systems for response

Major incidents will generally involve critical care. Recent examples include severe acute respiratory syndrome (SARS), train crashes, terrorist attacks, and natural catastrophes. These all place a sudden extra demand on critical care. Flu pandemics are a very real possibility in the near future and would potentially swamp critical care should they occur.

Advance planning for such events is the key to an effective response. This should include:
• Clear command and control structures.
• Effective and resilient communication channels.
• Planning to ensure resource availability: supplies, staff, facilities.
• Systems to review performance and learn from events.

Test runs of the major incident response plan

Different types of major incidents require different responses and planning. For instance, bomb blasts or bioterrorism will require a comprehensive command and control response that takes immediate effect within minutes of the alarm, and requires a high impact immediate response, which will peak early and become less intensive as patients either die or recover. Pandemics or epidemics have a slower onset, but a longer duration. Thus, planning for these must centre on being able to maintain staffing, staff morale, and protection of staff from infection, as well as ensuring other resource availability.

Understanding casualty numbers and demand for critical care

Conventional terrorist attacks (bombs, etc.) usually produce large numbers of casualties with relatively minor injuries, large numbers of fatalities, and a relatively small number of critically ill survivors. Following the attack on the World Trade Center in New York, only 10 of the 426 patients who attended hospital required intensive care. A review of multiple casualty trauma events in Jerusalem found less than 5% of patients required critical care. Thus, existing capacity and staffing are likely to be able to cope with casualty numbers, although the impact of multiple simultaneous admissions will require enhanced staffing levels and resources.

Modelling for an influenza pandemic, however, predicts that >171% of critical care capacity would be required to manage patient requirement over a 6-week period. Planning for pandemics therefore requires methods of increasing critical care capacity over a sustained period of time in the face of likely staff shortages due to increased sickness and stress levels, and a high likelihood of making unpleasant decisions with regard to denying admission.

Staff training and preparation

General introductory training to understand the response structure and the hospital's major incident plan is essential in dealing with any major emergency. Although the focus is likely to be the emergency department, critical care staff must be trained to provide an effective response.

Effective response training

This should include:
- Heightened disaster-response awareness.
- Enhanced skill sets
- Understanding of roles and responsibilities.
- Alternative communication methods.
- Self-preservation (personal safety) training.
- Experience in how to co-operate and co-ordinate during mayhem.

Initial training will help staff to understand the response processes in place, but simulations (either as table top exercises or as simulated events) are the most effective means of ensuring that staff engage and learn.

Training for terrorist events

Training should cover not only the processes for emergency response, but the systems used to triage patients, the types of injury and their management, and individual roles and general staff response to a major casualty event.

Different types of terrorist attack, including bomb blasts, chemical and nerve agents, and bioterrorism should all be covered.

Training for influenza pandemics

Advance training on personal protective equipment is an essential aspect of critical care training. This will include protective mask fit testing (to ensure that masks are effective), safety procedures for preventing exposure of other patients, and what to do if protection is breached.

Procedures to ensure that relatives are not exposed to infection, or do not expose staff and others to infection, must also be considered.

Blast injury

Victims of blast injuries experience trauma from a number of sources. The initial source is from the blast wave, and this is often accompanied by blunt or penetrating trauma associated with projectile debris from the explosive device or the surrounding area. Further injury (tertiary) can occur from being thrown against stationary objects or from building collapse. There may also be exposure to toxic or radioactive substances (quaternary injury).

The predominant injuries seen following bomb blasts are pulmonary, abdominal, orthopaedic (including soft tissue), neurological, and otological.

Blast wave or primary injury

Injuries are caused by the slamming effect of the high pressure energy wave impacting on the body. This causes injuries to hollow organs, such as ears, respiratory tract, and abdominal viscera. These injuries may have little in the way of external evidence of trauma so patients require careful assessment for any clinical manifestations (see Table 18.1).

Blast wave-related traumatic brain injury is also frequent and has the hallmark of diffuse brain injury. This is thought to be related to kinetic energy transfer of the blast pressure to the CNS.

Secondary injuries

These are commonly multiple, involving shrapnel wounds, traumatic amputations, fractures, and internal injuries. Victims may also receive extensive burns from the blast energy and blast-related fire. These injuries can lead rapidly to haemorrhagic shock and a severe systemic inflammatory response syndrome, and require immediate and effective treatment.

Management of blast injuries

- Immediate management will follow the ABCDE priorities of any acute trauma (see 📖 Initial management, p. 406). A primary assessment is needed to ensure that ABC are supported, followed by a thorough secondary assessment (see Table 18.1).
- **Airway:** should be secured by endotracheal intubation if there are signs of compromise, upper airway burns or smoke inhalation, or impending respiratory failure.
- **Breathing:** adequate arterial oxygen saturations should be maintained with additional inspired oxygen + mechanical ventilation. If there are concerns about pulmonary blast injury, care should be taken not to deliver too much fluid during resuscitation.
- **Circulation:** maintenance of an adequate circulating intravascular volume and organ perfusion, by filling against markers such as blood pressure, CVP, urine output, and metabolic acidosis. Hypotension requires correction usually with whole blood, clear fluids (colloid/crystalloid) and blood products to maintain haemostasis.

Table 18.1 Assessment of blast injury

Type of injury	Pathology	Clinical signs
Primary blast injury	Blast lung (alveolar rupture, pneumothorax, pulmonary contusion and haemorrhage)	Tachypnoea Hypoxaemia Cyanosis Wheezing Decreased breath sounds Haemoptysis Cough Chest pain Dyspnoea Haemodynamic instability
	Tympanic membrane rupture and damage	Deafness Bleeding from the ear
	Abdominal haemorrhage and perforation	Abdominal pain and rectal bleeding Liver or spleen lacerations Rebound tenderness Guarding Absent bowel sounds Signs of hypovolaemia Nausea and vomiting
	Traumatic brain injury	Loss of consciousness Headache Fatigue Poor concentration Lethargy Amnesia

Further information

Centers for Disease Prevention and Control (August 2008). Available at: http://www.bt.cdc.gov/masscasualties/explosions.asp

Serious infectious epidemics

This includes both flu pandemics and sudden serious infections, such as SARS. Pandemic flu could result from a new viral strain to which few people would be immune and would affect large numbers of the population. Traditional vaccinations, such as those made for seasonal flu, could not be developed in time to prevent large numbers of people becoming infected. Concern about avian flu (H5N1) is due to the possibility of mutation by this virus to become transmissible between humans. Currently, it is passed only from bird to bird, or from very close contact between humans and birds.

Definitions

• **Flu pandemic:** virulent human flu that causes a global outbreak or pandemic of serious illness.
• **SARS:** a virulent atypical pneumonia developed as the result of cross-over to humans of a coronavirus from palm civets in 2003 in China.

Critical care pandemic planning

One of the most important aspects of planning is determination of capacity and how capacity can be increased. Computer modelling for a flu pandemic suggests that an increase of up to 75% in critical care resources will be required during the initial 6 weeks. This is with a background of increased staff sickness or absence due to child care, etc. Guidance from the Department of Health suggests that approximately 50% of the population will develop symptoms, with up to 4% requiring hospital admission and 25% of hospital admissions expected to require level 3 critical care. In a population base of 56 million people, this equates to 30 000 critical care admissions. Is this sustainable?

Planning should focus on the ability to sustain a response over several weeks, and with a series of waves of patients lasting between 6 and 15 weeks for up to a year.

Managing the demand for critical care

A form of triage is necessary to ensure that the most appropriate patients receive critical care. This should apply to both patients with and without influenza.

Strategies to increase capacity within critical care should include:
• Identification of additional areas, such as theatre recovery areas, where critical care patients can be cared for.
• Identification of staff with basic skills who could work with critical care staff as a team in a pyramid-style grouping, overseen by trained critical care nurses.

- **Offering mass 'critical care':** provision on general wards and recovery units of a few key interventions, such as high flow oxygen therapy, to many patients, rather than comprehensive intensive interventions to a few.
- Prior discussion with staff about what is expected of them and how this would be managed.

Further information

Christian MD, Lapinsky SE, Stewart TE. (2007) Critical care pandemic preparedness primer. In: Vincent JL (ed.) *2007 Yearbook of Intensive Care Medicine*. Berlin: Springer, pp. 999–1010.

Haematology

Blood cells: types, terms, and normal values

Blood cell types
- Erythrocytes.
- Thrombocytes (platelets).
- Leukocytes:
  - neutrophils;
  - eosinophils;
  - basophils;
  - monocytes;
  - lymphocytes.

Terms associated with blood cells
- **Anaemia:** haemoglobin <11.5g/dl in the adult female or <13g/dl in the adult male.
- **Polycythaemia:** red cell count >6 × 10^{12}/l or Hb >18g/dl.
- **Leukopenia:** white cell count <4 × 10^9/l.
- **Leukocytosis:** white cell count >11 × 10^9/l.
- **Neutropenia:** neutrophil count <1.0 × 10^9/l.
- **Eosinophilia:** eosinophil count >0.4 × 10^9/l.
- **Lymphocytosis:** lymphocyte count >3.5 × 10^9/l.
- **Monocytosis:** monocyte count >0.8 × 10^9/l.
- **Agranulocytosis:** the bone marrow stops producing white cells, causing neutropenia/leukopenia. This leaves the body open to over-whelming infection. Often caused by irradiation, chemotherapy or drug toxicity (e.g. carbimazole).
- **Thrombocytopenia:** platelet count <150 × 10^9/l. Bleeding is unlikely to occur unless the count is <50 × 10^9/l. Results from increased destruction, increased consumption or decreased production of platelets.

Table 19.1 Normal values

Cell type	Normal adult value
Erythrocyte	Male: 3.8–5.6 × 10^{12}/l Female: 3.4–5. × 10^{12}/l
Thrombocyte	150–400 × 10^9/l
Leukocyte	4.0–11.0 × 10^9/l
Neutrophil	2.0–8.0 × 10^9/l
Eosinophil	0.1–0.5 × 10^9/l
Basophil	0.01–0.1 × 10^9/l
Monocyte	0.1–0.8 × 10^9/l
Lymphocyte	1.0–4.0 × 10^9/l

Erythrocyte disorders

Polycythaemia

An increase in red cell count >6 × 10^{12}/l or Hb >18 g/dl

Primary polycythaemia: blood cell mass (red cells, white cells, and platelets) increase due to excessive production in the bone marrow. The increased viscosity of the blood can cause cardiovascular, neurological, and vascular complications.

Treatment

Reduce viscosity of the blood by:
• Venesection to keep haematocrit <50%.
• Concurrent volume replacement with crystalloid.
• Aspirin to decrease platelet function and adhesion.
• Cytarbarine to reduce platelet production.
• Radioactive phosphorus or chemotherapy to depress bone marrow production.

Secondary polycythaemia: the red cell count increases in response to chronic hypoxaemia causing increased erythrocyte production (e.g. COPD, congenital cyanotic heart disease, adaptation to high altitude).

Sickle cell anaemia

Adult Hb (HbA) contains two alpha and two beta chains. There are two genes for the synthesis of each chain. Sickle cell Hb (HbS) contains two abnormal beta chains and is inherited as an autosomal dominant gene. When exposed to low oxygen tensions the red cells become deformed, rigid and sickle shaped. The cells can become lodged and aggregate in any part of the body causing ischemia or infarction. Abnormal cells are prematurely destroyed, resulting in a chronic, haemolytic anaemia.

Patients with sickle cell trait (<50% HbS) are usually symptom-free unless the oxygen tension is very low.

Sickle cell crisis

Acute haemolytic crises can occur from 6 months of age and may be precipitated by dehydration and hypoxia. This can result in:
• Anaemia.
• Jaundice.
• Tachycardia.
• Cardiomegaly.
• Splenic sequestration (causes spleen to enlarge, splenic function to deteriorate, and increase risk of overwhelming infection).
• Pulmonary sequestration causing hypoxaemia (can lead to rapid deterioration and death).
• Vaso-occlusion causing infarction of tissues (e.g. bone, spleen, gut, brain or lung) can cause severe pain. Often precipitated by cold, dehydration, infection, ischaemia.
• Haematuria.
• Swelling of toes and fingers.
• Fever.
• Abdominal pain.

Management
- Correction/prevention of hypoxaemia:
  - steady state values of Hb and oxygen saturation when the patient is clinically well should be used as a target for treatment. Hb levels in the steady state may be only 5–9g/dl;
  - monitor blood gases;
  - pulse oximetry (S_pO_2 may be <90% in the steady state);
  - oxygen therapy/respiratory support/mechanical ventilation.
- Rehydration:
  - fluid replacement (dilutes blood and decreases agglutination of sickled cells in small vessels);
  - NB. Fluid overload may precipitate heart failure in patients with cardiomyopathy (common problem in adult sickle cell patients).
- Analgesia: oral analgesia/anti-inflammatory drugs/opiates (e.g. PCA).
- Infection:
  - monitor temperature, white cell count, and markers such as CRP;
  - treat any underlying infection;
  - patients with splenic dysfunction are prone to infection with encapsulated organisms, e.g. *Pneumococcus* and *Meningococcus*, and may require long-term prophylactic penicillin.
- Blood transfusion: an exchange blood transfusion with fresh donor blood (e.g. 4 Units) is used to reduce levels of HbS during severe crises, e.g. acute haemolysis leading to a rapid drop in Hb, pulmonary, or cerebral crises, severe painful crises not responding to other therapy, or before elective surgery.

Leukocyte disorders

Neutropenia

Defined as a neutrophil count $<2 \times 10^9/l$. The risk of developing life threatening infection is higher with counts $<1 \times 10^9/l$ and such patients are often isolated until the marrow recovers. Patients are often asymptomatic until infection develops. Common initial infections include *Pneumococci, Staphylococci* and coliforms. After prolonged immunosuppression and repeated courses of antibiotics, *Pseudomonas*, fungi (candida, aspergillus,), TB, cytomegalovirus, and *Pneumocystis* infection may occur.

Causes

- Bone marrow failure (leukaemia, myeloma, lymphoma, chemotherapy, radiation).
- Systemic inflammation following severe infection or trauma (causes aggregation of neutrophils in vital organs).
- Infections (typhoid, brucellosis, viral, protozoal).
- Drug-related (e.g. carbimazole, sulphonamides).
- Destruction by neutrophil antibodies (e.g. SLE, rheumatoid arthritis).
- Deficiency of Vitamin B12 or folate, malnutrition.
- Hypersplenism (increased neutrophil destruction).

Management

- Discontinuation of implicated drug therapy.
- Protective isolation if neutrophil count $<1.0 \times 10^9/l$ (laminar flow air conditioning if available). Avoid uncooked foods, e.g. salads.
- Strict aseptic procedures.
- Minimize invasive procedures and practice strict infection control.
- Personal hygiene – skin, eye and mouth care. Nystatin mouthwashes for oral thrush, clotrimazole for fungal skin infections.
- Bone marrow biopsy and aspiration if no diagnosis has been made.
- Parenteral antibiotics (broad spectrum if no organism isolated).
- Regular surveillance for infection and specific treatment if identified.
- Growth factors, e.g. granulocyte-colony stimulating factor (G-CSF), to stimulate bone marrow.

Leukaemia

A neoplastic disorder of the blood cell-forming tissues (bone marrow, spleen, and lymphatic system) causing unregulated and prolific accumulation of white cells in the bone marrow, liver, spleen, and lymph nodes, and invasion of the gastrointestinal tract, meninges, skin, and/or kidneys.

Types

Classified according to the cell line involved; either acute or chronic.

Acute lymphatic leukaemia (ALL)

Common in children. A severe disease where lymph nodes, bone, and nervous tissue become infiltrated. Therapy aims to induce remission by cytotoxic drugs and irradiation of the CNS. 50% of children age 2–11 survive for 5 years.

Chronic lymphatic leukaemia (CLL)

Mainly in adults >50 years. Often symptom-free. Pleural or peritoneal effusions may develop. No treatment needed if asymptomatic. Chemotherapy or radiotherapy can reduce the size of swollen glands. 50% survive for 5 years.

Acute myeloid leukaemia (AML)

Affects any age, but more common in adults. Intensive chemotherapy regimens and bone marrow transplantation allow 30–50% to survive long-term.

Chronic myeloid leukaemia (CML)

Usually occurs in the 30–50 years age group. Insidious onset with fever and weight loss. Splenomegaly, hepatomegaly, and thrombocytopenia develop later with high white count. Survival with chemotherapy is about 3 years. With allogenic bone marrow transplantation, 50% may survive >5 years.

Thrombocyte disorders

Thrombocytopenia

Defined as a platelet count <150 × 10^9/l. Bleeding is unlikely to occur unless the count falls <50 × 10^9/l unless generalized infection is present. It is caused by increased destruction, increased consumption and/or decreased production of platelets

Causes of increased destruction/consumption of platelets

- Idiopathic thrombocytopenia purpura (ITP).
- Thrombotic thrombocytopenic purpura (TTP).
- Disseminated intravascular coagulation (DIC).
- Drugs (e.g. heparin causing heparin-induced thrombocytopenia syndrome (HITS).
- Sepsis.
- Haemorrhage.
- Autoimmune disorders (AIDS, malaria).
- Extra-corporeal circulation (e.g. dialysis).
- Hypersplenism.

Causes of decreased platelet production

- Drugs (e.g. chemotherapy).
- Uraemia.
- Megoblastic anaemia.
- Marrow infiltration, e.g. leukaemia, carcinoma, lymphoma.

Idiopathic thrombocytopenic purpura

Autoimmune disorder, where autoantibodies are directed against plate-lets, considerably shortening their lifespan. More common in young adults, particularly following respiratory or gastrointestinal viral infections. May be acute or chronic.

Manifestations include:
- Petechiae, multiple bruising, epistaxis.
- Low platelet count.
- Prolonged bleeding time, but normal coagulation times.

Treatment

There is no definitive treatment:
- In the acute form, steroids tend not to increase the platelet count, but may reduce the incidence of bleeding. High dose gamma globulin may be advocated in patients with bleeding complications.
- Platelet transfusions are generally avoided unless severe bleeding occurs.
- In the chronic form steroids may cause a rise in platelets.
- Blood transfusion if severe bleeding and anaemia.
- Intravenous immunoglobulin.
- Immunosuppression.
- Rituximab (an anti-CD20 monoclonal antibody that depletes B cells).
- Splenectomy, if unresponsive to medical management.

Thrombotic thrombcytopenic purpura, thrombotic microangiopathy and haemolytic uraemic syndrome

Thrombotic thrombocytopenic purpura (TTP) is a disorder character-ized by fever, thrombotic microangiopathy (TMA), haemolytic anaemia, neurological symptoms (including drowsiness, transient or permanent strokes, blindness), and renal dysfunction. TTP has many clinical similari-ties to haemolytic uraemic syndrome (HUS). However, HUS predomi-nantly affects the kidney (and children) and usually follows a diarrhoeal illness, while TTP more frequently affects the brain and adults. TTP is linked to a deficiency of ADAMTS-13 (a disintegrin and metallopro-tease with thrombospondin motifs 13) that cleaves von Willebrand factor (vWF), a multimeric protein released from stimulated endothelium that mediates platelet adhesion and aggregation. Deficiency thus results in persistence of these large vWG multimers that occlude the microcir-culation. ADAMTS-13 deficiency may be idiopathic or can occur during severe sepsis. Thrombotic microangiopathy (TMA) can occur with normal ADAMTS-13 levels – it may be idiopathic or triggered by infection, carci-noma, transplantation, autoimmune diseases, or drugs.

Symptoms
• Abdominal pain.
• Purpura.
• Fever.
• Hypertension.
• Neurological signs.
• Haematuria (may progress to renal failure).

Treatment
• Plasma exchange (using FFP to replace deficient ADAMTS-13).
• Steroids.
• Intravenous immunoglobulin.
• Immunosuppression.
• Rituximab (anti-CD20 monoclonal antibody that depletes B cells).
• Avoidance of platelet transfusion unless severe bleeding.

Drug-induced thrombocytopenia
Causes
Numerous drugs can cause thrombocytopenia including:
• Heparin.
• Quinine.
• Antituberculous drugs.
• Thiazide diuretics.
• Penicillins.
• Sulphonamides.
• Anticonvulsants.
• Chemotherapy.

Heparin-induced thrombocytopenia syndrome (HITS)
Antibodies generated during exposure to heparin affect platelet activation and cause endothelial dysfunction. Approximately 17% of patients treated with unfractionated heparin and 8% treated with low molecular-weight

heparin (LMWH) will form antibodies against complexes of platelet factor-4 (PF4) and heparin. However, most affected patients do not suffer clinical consequences, but up to 20% will develop thrombocytopenia, arterial, or venous thrombosis with, occasionally, significant thrombo-emboli, bleeding, and even death. It can rarely occur within hours of even transient exposure to heparinoids, but typically appears after 7–10 days' use.

HITS is responsible for only 0.3–0.5% of thrombocytopenia in the ICU. Much commoner aetiologies include sepsis, and immune-mediated, drug, transfusion, and foreign body (graft) reactions.

HITs is diagnosed by the presence of thrombocytopenia, prior exposure to heparinoids, and the laboratory detection of autoantibodies.

Treatment

Treatment of drug-induced thrombocytopenia is supportive and includes discontinuation of the offending drug. Platelet transfusions may be needed for active bleeding or if levels are very low. For HITS there should be total avoidance of heparin administration (including the small amounts used in arterial flush solutions). As up to 50% will develop a thrombo-embolic event when taken off heparin and not continued on any anticoagulation, an alternative anticoagulant should be commenced promptly. As thrombin generation plays a prominent role, direct thrombin inhibitors, such as lepirudin are often used, but these can cause bleeding for which there is no antidote. Heparinoids (e.g. danaparoid) can be substituted though crossreactivity can occur in up to 20% of cases. Low molecular weight heparin and warfarin are not generally used in the first instance.

Anticoagulation therapy

Used to prevent thrombus formation or extension of an existing thrombus. Haemorrhage is a potential complication. Patients being anticoagulated must be observed closely for signs of bleeding:

- Test urine daily for blood.
- Observe and test tracheal and nasogastric aspirate for blood.
- Observe cannulae sites, wounds, and drains for bleeding.
- Observe skin for purpura and bruising.
- Regular laboratory coagulation screens.
- Avoid vigorous endotracheal or nasogastric tube suction.
- Place lines and tubes either after cessation of anticoagulant for sufficient time, or after correction of coagulopathy.

Common anticoagulants

Heparin

Given intravenously, heparin has a rapid onset of action with a half-life of 90 min. Overdose can be reversed with protamine sulphate (1mg neutralizes 100IU of heparin).

Subcutaneous low molecular-weight heparin (e.g. enoxaparin, dalteparin) is now the treatment of choice for thromboprophylaxis, or for treatment of DVT, or pulmonary embolus (can be given iv or sc). It is also used for acute coronary syndromes. Fixed dosages are given and no laboratory monitoring is necessary.

Unfractionated heparin given by continuous infusion is recommended for patients in renal failure and for anticoagulation of extracorporeal circuits (e.g. haemofiltration, cardiopulmonary bypass). Dosage is monitored by the activated partial thromboplastin time (aPTT).

Warfarin

Given orally, it takes at least 3–5 days' loading to achieve full anticoagulation. Therefore, heparin cover should be provided for 72h when warfarin is commenced. Blood levels of free warfarin rise with some drugs (e.g. aspirin, amiodarone). Dosage is controlled using the international normalized ratio (INR) and a ratio of 2:3 is usually targeted for adequate anticoagulation. Excess levels are treated by reducing or temporarily discontinuing warfarin. If very high or symptomatic Vitamin K (may take 24h for effect and has a long-lasting effect thereafter preventing prompt re-institution of warfarin) or FFP can be given. For life-threatening bleeding, activated prothrombin complex concentrates (e.g. Octaplex®) should be given (in preference to FFP) in conjunction with a minimum dose of vitamin K 5mg iv.

Indications for use:
- Long-term thromboprophylaxis (e.g. atrial fibrillation, metal heart valves).
- Long-term anticoagulation for thrombosis/emboli.

Prostacyclin/epoprostenol (PGI₂) or prostin (PGE₁)

Given by iv infusion. Works by inhibiting platelet aggregation. Effect disappears within 30min of discontinuation. These drugs vasodilate, and can cause flushing, hypotension, and tachycardia.

Indications for use
- As an alternative to heparin in renal replacement therapy.
- Pulmonary hypertension.
- Poor gas exchange in ARDS (nebulized).
- Digital ischaemia (e.g. severe sepsis, autoimmune disease).

Thrombolytics, e.g. streptokinase, tissue plasminogen activator (tPA)

Used to break down a thrombus that has already formed. Allergic reactions can occur and are more likely with streptokinase. tPA and newer related agents (e.g. reteplase, tenecteplase) are easier to administer, but need to be given with heparin. Bleeding may be a major complication – correct with the antifibrinolytic agent, tranexamic acid plus FFP, cryoprecipitate, and blood transfusion as necessary.

Indications for use
- Acute myocardial infarction.
- Pulmonary embolism.
- May be infused locally for distal emboli (e.g. in leg).

Less frequently used anticoagulants

Direct thrombin inhibitors (e.g. lepirudin, argatroban)

Lepirudin is a recombinant form of hirudin (extracted from leeches), while argatroban is derived from arginine. Both form an irreversible complex with thrombin. These drugs are unrelated to and not affected by heparin. Antibody formation occurs in approximately 40% of patients treated with lepirudin >6 days. These drugs have long half-lives and as there are no antidotes, they are contraindicated in patients with active haemorrhage. Bivalirudin is related to hirudin but is reversible with a short half-life of only 25min.

Danaparoid

This is a heparanoid given intravenously with similarities to heparin. Its use is generally restricted to the treatment of heparin-induced thrombocytopenia syndrome and DVT prophylaxis, although there is a 10–20% risk of cross-reactivity. No antidote is available.

Clotting disorders

Disseminated intravascular coagulation

DIC is an excessive systematic activation of the coagulation cascade leading to excess generation of thrombin and fibrin within circulating blood leading to formation of microthrombi. The resulting depletion of clotting factors can lead to haemorrhage that may be relatively mild (e.g. into skin, haematuria, around catheter, and drain sites) or severe (e.g. major gastrointestinal bleed). It arises as a secondary complication of an underlying condition.

Disorders that may trigger DIC
- Infection (bacterial, viral, parasitic).
- Obstetric disorders (e.g. septic abortion, eclampsia, amniotic fluid embolism, placental abruption).
- Liver disorders (cirrhosis, cholestasis, acute hepatic necrosis).
- Malignant disease (carcinoma, leukaemia).
- Trauma (e.g. crush injuries, burns).
- Hypovolaemic shock.
- Pulmonary embolism, fat embolism.
- Organ transplant rejection.
- Heat stroke.
- Blood transfusion reaction.
- Extracorporeal circulatory bypass.
- Acute pancreatitis.
- Snake venoms.

Symptoms
- Haemorrhage.
- Respiratory failure due to haemorrhage, haemothorax, embolism.
- Renal failure due to microemboli or hypovolaemia.
- Cerebral ischaemia/infarction (haemorrhage, thrombus).
- Gastrointestinal haemorrhage.
- Small bowel infarction due to mesenteric embolus.
- Skin petechiae, purpura, bruising, and necrosis from decreased capillary refill and/or infarction.

Management
- Adequate fluid replacement and restoration of tissue perfusion.
- Treatment of underlying cause, e.g. sepsis.
- Transfusions of blood, FFP, platelets and cryoprecipitate as needed.
- Careful monitoring of haemodynamics and arterial blood gases.
- Observe endotracheal and nasogastric aspirate, urine and stool for blood.
- Observe skin and extremities.
- Regular blood tests particularly clotting screen (including fibrinogen, thrombin time and D-dimers).
- Heparin is not usually given and platelet transfusion avoided if not actively bleeding.

Laboratory values in DIC
- Prolonged prothrombin time >15s.
- Prolonged partial thromboplastin time >60–90s.
- Prolonged thrombin time >15–20s.
- Low fibrinogen levels <75–100mg/dl.
- Low platelet count (<20–75) × 10^9/l.
- High FDPs > 100mg/ml.
- Raised levels of D-dimers.
- NB. Not all results need be abnormal.

Uraemia

Can cause platelet dysfunction. Bleeding can be a serious consequence of severe renal failure.

Symptoms
- Prolonged bleeding time.
- Gastrointestinal bleeding.
- Epistaxis.
- Purpura.
- Pericarditis.
- Cerebral haemorrhage.

Treatment
- Blood transfusion.
- Desmopressin acetate will increase platelet adhesion, but should be used sparingly, e.g. for bleeding or prior to emergency surgery.
- Renal replacement therapy (use epoprostenol (prostacyclin), prostaglandin E1, or low-dose heparin to maintain patency of the circuit).

Liver disease

Bleeding associated with liver disease can be severe and difficult to manage.
- The liver produces nearly all the factors involved in the formation and control of coagulation (except factors IV and VIII).
- Fat-soluble vitamin K (necessary for the precursors of factors II, VII, IX, and X) may not be absorbed if cholestasis is present.
- DIC can be initiated or exacerbated by the release of tissue thromboplastin from damaged liver cells.
- PT and PTT are prolonged; low fibrinogen levels indicate severe disease or the presence of DIC.
- Fibrin degradation products may be elevated due to excessive fibrinolysis or because damaged liver cells fail to clear them from the blood.

Treatment
- Vitamin K.
- FFP and platelet transfusions to increase platelet levels and improve prothrombin time.
- Cryoprecipitate to increase fibrinogen levels.

Haemophilia

A sex-linked genetic disorder affecting men, but carried by women. Can cause severe bleeding from minor trauma, and disabling muscle and joint haemorrhages

- **Haemophilia A:** caused by deficiency of factor VIII.
- **Haemophilia B:** caused by deficiency of factor IX.

Treatment

- Administer purified factor VIII or IX concentrate (give prophylactically prior to surgery or dental extraction).
- Aim to raise the factor to above 30% of normal.
- Repeat infusions every 8–10hr as necessary.
- Never give aspirin as this impairs platelet function.
- Avoid intramuscular injections.
- Dental hygiene is important as extraction is hazardous.

Blood and blood component products

Blood and blood products

- All blood in Western Europe and in most of North America is now leukoreduced or depleted. Though initially intended to reduce the risk of prion transmission, its use is associated with decreased adverse reactions and improved outcomes in critically ill patients and those undergoing major elective surgery.
- Blood should be stored at 4°C in a dedicated blood fridge.
- Do not remove from fridge for more than 30min prior to use.
- Red cells may remain viable for up to 5 weeks, although oxygen carrying capacity decreases with age.
- Red blood cell transfusion contains no therapeutic amounts of clotting factors, apart from fibrinogen, and no viable platelets.

Stored whole blood
Used to restore red cell number and circulating blood volume in acute haemorrhage.

Packed red cells (red cell concentrate)
- Plasma is removed from whole blood leaving a concentrated solution of red cells to which 80ml of anticoagulant solution is added.
- Used in anaemic patients with chronic, persistent blood loss or bone marrow failure, or in heart failure patients to reduce risk of volume overload.
- Can be specifically CMV-negative or irradiated.
- Transfusion of 4ml/kg packed cells should raise Hb by ~1g/dl.

Frozen red cells
- Contains red cells, uncontaminated by other cells or plasma, in a suspending medium.
- Used in patients who have a rare blood group (blood is donated and then frozen for future use).
- Use within 12h of thawing.

Platelets
- Platelet concentrate is prepared in 30–50ml of donor plasma.
- Usually issued in pools of six packs or one combined pack.
- Once ready, platelet function is best preserved at room temperature.
- Use within 72h.
- Transfuse as rapidly as tolerated, complete infusion within 30min.
- Transfuse via a 170mm in-line filter; specific platelet giving sets are available.

Fresh frozen plasma (FFP)
- Plasma is separated and then frozen.
- Contains normal amounts of clotting factors.
- Use within 4h of thawing.
- Packs contain 150–250ml.
- Transfuse via a 170mm in-line filter as fast as patient can tolerate.

Cryoprecipitate
- Prepared from FFP.
- Contains factor VIII, fibronectin, and fibrinogen in 20ml donor plasma.
- Used to provide replacement factors in haemophilia and von Willebrand's disease, or in patients with major bleeding associated with hypofibrinogenaemia or uraemia.
- Prepared in pools of 6 Units.
- Transfuse through a 170mm in-line filter as rapidly as the patient's condition allows.

Adverse reactions to blood transfusions

Transfusion reactions due to pyrogens, allergens, bacteria, or incompatible blood usually occur within 20min of starting the transfusion. Monitoring (including haemodynamics and temperature) is essential throughout this period.

Febrile non-haemolytic reactions

Causes
- Incompatibility of donor red cells, white cells, platelets, or plasma proteins (main cause).
- Anti-HLA (human lymphocyte antibodies), granulocyte- and platelet-specific antibodies in the recipient as a result of sensitization during pregnancy or previous transfusions.
- Pyrogens (rare).

Symptoms
- Pyrexia.
- Urticaria.
- Pruritis.

Management
- Antipyretics (aspirin, paracetamol).
- Antihistamine (e.g. chlorpheniramine).
- Hydrocortisone.
- Continue transfusion slowly if only mild reaction.
- Stop transfusion if rigors or fever >38°C.
- Send implicated bag of blood to laboratory for examination.

Acute haemolytic reactions

Causes
- Incompatible ABO blood group.
- Incorrectly stored blood.
- Out-of-date blood.
- Over-heated blood.
- Frozen blood.
- Infected blood.
- Mechanical destruction of the red cells due to administering the infusion under pressure.
- Mixing of blood with hypotonic infusion fluids.

Symptoms
- Pain at infusion site.
- Pyrexia, facial flushing, rigors, nausea, vomiting.
- Dyspnoea.
- Headache, chest, abdominal and loin pain.
- Tachycardia and hypotension leading to circulatory collapse.
- Oliguria and renal failure.
- DIC (disseminated intravascular coagulation).

Management
- Stop blood transfusion immediately.
- Retain bag and return to the laboratory with samples of blood from patient to check blood group, FBC, coagulation screen, fibrinogen, urea and electrolytes, and direct antiglobulin test.
- Take blood cultures if sepsis is suspected.
- Take urine sample for haemoglobinuria.
- Full resuscitative measures may be required including ventilation.
- Continuous cardiovascular monitoring.
- 12-lead ECG.
- Maintain urine output >1ml/kg/h.
- if DIC develops, clotting factor replacement may be required.
- renal support if renal failure develops.

Circulatory overload

Can occur in the elderly or pregnant patient and those with abnormal cardiac or renal function. Such patients are less able to tolerate the fluid load associated with transfusion and can develop pulmonary oedema and heart failure.

Symptoms
- Dyspnoea, tachypnoea.
- Hypertension.
- Elevated JVP.
- Tachycardia.

Management
- Continuous cardiovascular monitoring.
- Diuretics.
- Avoid by administering diuretic at the beginning of transfusion and using red cell concentrate.

Transfusion-associated graft versus host disease

Rare, but usually fatal. Caused by engraftment of viable T lymphocytes, which cause widespread tissue damage. Can occur in immunosuppressed patients (e.g. bone marrow transplant recipients). Can be prevented by irradiating blood products (red cell, platelet and white cell) prior to transfusion.

Transfusion-related acute lung injury (TRALI)

This is associated with the presence of leukocyte antibodies in donor blood. Features typically occurring within 1–2h of transfusion. Include chills, fever, a non-productive cough, dyspnoea, cyanosis, hypotension unresponsive to fluid challenge (10–15%), or hypertension (15%). Radiological signs include bilateral pulmonary infiltrates and scattered opacities. Cardiac filling pressures are not raised.

In the USA, TRALI is estimated to occur once in every 5000 transfusions, although this is probably a serious underestimate in critically ill patients as the diagnosis depends on normal lungs prior to transfusion.

Hazards of blood transfusions

Bacterial contamination

Contamination of blood is rare, but may be lethal. Contaminants from the donor's skin can enter the blood during donation. Gram-negative bacteria grow slowly at $4°C$, but accelerate at room temperature. Onset of pyrexia and circulatory collapse can be rapid.

Transmission of disease

Donor selection criteria and testing of donor blood for infectious agents have decreased transmission of disease, but not completely eradicated it

Potential transmission includes:
- Hepatitis B and C.
- Cytomegalovirus (CMV).
- Malaria.
- HIV.

Hazards of massive blood transfusion

Defined as the transfusion of the patient's own volume of blood within a 24h period.

Hypothermia
- Stored blood is cold ($4°C$) and can rapidly cool the patient. Use a thermostatically-controlled blood warmer if giving more than several units of blood to a normothermic patient (may not be necessary if the patient is pyrexial).
- Hypothermia increases the risk of cardiac arrhythmias, reduces metabolism, and shifts the oxygen dissociation curve to the left.
- Citrate toxicity (q.v.) is more likely if the patient is hypothermic.

Acid-base and electrolyte disturbances
- Stored blood is acidic (pH 6.6–6.8) due to the citric acid used as an anticoagulant and lactic acid generated during storage. Both are metabolized by the liver in the well-perfused patient, but may cause a metabolic acidosis in the hypoperfused patient or the patient with liver failure. Monitor with regular acid-base measurements.
- The sodium content of whole blood and FFP is higher than in normal blood due to the sodium citrate anticoagulant. Monitor Na^+ (particularly in patients with renal failure and hypernatraemia).

Hypocalcaemia
- Stored blood contain anticoagulants such as citrate that can cause calcium depletion. Monitor ionized calcium levels and give supplements as necessary.
- Observe for tetany, muscle tremors, cardiac dysfunction, prolonged Q–T interval on ECG.

Haemostatic failure
- Stored blood contains no viable platelets and few clotting factors. Large transfusions may cause dilutional thrombocytopenia and an increased PT and aPTT.
- Give FFP according to the aPTT or, empirically, as 2 units per 10 units of blood transfused.

Haematological malignancy

Patients with life threatening, but potentially reversible complications can benefit from ICU admission. Reasons for admission include:
- Infection and sepsis.
- Haemorrhage.
- Cardiovascular disturbances, including arrhythmias.
- Graft versus host reactions.
- Tumour lysis syndrome.
- Hypercalcaemia.
- Fluid overload/renal failure.
- Respiratory failure.
- Following extensive surgical procedures.

Infection
- Such patients are often immunosuppressed and neutropenic, and thus at increased risk.
- Broad spectrum antibiotics suppress normal gut flora and can promote overgrowth of pathogenic Gram-negative organisms.
- Chemotherapy can cause ulceration of the G-I tract which can act as a focus for local colonisation
- Their immunosuppressed state increases the risk of opportunistic infections, including fungal (*Candida, Aspergillus*), viral (e.g. CMV, *Herpes simplex*) and protozoal (pneumocystis), as well as bacterial. Infection may result in septic shock, respiratory failure, or meningoencephalitis.
- Keep invasive procedures to a minimum; use tunnelled, large bore, soft Teflon catheters (e.g. Hickman) for iv drug administration.
- Maintain scrupulous infection control.

Haemorrhage
- Such patients are often thrombocytopenic due to bone marrow suppression/infiltration by tumour, cytotoxic drugs, and sequestration of platelets in spleen, or may have liver disease from the underlying tumour or as an adverse effect related to therapy.
- DIC may also be present secondary to infection or the malignancy.

Cardiac disturbances
- Commonest cause is cytotoxic drug therapy. Can cause congestive cardiac failure, direct endothelial damage, myocardial necrosis, cardio-myopathy, dysrhythmias.
- Cardiac tamponade from metastatic tumour, bleeding.
- Restrictive pericarditis (radiotherapy, tumour extending around heart).

Graft versus host disease
- Autoimmune reaction affecting allogenic bone marrow transplants.
- Immunocompetent donor T lymphocytes recognize the host histocompatibility antigens as 'foreign' and produce a cell-mediated reaction against sensitive tissue, e.g. skin, GI tract, liver, bone marrow. It can present with fever, diarrhoea, severe mucositis, skin rashes, hepatitis.
- Mortality is 25% – treat with steroids and supportive care.

Tumour lysis syndrome

- Rapid lysis of malignant cells by cytotoxic drugs results in large purine load with hyperkalaemia, hyperuricaemia, hyperphosphataemia, and acute renal failure.
- Keep patient well hydrated and maintain good diuresis.
- Give prophylactic rasburicase or allopurinol prior to cytotoxic therapy – prevents tissue urate deposition and renal calculi (secondary to raised uric acid levels).

Hypercalcaemia

- Causes include infiltration of bone by tumour cells or stimulation of osteoclastic activity by mediators (osteoclastic-activating factor).
- **Treatment:** rehydration, diuretics (prevents calcium re-absorption in Loop of Henlé), calcitonin (inhibits osteoclastic bone re-absorption), sodium etidronate.

Respiratory failure

May be due to:

- Infection.
- Drug-induced lung disease.
- Radiation pneumonitis.
- Pulmonary haemorrhage.
- Malignant lung disease.
- Tracheobronchial compression.
- ARDS (secondary to sepsis, pulmonary aspiration, haemorrhage).
- Pleural effusion.
- Fluid overload.
- Cardiac failure.
- Pneumothorax.
- Following diagnostic surgical procedures (e.g. mediastinotomy).

Following extensive surgical procedures

Radical surgery (e.g. pelvic clearance) can cause considerable blood loss with resultant hypovolaemia. ICU admission permits:

- Continuous haemodynamic monitoring.
- Optimal fluid replacement.
- Adequate analgesia.
- Respiratory support.

Immunological disorders

Organs and cells of the immune system: an overview

Organs

Lymph nodes
- Structures lying along the course of the lymphatic network and aggregated in particular locations.
- Immunologically filter lymph before returning it to the circulation.
- Comprised mostly of T and B cells, dendritic cells, and macrophages.

Bone marrow
Produces all immune cells by a process known as haematopoiesis.

Thymus
Produces mature T cells from immature thymocytes that have migrated from the bone marrow, then release them into the bloodstream.

Spleen
- Contains B and T lymphocytes, macrophages, dendritic cells, natural killer cells, and red blood cells.
- Acts as an immunological filter and destroys old red cells.
- Migratory macrophages and dendritic cells bring antigens to the spleen. An immune response is initiated when these antigens are presented to the appropriate B or T cells.
- B cells become activated and produce antibodies.

Cells

B cells
- Produce antibodies in response to foreign proteins of bacteria, viruses, and tumour cells.
- Antibodies circulate in blood and lymph; these specifically recognize and bind to particular proteins and mark it for destruction by others.
- Some antibodies combine with antigens, activating a cascade of proteins (complement system) that circulate in an inactive form in the blood. They help destroy foreign invaders and remove them from the body.
- Other types of antibodies block viruses from entering cells.

T cells
- Circulate in the blood and lymph.
- Mark antigens for destruction; attack and destroy diseased cells recognized as foreign.

There are two types of functionally different T cells:
- T helper cells (CD4 cells):
  - co-ordinate immune regulation;
  - augment or potentiate immune responses by secreting substances that activate other white cells and macrophages;
  - alert B cells to make antibodies;
  - influence the type of antibody produced;
- T killer cells (CD8 cells):
  - direct killing of tumour cells, virally infected cells and parasites;
  - important in down regulation of immune system.

Natural killer cells (NK cells)
- Similar to T killer cells.
- Directly kill certain tumours (melanomas, lymphomas) and cell infecting viruses (CMV, herpes).

Dendritic cells
- Originate in bone marrow and found in peripheral lymph nodes, thymus, spleen, and blood.
- Present antigens to responsive T and B cells.
- Bind high amounts of HIV.

Phagocytes and granulocytes
- Phagocytes are large white cells that engulf and digest foreign invaders.
- Granulocytes contain chemicals within granules that destroy micro-organisms and play a key role in acute inflammatory reactions.
- Phagocytes include monocytes (circulating in blood), macrophages (fixed in tissues) and neutrophils (in blood, but move into tissues).
- Macrophages scavenge, secrete powerful chemicals and activate T cells.
- Neutrophils are both phagocytes and granulocytes; eosinophils and basophils are granulocytes.

Cytokines
- Diverse and potent chemical messengers.
- Recruit other cells and substances by binding to specific receptors on target cells.
- Encourage cell growth, promote cell activation, direct cellular traffic, and destroy target cells including cancer cells.

Antibodies
- Belong to a family of large protein molecules called immunoglobulins.
- Have unique antigen-binding sites that allows an antibody to recognize a matching antigen.
- Nine classes of human immunoglobulins – IgG (4 types), IgA (2 types), IgM, IgE, and IgD.

See 📖 Chapter 16, pp. 389–404, for further information.

The immunocompromised patient

The immunocompromised patient exhibits reduced resistance to infection due to an abnormality in the immune system. Causes include:

- Extremes of age.
- Nutritional deficiencies (e.g. malnutrition):
  - reduces the number of T cells;
  - depresses antibody responses;
  - zinc deficiency (can cause lymphoid atrophy).
- Previous exposure to vaccination or infection.
- Autoimmune disorders (e.g. SLE, rheumatoid arthritis).
- Genetic disorders.
- Drug therapy:
  - H_2 blockers (e.g. ranitidine) – neutropenia;
  - antibiotics (e.g. chloramphenicol can cause neutropenia);
  - cardiovascular drugs (e.g. propranolol can cause neutropenia, while catecholamines increase anti-inflammatory mediator production);
  - non-steroidal anti-inflammatory drugs – neutropenia;
  - heparin – inhibits neutrophil adhesion;
  - propofol – inhibits B-cell proliferation, and reduces neutrophil chemotaxis;
  - specific immunosuppressive drugs (e.g. steroids, cytotoxic drugs, monoclonal antibodies).
- Specific infections (e.g. HIV).
- Major surgery or trauma:
  - suppresses T-cell proliferation;
  - burn injury causes reduction in natural killer cells and reduced neutrophil chemotaxis;
  - hypoxia stimulates prostaglandin E_2 and tumour necrosis factor-α production by macrophages.
- Acute/chronic renal failure:
  - reduced neutrophil bactericidal activity;
  - inappropriate macrophage activation;
  - impaired macrophage antigen presentation;
  - defective T-cell function.

Nursing the immunocompromised patient

- Strict infection control procedures.
- Protective isolation (preferably in a side-room with positive laminar flow and HEPA filtration) if neutropenic.
- Direct care equipment, such as stethoscopes, should be patient-specific.
- Consider use of anti-*Legionella* filters in water supply.
- Cannulae, catheters, disposables changed according to unit protocols.
- Microbiological screening if there is a deterioration in condition.
- Minimize invasive procedures and manipulations – use non-invasive monitoring where possible.

- Observe iv cannulae insertion sites, wounds, drains, and secretions for signs of infection.
- Follow unit protocols for use of prophylactic antibiotics – avoid overuse.

See 📖 Chapter 19, pp. 445–470, for further information.

Human immunodeficiency virus

A retrovirus that causes autoimmune deficiency syndrome (AIDS). Following the initial infection, viral replication continues with progressive destruction of CD4 lymphocytes. Eventually, production of new CD4 cells cannot match their rate of destruction and the clinical picture of AIDS develops.

Admission to the critical care unit

May be due to:
- Infection (bacterial, fungal, protozoal, viral).
- Co-infections (e.g. hepatitis B and C, causing liver failure, TB).
- Acute respiratory failure.
- Altered conscious level or intractable seizures secondary to neurological manifestations (e.g. CNS toxoplasmosis, CNS lymphoma, cryptococcal meningitis).
- Surgical or medical issues unrelated to the HIV infection.

Complications of HIV infection

Respiratory

See Table 20.1 for causes of respiratory failure. The commonest cause is *Pneumocystis carinii*.
- A fungus, transmitted through air, causing upper and lower respiratory tract infection.
- Patient presents with fever, tachycardia, and cough.
- Exertional dyspnoea develops with severe tachypnoea and hypoxia.
- Pneumatoceles (air filled cysts) on CXR predispose to pneumothorax.
- Treatment is by antibiotics (e.g. high-dose co-trimoxazole, high-dose steroids and, if needed, ventilatory support).

Neurological

HIV is a neurotrophic virus that can cause:
- Acute myelopathy.
- Encephalopathy.
- Meningitis.
- Cerebral mass lesions.
- Secondary brain infection, e.g. toxoplasmosis.

Gastrointestinal
- CMV-related peritonitis from small bowel or colonic enteritis.
- AIDS cholangiopathy causing biliary sepsis.

AIDS related malignancies
- Karposi's sarcoma.
- Lymphomas.
- Cervical carcinomas related to human papilloma virus.
- Hepatitis B related carcinomas.
- Non-Hodgkin's lymphoma.

Table 20.1 Other causes of respiratory failure in HIV disease.

Bacterial pneumonia	Streptococcus pneumoniae Staphylococcus aureus Hamophilis influenzae Pseudomonas species (e.g. Serratia marcescens)
Atypical pneumonia	Mycobacterium tuberculosis Mycoplasma pneumoniae
Fungal pneumonia	Cryptococcus neoformans Histoplasma capsulatum Coccidiodes immitus Aspergillus fumigatus
Cytomegalovirus pneumonia	
Lymphocytic interstitial pneumonia	
Toxoplasmosis gondii pmeumonitis	
Non-Hodgkin's lymphoma and pulmonary Karposi's sarcoma	

Reproduced with permission from *Critical Care Nursing*, Adam and Osborne (2005), Oxford University Press.

Further information

Adam SK, Osborne S. (2005) *Critical Care Nursing*. Oxford: Oxford University Press.

Systemic lupus erythematosus (SLE)

A chronic, potentially fatal, auto-immune disease, which varies from a mild episode to severe disease affecting multiple organs. It most commonly affects young women and, in particular, those of West-Indian origin. The aetiology is unknown, but results in:

- Production of anti-nuclear antibodies.
- Generation of circulating immune complexes (a network of several antigens and antibodies cross-linked to form a large mass that, if trapped in the tissue, can initiate further inflammatory reaction).
- Activation of the complement system.
- Thrombosis, immune complex, and white cell deposition causing recurrent vascular injury.
- Cytotoxic antibodies that mediate autoimmune haemolytic anaemia and thrombocytopenia.
- Antibodies to specific cellular antigens that disrupt cell function (the main causes of admission to the critical care unit are infection, renal failure, and emboli).

Manifestations of systemic lupus erythematosus

Skin and mucosa

- Photosensitivity with flushing on cheeks and bridge of nose (butterfly rash).
- Rashes and skin lesions on sun-exposed parts of the body, urticaria.
- Alopecia (hair loss).
- Mucosal ulcers on soft and hard palate and nasal septum.
- Conjunctivitis.

Musculoskeletal

- Joint pain.
- Arthritis.
- Myalgia.
- Myositis.
- Bone necrosis (hips and shoulders).

Renal

- Lupus nephritis (persistent inflammation of the kidney).
- Renal failure that may require dialysis or transplantation.

Haematological

- Anaemia.
- Leucopenia.
- Autoimmune thrombocytopenic purpura.
- Venous or arterial thrombi (causing strokes and pulmonary emboli).
- Reduced platelet level.
- Antibodies can form against clotting factors and may cause significant bleeding.
- Prolonged activated partial thromboplastin time.

Cardiac

- Endocarditis.
- Myocarditis.

- Pericarditis.
- Cardiac tamponade from pericardial effusions (rare).
- Chest pain.
- Arrhythmias.

Lung
- Inflammatory serositis causing pleurisy.
- Pleural effusion.
- Inflammatory pneumonitis.
- Interstitial pulmonary fibrosis.
- Pulmonary hypertension.
- Pulmonary alveolar haemorrhage.
- Phrenic nerve palsy.

Central nervous system
- Isolated nerve palsies.
- Cerebral dysfunction manifesting as psychosis, personality disorder, coma, organic brain syndrome, dementia.
- Cerebrovascular accidents.
- Seizures.

Gastrointestinal
- Peritonitis.
- Ascites.
- Pancreatitis.
- Mesenteric ischaemia.
- Inflammatory liver disease.
- Splenomegaly.

Treatment
- Steroids, such as prednisolone, or pulsed methylprednisolone/immuno-supressive drugs, such as azathioprine or cyclophosphamide.
- Cessation of drugs that may induce SLE (e.g. procainamide, hydralazine, isoniazid).
- Supportive therapy (respiratory support, dialysis).
- Antibiotics for infections.
- Plasma exchange or intravenous immunoglobulin may be useful for pulmonary haemorrhage.
- Long-term anticoagulation (to prevent thrombi and emboli).

Rheumatoid arthritis

A chronic, inflammatory disease of unclear aetiology. There is evidence of genetic predisposition and that it is immune mediated. It is still unclear if it is a primarily autoimmune disease or whether the initiating agent is infectious, a self-antigen, or both. Admission to critical care is usually due to pulmonary involvement or complications of treatment (e.g. renal failure, bleeding disorders, immunosuppression).

Symptoms

- Pain, swelling, and stiffness of joints, particularly hands and feet.
- Tendons, muscle, ligaments, and fascia can be affected causing deformities (e.g. ulnar deviation of fingers, 'z' deformity of thumbs).

Manifestations

Respiratory

- Pleurisy.
- Pleural effusion.
- Fibrosing alveolitis.
- Laryngeal nodules (may present problems during intubation).
- Pulmonary hypertension.
- Bronchiectasis.
- Pulmonary vasculitis.
- Interstitial pneumonitis and fibrosis (rheumatoid lung).

Cardiac

- Pericarditis.
- Conduction defects.
- Mitral valve disease.

Neurological

- Compression of cervical spinal cord.
- Instability of cervical spine (may preclude extension of the neck for endotracheal intubation).
- Entrapment of peripheral nerves and compression of nerve roots.
- Peripheral neuropathy.

Skin

- Cutaneous vasculitis.
- Palmar erythema.
- Pyoderma gangrenosum.

Other

- Splenomegaly.
- Anaemia.
- Lymphadenopathy.
- Carpal tunnel syndrome.
- Osteoporosis.
- Amyloidosis.
- Eye disorders – episcleritis, scleritis, keratoconjunctivitis sicca.

Management

- Non-steroidal anti-inflammatory drugs (e.g diclofenac, ibuprofen).
- Steroids for rheumatic interstitial lung disease to prevent development of fibrosis.
- Cytotoxic drugs (e.g. methotrexate, cyclophosphamide, azathioprine) – use may be limited by side effects.
- Gold injections.
- Anti-TNF antibody.
- Anti-CD20 antibody (rituximab) in severe cases.
- Physiotherapy, occupational therapy.
- Surgery to improve function.
- Household and personal aids.
- Monitor drug therapy closely for side effects.
- Care must be taken with rolling the patient (especially if they are unconscious) if the cervical spine is unstable.

Vasculitic disorders

Wegener's granulomatosis
Characterized by necrotizing vasculitis, affecting small- and medium-sized vessels (nose, eyes, lungs, kidneys). Auto-antibodies are directed against white blood cells and bind to epithelial cells, forming immune complexes. These accumulate in the tissues leading to granulomatous inflammation of the vessels. Blood flow is reduced to organs and tissues.

Symptoms
- Cold–like symptoms, fever, weight loss, malaise, myalgia.
- Sinusitis and purulent, bloody nasal discharge.
- Epistaxis.
- Destruction of nasal cartilage, septal perforation.
- Subglottal stenosis (may cause difficulty in endotracheal intubation).
- Haemoptysis (from laryngeal and pulmonary ulcers).
- Pulmonary haemorrhage (due to necrotizing capillaries).
- Pleurisy, pneumonia, cavitating granulomatous lung masses.
- Renal failure (secondary to necrotizing glomerulonephritis).
- Conjunctival haemorrhage, keratitis, ocular muscle paralysis.

Treatment
- Immunosuppressive drugs (e.g. corticosteroids, cyclophosphamide).
- Balloon dilatation and stent insertion for tracheobronchial stenosis.

Goodpasture's disease
Caused by antiglomerular basement membrane antibodies (anti-GBM) binding to the glomerulus and alveolus. Patients present with glomerulonephritis and/or pulmonary haemorrhage (particularly in patients who smoke).

Treatment
- Daily plasma exchange to remove anti-GBM antibodies.
- Corticosteroids.
- Cyclophosphamide.

Polyarteritis nodosa
A necrotizing vasculitis causing segmental inflammation, and necrosis of small- and medium-sized arteries. Secondary thrombosis and occlusion of the vessels leads to ischaemia and infarction of multiple organs. Small aneurysms develop in weakened tissue walls. Healing can result in fibrosis.

Symptoms
Gastrointestinal
- Abdominal pain.
- Nausea, vomiting.
- Bloody diarrhoea.
- Bleeding into retroperitoneal space.
- Mesenteric artery thrombosis.
- Bowel infarction.

Cardiovascular
- Hypertension.
- Myocardial infarction.
- Pericarditis.
- Heart failure.

Neurological
- Sensory changes – numbness, tingling.
- Headaches.
- Strokes.
- Seizures.

Renal
- Oliguria.
- Renal failure.

Other
- Fever.
- Weakness, myalgia, arthralgia.
- Skin lesions, palpable nodules along tract of affected blood vessels.
- Weight loss.
- Oedema.
- Focal ischaemia.
- Bronchospasm.

Treatment
- Renal replacement therapy.
- Corticosteroids (high doses, long-term).
- Cyclophosphamide.

Anaphylactic and anaphalactoid reactions

Anaphylactic reaction

A potentially life-threatening, systemic reaction that occurs after re-exposure to an antigen. It is IgE-mediated, causing immediate release of potent mediators (e.g. histamine, kinins, leukotrienes) from tissue mast cells and peripheral basophils causing:

- Increased mucus production.
- Pruritus.
- Increased vascular permeability.
- Smooth muscle constriction.

Anaphylactoid reaction

Symptomatically indistinguishable from anaphylactic reactions, but is not IgE mediated. Mast cells are induced to react:

- By exercise or stress.
- By some drugs (e.g. aspirin, opiates).
- Following complement activation by immune complexes.

Causes of anaphylactic and anaphylactoid reactions

- Foods (e.g. nuts, shellfish, eggs, milk).
- Venoms (e.g. bee sting).
- Vaccines.
- Latex.
- Drugs (e.g. opiates, antibiotics, non-steroidal anti-inflammatory drugs).
- Blood and blood products.
- Immunoglobulins.
- Radiocontrast media.
- Dextran.

Symptoms

Can occur within seconds of exposure and the reaction is variable.

Skin

- Flushing.
- Urticaria.
- Pruritus.
- Angioedema.

Gastrointestinal

- Diarrhoea, nausea, vomiting.
- Abdominal cramps.

Respiratory

- Nasal congestion.
- Stridor.
- Upper airway obstruction (oedema of tongue, glottis, larynx).
- Severe bronchospasm and laryngospasm.
- Pulmonary oedema.

Cardiovascular
- Vasodilation.
- Myocardial ischaemia.
- Arrhythmias.
- Hypotension and cardiovascular collapse.
- Cardiac arrest.

Other
- Rhinitis.
- Conjunctivitis.
- Coagulopathy.

Management of a severe reaction

Primary management
- Remove causative agent.
- Maintain adequate airway:
  - 100% oxygen;
  - endotracheal intubation if breathing inadequate;
  - cricothyroidotomy or emergency tracheotomy if upper airway obstruction.
- Give adrenaline (epinephrine) 0.05–0.2mg iv if iv access available. If circulatory or airway access are compromised, give im (0.5mg given as 0.5ml of a 1:1000 solution) if no iv access. Both may need to be repeated if hypotension or airway compromise is ongoing. Nebulized bronchodilators (e.g. salbutamol) for bronchospasm.
- Nebulized adrenaline (epinephrine) can be given for laryngospasm, bronchospasm, and laryngeal oedema.
- Commence CPR if necessary.
- Establish venous access and rapidly infuse fluid – ideally colloid.
- Continue to administer adrenaline (epinephrine) if hypotension persists (preferably by iv infusion).

Secondary management
- Antihistamines (e.g. chlorphenamine, 10mg iv).
- Steroids (e.g. hydrocortisone, 100–200mg iv).
- If ongoing hypotension, continue delivery of iv colloid.
- Continuous cardiovascular monitoring, pulse oximetry.
- 12-lead ECG.

Metabolic disorders

Phaeochromocytoma

A tumour of chromaffin cells, where high levels of adrenaline (epinephrine) and noradrenaline (norepinephrine) are secreted. It usually originates in the adrenal medulla, but can occur anywhere along the sympathetic chain (aorta, bladder, pelvis, abdomen, thorax). The secretion of catecholamines is usually intermittent causing acute attacks of severe hypertension; between attacks the blood pressure may be only slightly raised. Depending on the type of catecholamine secreted, it may present as episodes of hypotension, which can be mistaken for septic shock.

Clinical features

- Severe hypertension (systolic can rise up to 300mmHg).
- Severe hypotension (occasional presentation).
- Tachycardia.
- Pulsating headaches.
- Hyperglycaemia.
- Blurred vision.
- Bowel disturbances.

Diagnosis

- Blood catecholamine levels.
- Computed tomography.
- 24h urinary vanillylmandelic acid (VMA), a metabolic product of catecholamines (not useful in critical illness, where levels are increased anyway).
- MIBG (meta-iodobenzyl guanidine) radionuclide scan.

Treatment

- Control of high blood pressure using alpha- and beta-adrenergic blocking agents. Alpha-blockade should begin before beta-blockade, or a severe hypertensive crisis can be precipitated. Phentolamine or phenoxybenzamine are commonly used for alpha blockade, and propanolol for beta blockade. Alternatively, labetalol can be used as it has both alpha- and beta-blockade effects. During a severe hypertensive crisis, a sodium nitroprusside infusion can be used to facilitate blood pressure control.
- Surgical removal.

Management

- Continuous monitoring of BP and heart rate.
- Titration of antihypertensive drugs according to blood pressure.
- Blood glucose monitoring.
- Post-operative care as for any major abdominal surgical operation.
- Adequate fluid loading prior to and during surgery will reduce the likelihood of post-operative hypotension.

Actions of adrenaline (epinephrine)

- Constricts blood vessels in skin and mucosa.
- Dilates blood vessels in skeletal muscle, brain, myocardium, and eye.
- Bronchodilates.
- Increases heart rate, cardiac output and BP (although may also cause a drop in BP).
- Converts liver glycogen to glucose.
- Stimulates fatty acid oxidation.
- Stimulates glycolysis and may cause a lactic acidosis.

Actions of noradrenaline (norepinephrine)

- Constriction of arterioles and veins (except in crucial areas where adrenaline counteracts this effect).
- Raises BP.

Addison's disease

Results from a chronic deficiency of adrenal cortical hormones. Can be due to absence, atrophy, or disease of the adrenal cortex or occur secondary to hypopituitarism. The symptoms reflect the lack of cortisol, aldosterone and androgens (see 📖 Relative adrenal insufficiency, p. 491).

Diagnosis

- Low serum sodium.
- High serum potassium and urea.
- High serum ACTH levels.
- Positive Synacthen (ACTH) stimulation test.

Treatment

Lifelong cortical hormone replacement therapy.

Addisonian crisis

A life-threatening condition that develops if an acute demand for cortisol cannot be met (e.g. during sepsis, chest infection, pulmonary embolism). The patient progresses to complete circulatory collapse unless immediate treatment is instituted.

Features of an Addisonian crisis

- Severe hypotension.
- Tachycardia.
- Dysrhythmias – particularly atrial fibrillation.
- Hyponatraemia.
- Hyperkalaemia.
- Uraemia.
- Hypoglycaemia.

Management of an Addisonian crisis

- Continuous monitoring of vital signs.
- 12-lead ECG.
- Correct hypovolaemia according to monitored variables (CVP, SV).
- If hypotension or low cardiac output persist, despite adequate filling, inotropic support will be required.
- Monitor blood glucose levels: correct hypoglycaemia with infusions of hypertonic glucose (via a central venous catheter).
- Administer cortisol (iv hydrocortisone initially).
- Monitor urine output: long periods of hypotension and hypovolaemia may precipitate renal failure.
- Monitor and correct blood urea and electrolytes.
- Oxygen requirement and ventilatory support will be dictated by the patient's condition and blood gas analyses.
- Monitor core temperature and maintain normothermia.
- Identify sources of infection by appropriate cultures. Treat accordingly.

Relative adrenal insufficiency

This may occur with critical illness and is usually manifest as catecholamine-unresponsive hypotension. It is usually diagnosed by an inadequate rise in cortisol (<250nmol/l) in blood taken 60min after injection of 250 micrograms ACTH. Hydrocortisone treatment will improve the blood pressure in such patients, but its benefit on outcome is uncertain.

Effects of lack of aldosterone

- Polyuria, dehydration, thirst.
- Hyponatraemia.
- Hyperkalaemia.
- Hypotension (often postural).
- Cardiac dysrhythmias.

Effects of lack of cortisol

- Muscle weakness, fatigue, weight loss.
- Hypoglycaemia.
- Gastrointestinal disturbances (nausea, vomiting, diarrhoea, abdominal pain).
- Emotional disturbances (irritability, depression).
- Low resistance to infection, inability to cope with any type of stress.

Effects of lack of androgens

- Loss of body hair.
- Loss of libido.

Hypothyroidism: myxoedema

Caused by decreased thyroid hormone [levothyroxine sodium (thyroxine sodium, T4) and liothyronine sodium (L-Tri-iodothyronine sodium, T3)] secretion. Can be classified as:
- **Primary:** due to disease of the thyroid.
- **Secondary:** the anterior pituitary secretes insufficient TSH.
- **Tertiary** – the hypothalamus does not secrete enough TRH.

Causes
- Previous surgery to the thyroid (partial or complete thyroidectomy).
- Secondary to ^{131}I therapy for hyperthyroidism.
- Spontaneous – the gland atrophies.
- Hashimoto's thyroiditis – autoimmune destruction of thyroid tissue.
- Disease or surgery of the anterior pituitary or hypothalamus.

Clinical features
- Bradycardia.
- Decreased cardiac contractility and low cardiac output.
- Slow mental function, dementia.
- Hoarse voice, slurred speech.
- Fatigue, excessive sleep.
- Constipation.
- Weight increase.
- Dry, scaly skin.
- Oedema of the hands, puffy face, peri-orbital oedema, eyebrow loss.
- Coarse, easily broken hair.
- Poor wound healing.

Treatment
Identify the cause. Give oral levothyroxine sodium (thyroxine sodium, T4) supplements. If the hypothyroid state continues, myxoedema coma can result.

Myxoedema coma
Precipitating factors
- Infection.
- Trauma.
- Cerebrovascular accident.
- Myocardial infarction.
- Drugs with an antithyroid action (e.g. lithium, amiodarone).

Features
- Decreased conscious level.
- Hypoventilation.
- Hypotension and bradycardia.
- Hypoglycaemia.
- Hypothermia.
- Hyponatraemia.
- Convulsions.
- Ileus due to decreased gut motility.

Management
- Continuous monitoring of vital signs, 12-lead ECG.
- Respiratory support.
- Fluid management for hypotension.
- Monitor urine output, treat oliguria with cautious rehydration if hypovolaemic.
- Monitor blood glucose, correct hypoglycaemia with glucose infusions or boluses of 50% glucose.
- Monitor core temperature, rewarm (0.5–1.0°C/h) until normothermic.
- Neurological observations, observe for seizures, maintain patient safety.
- Monitor blood electrolytes, correct hyponatraemia.
- Nasogastric tube.
- Identify precipitating factors.

Return to euthyroid state
Levothyroxine sodium (thyroxine sodium) supplements will be required, but the sudden introduction of high plasma levels of levothyroxine sodium (thyroxine sodium) can be dangerous. The abrupt increase in metabolism can cause angina, myocardial infarction, and arrhythmias. Levothyroxine sodium (thyroxine sodium, T4) should thus be administered in small quantities initially, then gradually escalated. Corticosteroids are usually given as well.

Sick euthyroid (low T3) syndrome

Can occur within hours or days of the onset of critical illness. Instead of T4 being metabolized to 'active' T3, a different iodine atom is cleaved resulting in the formation of the inactive 'reverse' T3 (rT3). TSH levels are often elevated, but may sometimes be depressed. The relevance of the syndrome is its direct association with a poor prognosis. There is no benefit (and even harm) in administering thyroid hormones.

Hyperthyroidism: thyrotoxicosis

Results from excess secretion of thyroid hormones (T3 and T4). Admission to the critical care unit may be necessary for control of rapid atrial fibrillation requiring cardioversion (if unresponsive to anti-arrhythmics), severe heart failure or a thyroid crisis.

Causes
- Primary disease of the thyroid gland.
- Secondary to a pituitary tumour (produces excess TSH).
- Excess levothyroxine sodium (thyroxine sodium) medication.

Clinical features
- Increased heart rate, cardiac output and BP.
- Tachyarrhythmias (e.g. atrial fibrillation).
- Hyponatraemia (if excess sweating, diarrhoea, pyrexia).
- Goitre – may cause swallowing or breathing difficulties.
- Nausea, vomiting, diarrhoea.
- Weight loss.
- Nervousness, agitation, confusion, hyperactivity, tremors.
- Frequent micturition.
- Exophthalmus, corneal ulceration.
- Increased body temperature, moist skin.
- Heat intolerance.

Treatment
- Beta-blockers (e.g. propranolol) to reduce sympathetic activity.
- Anti-thyroid drugs (e.g. carbimazole) to interfere with the synthesis of thyroid hormones. Iodine solution is given as a short-term treatment in thyrotoxic crisis or prior to surgery.
- Radioactive iodine (^{131}Iodine) destroys the thyroid cells, and reduces its vascularity and size.
- Surgery to remove part of the gland.

Thyroid crisis
A rare, exaggerated, and life-threatening form of hyperthyroidism that can occur at any age. Mortality is 15–20%. Patients are often undiagnosed or have inadequately treated hyperthyroidism. Predisposing factors are usually required to trigger the crisis.

Predisposing factors
- Infection.
- Trauma.
- Myocardial infarction.
- Cerebrovascular accident.
- Eclampsia, labour.
- Radioactive iodine if given to patients who are not euthyroid.

Clinical features

- Hyperpyrexia (>40°C).
- Cardiac failure.
- Tachyarrhythmias (atrial and ventricular).
- Extreme agitation, tremors, and confusion, which may lead to convulsions and coma.
- Epigastric pain, vomiting, diarrhoea.
- Liver dysfunction, jaundice.
- Increased sweating.

Management

Aimed at reducing the effects of the thyroid hormones and supportive treatment until these are under control. Before treatment begins, blood samples are taken for measurement of TSH, and free, and total T3 and T4.

- Continuous ECG and BP monitoring, 12-lead ECG.
- Anti-arrhythmics (e.g. amiodarone); cardioversion if indicated.
- Monitor serum potassium, correct hypokalaemia.
- Beta blockade (e.g. propranolol).
- Hydrocortisone.
- Monitor CVP and cardiac output and correct hypovolaemia.
- Treat heart failure (nitrate infusions, CPAP etc.).
- Monitor core temperature and undertake active cooling if appropriate.
- Monitor blood glucose and correct hypoglycaemia.
- Sedation (e.g. haloperidol, benzodiazepines) for agitation.
- Observe for and treat any seizures, maintain patient safety (cot sides, airway control).
- Monitor respiratory rate, oxygen saturation, and blood gases.
- Oxygen therapy or respiratory support to maintain patent airway and prevent hypoxaemia.
- Eye care: frequent application of hypromellose eye drops or artificial tear solution to protect exposed cornea.

Hypocalcaemia

Causes

- Hypomagnesaemia.
- Critical illness (sepsis, trauma, burns).
- Acute pancreatitis.
- Osteomalacia.
- Over-hydration.
- Massive blood transfusion (chelating effect of citrate anticoagulant).
- Hyperventilation (respiratory alkalosis may reduce ionized plasma calcium fraction).
- Malnutrition.
- Hypo-albuminaemia (diminished calcium binding sites).
- Associated with hyperphosphataemia:
  - hypoparathyroidism;
  - renal failure;
  - rhabdomyolysis.

Clinical features

- Tetany, muscle twitching, facial spasms, carpopedal spasm.
- Paraesthesiae (tingling) of mouth and extremities.
- ECG changes: prolonged Q-T interval
- Muscle weakness.
- Hypotension.
- Seizures.
- Cataracts, changes to teeth, nails, hair (long-term).

Management

- If symptomatic (usually when total plasma calcium levels <2mmol/l or ionized fraction <0.9mmol/l), give 5–10ml 10% calcium chloride iv over 2–5min.
- If asymptomatic, give calcium supplements orally.
- Correct hypomagnesaemia or hypokalaemia.
- If respiratory alkalosis is present, adjust ventilator settings or, if breathing spontaneously and hyperventilating, calm/sedate and rebreathe into a bag.
- Continuous ECG monitoring.
- Observe for dysrhythmias.
- Monitor blood pressure.
- Protect patient from potential injury in the event of seizures (cot sides).

Hypercalcaemia

Causes

- Hyperparathyroidism.
- Malignancy (bony metastases, myeloma).
- Sarcoidosis.
- Excess calcium, vitamin D, or synthetic analogues (usually iatrogenic).
- Rarely, late diuretic phase of acute renal failure, hyperthyroidism, Addison's disease.
- Drug-related, e.g. lithium, thiazide diuretics.
- Immobility and prolonged bed-rest (particularly relevant in long-term ICU patients).

Clinical features

- ECG changes (short Q–T interval, long P–R interval, AV block, AF).
- Hypertension.
- Drowsiness, coma.
- Abdominal pain, pancreatitis, peptic ulceration.
- Anorexia, thirst, constipation.
- Muscle weakness, general malaise, myalgia.
- Headaches, confusion.
- Bone pain, joint effusions.
- Nausea, vomiting.
- Conjunctivitis (due to calcium deposits on the cornea).
- Ureteric stones (may cause obstructive uropathy).
- Damage to renal tubular mechanism causing renal failure.

Management

Symptomatic hypercalcaemia requires prompt treatment:
- Continuous ECG monitoring, 12-lead ECG.
- Observe for and treat dysrhythmias.
- Monitor blood pressure and give antihypertensive therapy as indicated (e.g. calcium antagonists).
- Monitor haemodynamics and treat hypovolaemia.
- Monitor urine output, plasma electrolytes, Ca^{2+}, PO_4, Mg^{2+}, arterial pH, and bicarbonate.
- Reduce plasma calcium level:
  - rehydration followed by low dose iv furosemide – increases calcium excretion by the kidneys;
  - glucocorticoid therapy (hydrocortisone, dexamethasone) – reduces intestinal absorption of calcium;
  - calcitonin – inhibits osteoclastic activity (short-lived action);
  - haemodialysis/haemofiltration – use calcium-free dialysate;
  - biphosphonates (e.g. pamidronate) – inhibits osteoclastic activity, only use after specialist advice due to toxic effects.

Functions of calcium

- Formation and maintenance of bones and teeth: 99% of calcium is stored in bones and teeth, 1% in soft tissues and blood.
- Transmission of nerve impulses:
  - triggers the release of neurotransmitter substances;
  - at low calcium levels nerve fibres become more permeable to sodium ions and become partially depolarized; these fibres then transmit repetitive and uncontrolled impulses to the muscles resulting in spasm (tetany); increased calcium levels depress neuronal activity and the membranes will not depolarize easily.
- Blood clotting: essential for the formation of fibrin and for the clotting cascade.
- Muscle contraction:
  - the flow of calcium and sodium is essential for muscle contraction;
  - calcium facilitates the interaction of myosin and actin;
  - when impulses pass through cardiac muscle, small amounts of calcium ions are released from the sarcoplasmic reticulum within the muscle cells; this initiates the contractile process though binding of actin-myosin cross-bridges – if only small amounts of ionized calcium are available, the intensity of the contraction is reduced.
- Decreases the permeability and increases the strength of capillary membranes: at low calcium levels these become friable with increased permeability to fluid.
- Regulates cellular metabolism (binds calmodulin – a protein that regulates a variety of enzymatic processes).

Diabetic ketoacidosis

May present in a newly-diagnosed diabetic patient or follow an acute insult in a known diabetic.

Predisposing factors
- Infection (e.g. chest, urine, infective gastroenteritis).
- Myocardial infarction.
- Thrombo-embolism.
- Not taking prescribed insulin.

Clinical features
- Hyperglycaemia: due to lack of insulin.
- Dehydration and hypovolaemia: due to osmotic diuresis.
- Electrolyte depletion: due to polyuria.
- Ketoacidosis: due to excess fat metabolism with ketone production.

Management
- Continuous cardiovascular monitoring, 12-lead ECG.

Airway protection
- If conscious level is decreased, endotracheal intubation ± mechanical ventilation may be required.
- If breathing spontaneously, monitor respiratory rate and give oxygen therapy as indicated by arterial blood gases/pulse oximetry.
- Monitor blood gases and potassium.
- Insert nasogastric tube (high risk of aspiration due to gastric atony).

Rehydration
- Correct hypovolaemia promptly to maintain organ perfusion.
- Average requirements are 5–10l in first 24h. This should be directed by appropriate monitoring (e.g. BP, CVP, ±SV, urine output), but excessive, rapid infusion should be avoided.

Correct hyperglycaemia
- Measure blood glucose levels regularly – initially hourly.
- Continuous infusion of insulin, titrated against blood glucose level.
- Aim for smooth, slow return to normal over the next 24–48h (2–4mmol/h reduction in blood glucose). Avoid over-rapid reduction.
- Continue insulin when normoglycaemia is achieved. To prevent hypoglycaemia, glucose can be given iv, and/or enteral nutrition commenced, and/or the patient may be able to eat and drink.
- Test urine regularly for glucose and ketones.

Electrolyte depletion
- Although the patient is usually hyperkalaemic, potassium levels may fall rapidly with insulin and fluid.
- Monitor potassium levels 1–2 hourly initially, give iv supplements accordingly (usually 5–20mmol/h are required).
- Observe ECG for dysrhythmias.
- Measure serum phosphate and magnesium on admission and thereafter daily until normal. Give supplements as required.

Metabolic acidosis due to ketosis
- Measure blood gases regularly – initially hourly.
- The acidosis usually corrects with insulin and fluid replacement.
- Consider other causes if not correcting, e.g. sepsis-induced lactic acidosis.

Prevention of thrombo-embolism
- Passive limb movements if immobile.
- Prophylactic subcutaneous heparin.
- Elasticated thrombo-embolism stockings.

Identify and treat predisposing factors
For example:
- Exclude myocardial infarction (12-lead ECG, troponin).
- Seek, culture, and treat potential infection.

Hyperosmolar, hyperglycaemic states

Most commonly occurs in elderly, previously undiagnosed diabetics and is often triggered by a predisposing factor. Mortality is much higher than DKA and is usually from thrombo-embolism as the duration of illness and severity of volume loss is usually greater. It differs from DKA in that the level of free fatty acids and counter-regulatory hormones are lower. This is probably due to sufficient insulin still being secreted to prevent lipolysis (and, hence, ketosis), but not hyperglycaemia.

Predisposing factors

- Infection.
- Trauma (including burns).
- Myocardial infarction.
- Pancreatitis, hepatitis.
- Renal failure.
- Hypothermia.
- Carbohydrate overload (enteral feeding, dextrose solutions).
- Drugs [e.g. phenytoin, thiazides (may inhibit insulin release), glucocorticoids, growth hormone (stimulate gluconeogenesis)].

Management

Similar to DKA (see 📖 Diabetic ketoacidosis, p. 500). The principal differences are:

Conscious level

- Coma may last up to a week and, therefore, active management may need to be much longer.
- Early endotracheal intubation is often required to protect airway or support respiration.

Insulin therapy

- Commence insulin infusions at a lower dose (1–2Units/h) as patients are more sensitive to insulin.
- Aim to reduce blood glucose level by 2–4mmol/h over 36–48h.

Fluid replacement

- Dehydration is usually more severe and hypovolaemic shock may be present. Colloid is given initially to resuscitate, but the overall rate of rehydration should be slower than for DKA.
- Plasma sodium level is usually elevated, although total body sodium is grossly depleted. Sodium chloride 0.9% (or 0.45%) is usually used for volume replacement, with added potassium.
- Titrate fluid replacement against cardiovascular parameters with care as the patients are often elderly with pre-existing cardiac or renal dysfunction.

Prophylactic anticoagulation

- Pulmonary embolus is the major cause of mortality due to prolonged immobility and hyperviscosity of the blood.
- Anticoagulation with heparin is essential (high-range prophylactic dose of subcutaneous low molecular weight or iv heparin).

Hypoglycaemia

Low blood glucose level.

Causes

- Diabetic patients controlled by insulin or oral sulphonylurea hypoglycaemics (e.g. glibenclamide) with inadequate carbohydrate intake.
- Liver failure (depletion of glycogen stores).
- Insulin or sulphonylurea excess (deliberate or accidental).
- Drugs (quinine, aspirin).
- Rarely, Addison's disease, hypopituitarism, insulinoma.

Clinical features

- Coma.
- Seizures, focal neurological signs.
- Irrational behaviour, agitation.
- Tachycardia.
- Slurred speech.
- Sweating.
- Cool, moist skin.
- Faintness.
- Hunger.
- Headache.

Management

Treatment must be rapid as hypoglycaemia can cause irreversible brain damage.

- Monitor blood glucose level frequently.
- Administer aliquots of 20–50ml iv of 50% glucose every few minutes, rechecking the glucose level between each aliquot until normoglycaemia restored.
- A continuous infusion of 10, 20, or 50% glucose may be required if hypoglycaemia persists.
- Continue to monitor blood glucose levels regularly, particularly if an insulin overdose (may be long-acting insulin) or in conditions that precipitate hypoglycaemia (e.g. liver failure).
- Glucagon 1mg may be given im or sc if no venous access is available or if the patient is still conscious, glucose gel (40% glucose) can be given to be absorbed through the oral mucosa.

Diabetes insipidus (DI)

Inadequate secretion of anti-diuretic hormone (ADH) in response to increased plasma osmolality.

Causes
- **Central DI** (damage to hypothalamus or posterior pituitary gland):
  - neurosurgery;
  - head injury;
  - hypoxic brain injury;
  - pituitary tumour;
  - infarction of the pituitary;
  - meningococcal meningitis.
- **Nephrogenic DI** (decreased response of kidney to ADH):
  - polycystic kidney disease;
  - sickle cell disease;
  - drugs (e.g. tetracycline, lithium).
- **Gestational DI:** pregnancy.

Clinical features
- Thirst.
- Polyuria (6–30l/day).
- Fluid loss – may cause severe hypovolaemic shock.
- Hypernatraemia causing delirium, lethargy, convulsions, and coma.

Management
- Monitor cardiovascular variables.
- Monitor urine output.
- Fluid replacement:
  - rapid fluid replacement in hypovolaemic shock to restore circulatory volume;
  - replace volume of previous hours urine output with 5% dextrose or 4% dextrose with 0.18% NaCl + allow the patient to drink freely.
- For cranial DI, replacement therapy with desmopressin (10–40 micrograms daily, intranasally, in divided doses or 1–2 micrograms iv bd). Partial CDI may respond to drugs that increase the rate of ADH secretion or end-organ responsiveness to ADH, e.g. chlorpropamide, hydrochlorthiazide.
- For nephrogenic DI, manage with a low salt diet and thiazides. High dose desmopressin may be effective. Consider removal of causative agents, e.g. lithium, demeclocycline.

Obstetric emergencies

Pre-eclampsia and eclampsia

This is a progressive disorder characterized by hypertension and proteinuria presenting during the latter half of pregnancy, or during or postpartum. Eclampsia is the same condition but associated with seizures.

Clinical features of pre-eclampsia

Cardiovascular
- Hypertension.
- Thrombocytopenia.
- Prolonged clotting time.
- Increased Hb and packed cell volume.

Renal
- Proteinuria.
- Hyperuricaemia.
- Oedema.
- Elevated urea and creatinine.

Neurological
- Headaches.
- Visual disturbances.
- Hyper-reflexia.

Hepatic
- Elevated LFTs.
- Epigastric pain.
- Nausea and vomiting.

Utero-placental
- Reduced foetal growth.
- Possible uterine death.

Complications
- Eclampsia.
- Renal failure.
- HELLP syndrome.
- Hepatic rupture.
- Cerebral haemorrhage.
- Cerebral oedema.
- DIC.
- Pulmonary oedema.
- ARDS.
- Placental abruption.

Management
- Haemodynamic monitoring.
- Ensure adequate volume resuscitation.
- Antihypertensive drug therapy (labetolol, nifedipine, hydralazine).
- Monitor urine output, the level of proteinuria, and fluid balance.
- Observe for neurological disturbances.
- Treat seizures with magnesium sulphate infusion and benzodiazepines.

- Consider prophylactic magnesium infusion (monitor respiratory rate and levels as magnesium is a CNS depressant – respiratory arrest can occur at levels above 5mmol/l).
- Avoid excess sedation, however, continual seizures may require elective intubation and ventilation.
- Monitor blood electrolytes, glucose, clotting studies.
- Observe for bleeding – correct coagulopathy with FFP, cryoprecipitate, and other blood products.
- Consider early foetal delivery.

Attempts may be made to prolong the pregnancy if considered safe for the mother, but the only definitive treatment for eclampsia is foetal delivery. Hypertensive crises and seizures may continue for 48h post-partum. A spontaneous onset diuresis usually heralds recovery.

Massive obstetric haemorrhage

Risk factors
- Antepartum haemorrhage.
- Multiparous.
- Pre-eclampsia.
- Previous post-partum haemorrhage.
- Multiple pregnancy.
- Previous Caesarian section.
- Large baby.
- Fibroids.
- Placental site disorders, e.g. placenta previa.

Causes
- Tears of uterus, cervix, vaginal wall.
- Uterine atony (inability to contract).
- Retained placenta or placental fragments.
- Coagulation defects.

Management
- Resuscitation – the same principles apply as for the management of any case of haemorrhagic shock. Massive blood transfusion may be required with replacement of clotting products.
- Haemodynamic monitoring.
- Identify cause of bleeding.
- The contents of the uterus must be emptied – achieved in the third stage by early clamping of the cord, prophylactic administration of an oxytoxic drug, and controlled cord traction. Prostaglandin F2α injected locally into the uterus can stimulate uterine contraction and may avoid the need for surgery.

If bleeding persists further techniques include:
- Vaginal packing.
- B-lynch suture.
- Foley catheter or Sengstaken–Blakemore tube used as a tamponade.
- Laparotomy and direct ligation of the uterine vessels or internal iliac artery.
- Radiographic embolization.
- Hysterectomy.

Following resuscitation monitor for the complications of massive blood loss (ARDS, renal failure, DIC).

Amniotic fluid embolism (AFE)

AFE is the entrance of amniotic fluid, containing foetal cells and debris, into the maternal circulation. However, it may not be the amniotic fluid *per se*, but the woman's individual response to amniotic fluid that is the crucial factor in the development of the syndrome.

The release of soluble mediators into the maternal circulation results in a syndrome of haematological and cardiovascular manifestations. There are two phases. In the first, pulmonary artery spasm with pulmonary hypertension occurs, leading to right heart failure and hypoxaemia. Hypoxaemia causes myocardial and pulmonary damage, the left ventricle fails and pulmonary oedema may develop.

In the second phase, non-cardiogenic pulmonary oedema develops due to increased alveolar capillary permeability. There may also be a haemorrhagic phase characterized by massive haemorrhage, uterine atony, and DIC.

Features
- Sudden dyspnoea in late stages of labour or shortly after birth.
- Hypotension.
- Hypoxaemia.
- Cardiorespiratory arrest.
- Seizures.
- Pulmonary oedema/ARDS.
- DIC causing massive haemorrhage.

Management
- Cardiopulmonary resuscitation.
- Maintain oxygenation – intubation and ventilation are usually necessary.
- Haemodynamic monitoring and restoration of blood pressure – rapid volume infusion and inotropic support (blood transfusion if haemorrhage).
- Correct coagulopathy (platelets, cryprecipitate, FFP).
- Expedite delivery (caesarian section) and control haemorrhage (surgery if indicated).
- Renal support may be required.

HELLP syndrome

This syndrome is characterized by haemolysis, elevated liver enzymes and low platelets.

Diagnosis

- Thrombocytopenia (from increased platelet consumption) although PT and APTT times are often normal, unlike DIC. The platelet count falls <100 × 10^9/l.
- Hepatic dysfunction (periportal necrosis and hyaline deposits in the sinusoids), hyperbilirubinaemia, LDH>600U/l, AST>70U/l.
- Micro-angiopathic haemolysis (from destruction of red cells as they pass through damaged small vessels).

Clinical features

- Nausea and vomiting.
- Generalised oedema.
- Epigastric or right upper quadrant pain.
- Malaise.
- Hypertension (less common).

Management

- Resuscitation and monitoring.
- Observe for signs of haemorrhage.
- Transfusion of platelets, red cells, FFP, cryoprecipitate.
- Plasma exchange.
- Urgent Caesarean section.
- Surgical repair if liver ruptures.

Complications

- Liver haemorrhage, necrosis or rupture.
- Encephalopathy.
- Generalized haemorrhage.

Cardiac arrest in the pregnant patient

Cardiac arrest occurs in approx 1 in 30 000 pregnancies. The life of the mother usually takes precedence over the foetus.

Major causes

- Venous thrombosis.
- Severe pregnancy induced hypertension (pre-eclampsia/eclampsia).
- Amniotic fluid embolism.
- Sepsis.
- Haemorrhage (e.g. post-partum haemorrhage, placenta previa, placental abruption, profound coagulopathies, intracerebral haemorrhage).
- Trauma.
- Congenital/acquired heart disease.
- Iatrogenic (anaesthetic complications, drug allergy, hypermagnesaemia).

Physiological changes

Normal physiological changes of pregnancy must be taken into account during resuscitation, e.g.:
- Increase in circulating blood volume.
- Increase in cardiac output (the foetus receives 30% of cardiac output).
- Aortocaval compression by the uterus from 20 weeks' gestation onwards.
- Supine hypotensive syndrome (syncope, hypotension, bradycardia) due to decreased venous return caused by inferior vena cava compression. Moving the patient from supine to the left lateral decubitus position can increase CO by 25–30%.
- Increase in resting oxygen consumption and minute ventilation.
- Mild compensated respiratory alkalosis.
- Diaphragmatic elevation causing decreased functional residual capacity.

CPR and advanced life support

The algorithms of basic and advanced life support (ACLS) should be followed with the following exceptions:
- Rapid endotracheal intubation to avoid hypoxaemia (also increased risk of gastric aspiration).
- After 20 weeks gestation CPR must be carried out with the patient in the left lateral decubitus position – ideally at a 27° tilt (achieved by a Cardiff wedge, foam wedge, or pillow under the left hip, manual displacement of the uterus to the left and upwards).
- Cautious use of sodium bicarbonate.
- If gestation is > 24 weeks, emergency Caesarean section is indicated within 4min of maternal cardiac arrest if a circulation is not restored – aiming for delivery of the child within 1 further minute.

The same medication and defibrillation protocols for ACLS should be followed for both pregnant and non-pregnant patients.

The pregnant patient in the critical care unit

The normal physiological changes in pregnancy both stress and limit the response to an acute illness. Although some conditions are unique to pregnancy, other pre-existing medical conditions may complicate its course. A collaborative approach is vital between the critical care and obstetric teams.

Commonest causes of admission

- Pre-eclampsia/eclampsia.
- Post-partum haemorrhage.
- Placental abruption/placenta previa.
- Infection.
- Anaesthetic-related complications.
- Cardiac complications.
- Gestational diabetes.
- Acute renal failure.
- Cerebral vascular accident.
- Amniotic/blood clot embolism.

The extent of invasive monitoring will depend on the condition of the mother, but clinical interventions and treatments (including medications) must be carefully considered as they can have profound effects on the foetus depending on the trimester and drug dosage (Table 22.1).

Table 22.1 Effects of commonly used drugs on the foetus

Drug	Potential affect on foetus
Amiodarone	Bradycardia
Bretylium	Decreased uterine blood flow
Lidocaine	Bradycardia
Phenytoin	Teratogenic
Atenolol	Bradycardia
Esmolol	Decreased uterine blood flow, hypoxia, bradycardia
Propranolol	Bradycardia
Diltiazem	Teratogenic
Verapamil	Decreased uterine blood flow, hypoxia
Digoxin	Foetal toxicity, neonatal death

Maintaining foetal oxygenation

- Maintain adequate maternal cardiac output and blood pressure.
- Maintain maternal Hb >10g/dl.

- Maintain oxygen saturation >95%.
- Nurse in lateral position to prevent aortocaval compression – if not feasible a right or left hip wedge should be used.
- Minimize uterine activity (iv fluid volume, salbutamol, $MgSO_4$).

Electronic foetal monitoring (EFM)

Interpretation of EFM will be made by a midwife or obstetrician. The mother's condition and gestation determines if it is continuous or intermittent:

- Normal baseline foetal heart rate (FHR) is 110–160bpm.
- <110bpm for ≥10min is considered bradycardia.
- >160bpm for ≥10min is considered tachycardia.
- Tracings are interpreted relative to uterine activity.
- Decelerations or decreases from the baseline rate can suggest foetal compromise (e.g. hypoxaemia).
- Abnormal FHR tracings require interventions as appropriate (e.g. lateral position changes, IV bolus, increased oxygenation).

Preparation for emergency Caesarean section

At >24 weeks' gestation, Caesarean section must be carried out within 4min of maternal cardiac arrest if circulation cannot be restored, aiming for delivery within a further minute. A contingency plan should be in place for high-risk patients to have the necessary equipment and personnel promptly available for delivery of the foetus in the ICU. The plan should include:

- A method of contacting the obstetrician/perinatal team/neonatal resuscitation team for immediate attendance.
- Operation pack for Caesarean delivery.
- Theatre lights.
- Diathermy.
- Neonatal resuscitation equipment and drugs, Resuscitaire, suction.
- Neonatal monitoring equipment.

Chapter 23

Poisoning

General principles

Poisoning can be acute or chronic, intentional or accidental. It can result from:
- Ingestion.
- Injection.
- Inhalation.
- Exposure of body surfaces (skin, eyes, mucous membranes).

In patients presenting with an altered conscious level, other causes must be considered (e.g. meningoencephalitis, head injury, stroke, hypoglycaemia, hepatic encephalopathy).

The consequence of poisoning depends on:
- The patient's age, size and general health.
- The drug or substance.
- The route.
- How long ago the drug was taken or the period of exposure.
- The quantity of the poison.
- Other substances taken at the same time (e.g. alcohol).

Diagnosis

History

Obtained from:
- Evidence of empty bottles, syringes, drugs, suicide note.
- Patient, relatives, ambulance personnel, friends, GP.
- Medical history (e.g. depressive illness).
- Supervisors and co-workers in potential workplace exposure in order ascertain the use of any industrial chemicals or gases.

Physical examination

Signs may be suggestive of particular substances, e.g.
- Toxidromes: a collection of characteristic signs and symptoms elicited by a particular substance when taken in excess (see ▢ Toxidromes, p. 520).
- Breath odour:
  - cyanide – bitter almonds;
  - phenol, salicylates, isopropyl alcohol – acetone;
  - heavy metals, organophosphates - garlic.
- Needle tracks, venepuncture marks from recreational drug use.
- Colour of skin/mucous membranes (jaundice, cherry red, cyanosed).
- Presence of rashes/blisters.

Investigations

Urgent laboratory measurement of blood levels is usually limited to paracetamol and salicylate. Variably, hospital laboratories can measure some other drug levels 'out-of-hours', including digoxin, lithium and phenytoin, in order to direct management. Bedside kits can detect recreational drugs, including opiates and cannabis. A more comprehensive drug screen can be carried out, if required, by a specialized Poisons Unit. Blood, urine, and gastric aspirate/vomitus should be taken and sent to the laboratory.

Additional investigations to be considered include:
- Blood glucose.
- Urea and electrolytes.
- FBC.
- Clotting screen.
- Osmolality.
- LFTs.
- Urinalysis.
- Arterial blood gases (if CO poisoning suspected, use a co-oximeter to measure oxygen saturation as it can identify the concentration of carboxyhaemoglobin).
- 12-lead ECG.
- CXR if indicated (aspiration is common, pulmonary oedema may occur with salicylate and heroin poisoning).

Conditions requiring admission to the critical care unit

- Cardiovascular instability: hypo/hypertension, cardiac arrhythmias, heart failure.
- Reduced conscious level (e.g. GCS ≤ 8 or continuing to fall).
- Repeated or prolonged seizures.
- Need for endotracheal intubation ± mechanical ventilation.
- Need for specialist support: e.g. haemo(dia)filtration, haemoperfusion, temporary pacing.
- Management of bleeding (e.g. from warfarin overdose).

Management of poisoning

Initial management

- Maintain a patent airway: if comatose, no cough or gag reflex. Endotracheal intubation and ventilation will be required.
- Give oxygen therapy to maintain arterial Hb saturations at 95–98%.
- Assess the haemodynamic status of the patient: cardiopulmonary collapse may require urgent intervention. Monitor HR, BP, and oxygen saturation. Establish venous access, correct hypovolaemia, and treat excessively high or low blood pressures.
- Recognize and promptly manage seizures.
- Perform bedside glucose test and treat hypo- (or hyper-)glycaemia.
- Perform thorough neurological assessment and institute regular neuro-monitoring with GCS scoring.
- Monitor core temperature and treat hyper- or hypothermia.
- Check limbs, buttocks, back for evidence of compartment syndrome, and blood/urine for rhabdomyolysis.
- Examine skin for signs of injury, blisters, or venepuncture marks.
- Regularly re-assess patient.

Decreasing further poison absorption

Gastric lavage and emesis are rarely used due to doubts over their efficacy and the risk of serious complications.

Activated charcoal

- Prevents absorption from stomach.
- Give 1g/kg charcoal orally or via NG tube.
- Ideally give as early as possible after ingestion of substance, but can be effective up to 24h post-ingestion.
- Effective for benzodiazepines, anticonvulsants, antihistamines, phenothiazines, tricyclics, and theophylline – does not work for heavy metals (e.g. iron).
- Airway must be protected as there is a risk of aspiration.
- Do not give to patients with an ileus.

Whole bowel irrigation

- A solution of polyethylene glycol given orally or via NG tube at 2l/h until rectal effluent runs clear.
- Used for substances such as enteric-coated preparations, those for which activated charcoal is ineffective, and for intact elimination of packets of cocaine or heroin.
- Do not use in patients with an unprotected airway, ileus, bowel obstruction, or perforation.

Increasing excretion of poison

Forced diuresis

Large volumes of iv fluid are infused with diuretics to promote urinary excretion. Contraindicated in the presence of impaired renal function or heart failure:

- Maintain urine output >200ml/h.
- Avoid excess positive fluid balance.
- Monitor blood electrolytes and magnesium.
- For forced alkaline diuresis (used for acid poisons such as aspirin) infuse aliquots of 8.4% sodium bicarbonate to maintain urinary pH > 7. If pH >7.5 alternate with 0.9% saline or 5% glucose.
- For forced acid diuresis (used for soluble alkaline drugs) use 5% dextrose with added ammonium chloride to maintain urinary pH near to 6.5.

Extracorporeal elimination

- Haemodialysis, haemofiltration/diafiltration, haemoperfusion.
- Effective for removal of small molecule poisons with limited protein binding (e.g. methanol, ethylene glycol, lithium, theophylline).

Antidotes/ alteration of drug metabolism

Specific antidotes can be given for certain poisons, e.g. naloxone for opiates, flumazenil for benzodiazepines, ethanol for methanol, N-acetylcysteine for paracetamol.

Continued supportive therapy

Respiratory

- Maintain patent airway (positioning, oropharyngeal airway, endotracheal intubation, suctioning).
- Respiratory support (O_2, CPAP, ventilation).
- Monitor blood gases, pulse oximetry.

Cardiovascular

- Continuous haemodynamic monitoring.
- 12-lead ECG and monitor for arrhythmias.
- Monitor for and correct hypovolaemia.
- Inotropic support if required.

Neurological

- Neurological assessment and observations until conscious.
- Monitor for and treat convulsions.
- Exclude hypoglycaemia, hypercapnia, and other metabolic causes if obtunded.

Renal

- Maintain adequate volaemia and urine output.
- Urinalysis.
- Monitor urea, electrolytes, and creatinine.

Other

- Monitor blood glucose.
- Monitor core temperature.

Toxidromes

- A collection of characteristic signs and symptoms elicited by a particular substance when taken in excess.
- Based on the pharmacology and physiological effects of the substance.
- Recognizing a toxidrome guides treatment without specific knowledge of the substance.

Table 23.1 Common toxidromes

Toxidrome	Signs and symptoms	Example of drugs
Anticholinergic	Hypertension Tachycardia Dilated pupils Hyperthermia Delirium Dry, flushed skin Urinary retention Seizures Coma Psychosis	Atropine Antihistamines Psychoactive drugs
Cholinergic	Bradycardia Hypotension Tachypnoea Confusion Seizures Sweating Vomiting Lacrimation Defaecation Fasciculations Dilated pupils	Organophosphates Nerve agents (e.g. sarin) Common pesticides
Sedative/hypnotic	Respiratory depression Slurred speech Depressed mental state Ataxia	Barbiturates Ethanol Anticonvulsants Benzodiazepines Some antidepressants
Opioid	Respiratory depression Depressed mental state Bradycardia Hypotension Pinpoint pupils	Morphine Heroin Fentanyl Codeine

Salicylate poisoning

Most common cause is ingestion of aspirin, less commonly by ingestion of oil of wintergreen (used in liniments) or methyl salicylate. Toxic blood level is >150mg/kg.

Salicylates impair cellular respiration by uncoupling oxidative phosphorylation, stimulating the respiratory centre in the medulla, and interfering with lipid, amino acid and carbohydrate metabolism. They may also cause gastrointestinal erosions, bleeding, ulceration, and (rarely) perforation, plus renal or liver failure

Symptoms

Mild to moderate poisoning(150–300mg/kg)
- Vertigo.
- Tinnitus.
- Diarrhoea.
- Vomiting.
- Headache.
- Confusion.
- Tachycardia.
- Hyperventilation.

Severe poisoning (300–500mg/kg)
- Altered mental state (delirium, hallucinations, coma).
- Acid-base disturbances (respiratory alkalosis due to central stimulation followed by metabolic acidosis due to the acidic nature of the drug and increased metabolic rate).
- Pulmonary oedema.
- Seizures.
- Gastrointestinal bleeding.
- Liver failure.
- Acute renal failure.
- Respiratory failure.
- Rhabdomyolysis.
- Hypoglycaemia.
- Hyperthermia.
- Dehydration and electrolyte imbalance (renal Na^+, K^+, and water loss is increased).

Investigations

- Serum salicylate levels (serial levels determine if absorption is continuing).
- Arterial blood gases.
- Blood glucose.
- Coagulation studies (including INR).
- Urea, creatinine and electrolytes.
- LFT's.
- Serum CK and urine myoglobin if rhabdomyolysis is suspected.

Management

- Activated charcoal to prevent absorption (give as soon as possible after acute ingestion).
- Urinary alkalinization increases elimination – aim for urine pH 7.5–8.0.
- Some authorities still recommend a forced diuresis – aim for urine output 2–3ml/kg/h, although the evidence for any benefit over urinary alkalinization is weak.
- Correct dehydration.
- Avoid fluid overload (particularly in the elderly or those with cardiac or renal disease).
- Monitor electrolytes – give K^+ supplements as required.
- Monitor blood glucose – treat hypoglycaemia.
- Observe for seizures – treat with benzodiazepines.
- Monitor core temperature – active cooling if hyperthermic.
- Haemodialysis if renal failure, refractory acidosis, coma, seizures, pulmonary oedema or serum salicylate level >6.2mmol/l.

Paracetamol poisoning

Hepatic glucuronide and sulphate are depleted following a paracetamol overdose with a consequent increase in P450 catalysed oxidation. This leads to increased production of a reactive arylating metabolite (N-acetyl-p-benzoquinone imine – NAPQI). NAPQI is usually rendered non-toxic by conjugation with glutathione, but this is reduced following overdose. NAPQI causes cellular damage and hepatic necrosis.

Toxic effects are serious or fatal at 150mg/kg in adults, or around 75mg/kg in those with impaired hepatic metabolism, e.g.

- **Malnutrition:** decreases glutathione stores.
- **Alcoholism:** decreases glutathione stores.
- **HIV infection:** decreases glutathione stores.
- **Chronic disease:** decreases glutathione stores.
- **Enzyme inducing drugs** (e.g. rifampicin, barbiturates, carbamazepine, ethanol, phenytoin): increase P450 activity.

Symptoms

Patients are often asymptomatic for the first 24h or experience non-specific abdominal pain, nausea, and vomiting. After 24h hepatic necrosis develops causing elevated transaminases, jaundice, and right upper quadrant pain. This can progress to:

- Encephalopathy.
- Oliguria.
- Hypoglycaemia.
- Hypotension.
- Lactic acidosis.
- Coagulopathy.
- Acute liver failure (at day 2–7).
- Renal failure (at about day 3).

Investigations

- Serum paracetamol levels: take first sample as soon as possible after 4h of ingestion.
- Urea, creatinine, and electrolytes: if needed, repeat 12-hourly.
- LFTs: if needed, repeat 12-hourly (ALT >1000IU/l indicates severe liver damage).
- Clotting screen: monitor INR (perform 12-hourly if needed).
- FBC.
- Arterial blood gases.
- Regular blood glucose.

Management

- Consider activated charcoal (50mg) if more than 150mg/kg paracetamol or 12g, whichever is the smaller, has been ingested and if it can be given within 1 hour of the overdose.
- Monitor urine output.
- Hourly blood glucose measurement - treat hypoglycaemia.
- Renal support if renal failure.
- Oral methionine or *n*-acetylcysteine (NAC).

NAC (and methionine) act as a precursor for glutathione, promoting normal conjugation of the remaining paracetamol. Its protective effect is greatest within 12h of ingestion, but can decrease mortality in late-presenting patients up to 36h. Protection is most effective if given within 8h of ingestion.

Start NAC
- If paracetamol levels at 4h exceed the treatment line (q.v.).
- Immediately if more than 150mg/kg has been ingested.
- The overdose is staggered or time of ingestion is uncertain.
- The patient is a late presenter (>24h) with detectable paracetamol levels or elevated transaminase levels.
- Evidence of severe toxicity regardless of time of overdose.
- High risk patients with depleted glutathione or on enzyme-depleting drugs.
- **Liver transplantation:** contact Regional Liver Centre. Consider if:
  - pH< 7.3 or arterial lactate >3.0 after fluid resuscitation;
  - creatinine >300µmol/l;
  - PT >100.
  - INR >6.5.
  - grade III/IV encephalopathy in a 24h period.

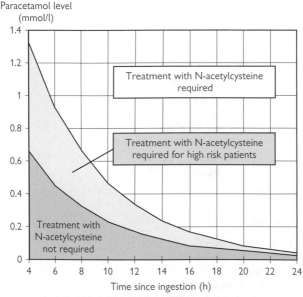

Fig. 23.1 Treatment with *n*-acetylcysteine. Reproduced with permission from *Oxford Handbook of Critical Care* 2nd edition, Singer and Webb (2005), Oxford University Press.

Further information

Singer M and Webb AR. (2005) *Oxford Handbook of Critical Care*, 2nd edn. Oxford: Oxford University Press.

Carbon monoxide poisoning

CO is a colourless, odourless gas produced by the incomplete burning of organic compounds. CO has a greater affinity for haemoglobin than oxygen, forming carboxyhaemoglobin. The oxyhaemoglobin dissociation curve is shifted to the left, decreasing release of oxygen at the tissues. CO also binds to myoglobin with even greater affinity than Hb, further exacerbating tissue hypoxia.

The elimination half-life from blood is:
- 4.5h at room air.
- 1.5h on 100% oxygen.
- 15–23min in 2.5atm hyperbaric oxygen.

CO also competes with oxygen for binding to the haem moiety within cytochrome oxidase, the last part of the mitochondrial electron transport chain responsible for generating most of the body's ATP. As mitochondrial pO_2 levels are much lower than arterial levels, the CO is harder to displace, thus the rationale for hyperbaric treatment.

Symptoms
- Headache.
- Nausea.
- Vomiting.
- Tiredness and weakness.
- Confusion/memory disturbance/amnesia.
- Abdominal pain.
- Co-ordination problems.
- Angina (if pre-existing heart disease).
- Dyspnoea.
- Loss of consciousness.
- Coma.
- Seizures.
- Classic cherry-red appearance of skin and mucosa rarely occurs – usually pallor.
- Tachycardia.
- Hypotension or hypertension.
- Hyperglycaemia.
- Hypokalaemia.
- Hyperthermia.
- Bright red retinal veins.
- Papilloedema.
- Retinal haemorrhages.
- Non-cardiogenic pulmonary oedema.

Complications
- Myocardial depression/ischaemia/infarction.
- Cardiac arrhythmias secondary to hypoxia or myocardial injury.
- Non-traumatic rhabdomyolysis.

- Renal failure (secondary to myoglobinuria from rhabdomyolysis).
- Cerebral oedema.
- White matter demyelination.
- Permanent brain damage/long-term neuropsychiatric sequelae.

Investigations
- Carboxyhaemoglobin (HbCO) levels: measure on co-oximeter.
- Arterial blood gases:
  - metabolic acidosis may be present secondary to lactic acidosis;
  - NB: oxygen saturation is inaccurate when calculated from P_aO_2 (most blood gas machines) or pulse oximetry.
- Troponin.
- Creatinine kinase and urine myoglobin.
- FBC, U&Es, LFTs, glucose.
- 12-lead ECG.
- Urinalysis – positive for albumin and glucose in chronic intoxication.
- Chest X-ray.
- CT head if coma or unresolving CNS symptoms.

Management
- 100% oxygen.
- Ventilatory support as required.
- Continue 100% oxygen until HbCO levels are <10%.
- Hyperbaric oxygen (if feasible) if HbCO levels >25%. Benefits have been shown in long-term cognition.
- Continuous haemodynamic monitoring.
- Serial neurological assessments.
- Monitor electrolytes – correct hypokalaemia.
- Monitor blood glucose.

Tricyclic antidepressant poisoning

These are rapidly absorbed and then metabolized in the liver. Conjugates are then excreted renally. Impaired renal function may prolong toxicity. They have long elimination half-lives (often >24h).

Symptoms

Toxic effects are related to:
- Anticholinergic effects:
  - dry mouth, blurred vision;
  - urinary retention;
  - agitation, hallucinations;
  - depressed mental state;
  - pyrexia;
  - delayed gastric emptying.
- Direct alpha blockade: vasodilation causing profound hypotension.
- Inhibition of noradrenaline (norepinephrine) and serotonin reuptake: hypokalaemia.
- Blockade of fast sodium channels in myocardial cells causing depression of myocardial contractility and arrhythmias.

Cardiovascular effects
- Prolonged PR and QT interval, widened QRS.
- Unstable ventricular arrhythmias/asystole.
- Heart block.
- Sinus tachycardia.
- Hypotension.

CNS effects
- Drowsiness, coma.
- Rigidity.
- Extrapyramidal signs.
- Ophthalmoplegia.
- Respiratory depression (causing hypoxia).
- Delirium.
- Seizures.

Investigations
- U&Es, LFTs.
- Arterial blood gases.
- Toxicology screen is not particularly helpful as serum tricyclic antidepressant levels do not correlate with toxic effects. The high degree of protein binding and their lipophilic nature means that tissue levels are often much higher than serum levels of free drug.
- 12-lead ECG.
- Chest X ray.

Management
- Activated charcoal to reduce absorption.
- Respiratory support:
  - monitor respiratory rate;
  - oxygen therapy;

- • intubate to protect airway if obtunded/comatose;
  - • mechanical ventilation for severe respiratory depression.
- Continuous haemodynamic monitoring: treat hypotension with fluid ± inotropes (use agents with alpha-adrenergic effects).
- Continuous ECG monitoring: observe for arrhythmias. Correct hypotension, hypoxia, and acidosis, and consider magnesium therapy before using anti-arrhythmics, as these may potentially worsen myocardial depression (e.g. beta blockers) and/or further prolong the QT interval (e.g. amiodarone), increasing the risk of serious ventricular arrhythmias. Monitoring should continue for 24h after patient is symptom-free.
- Serum alkalinization using sodium bicarbonate to attain a blood pH 7.45–7.55 – this increases protein binding, decreases QRS width, stabilize arrhythmias and can raise BP. Administer sodium bicarbonate as an initial slow bolus of 1–2mEq/kg body weight (70–140ml of 8.4% solution for a 70kg adult) through a central venous catheter, followed by an infusion.
- Observe for seizures: treat with benzodiazepines, if necessary.
- Urinary catheter to relieve retention and monitor output.

Illicit drug overdose

Street drugs are often 'cut' with various contaminants. Purity, and hence dosage, is difficult to determine. Allergic reactions can also occur to the cutting agents (e.g. quinine). Management is largely supportive:

Management of illicit drug overdose

- **Respiratory:** monitor respiratory rate, endotracheal intubation may be required for airway protection ± mechanical ventilation.
- **Neurological**: assess conscious level, observe for and treat seizures.
- **Cardiovascular:** continuous cardiac monitoring, treatment of hypertension/hypotension.
- **Renal:** monitor urine output, renal support if required.
- **Active cooling if hyperthermic**: dantrolene may be considered if core temperature exceeds 40°C.
- **Specific antidotes** exist for some of these agents, e.g. naloxone for opiates and flumazenil for benzodiazepines. Short-term reversal may be useful for diagnostic purposes or for life-threatening situations where respiratory support is not immediately available. The half-lives of these drugs are short, so the patient may deteriorate within minutes. Longer-term infusions are very expensive so, in general, such patients are intubated ± ventilated until the airway, respiratory, and neurological depressant effects of the overdose have worn off. Sudden reversal of the neurological depression with flumazenil or naloxone may precipitate seizures, so these drugs should generally be avoided if the patient has a history of epilepsy or presents with seizure activity.

Illicit drugs

Cocaine

A potent central nervous system stimulant. Crack cocaine is made from cocaine 'cooked' with ammonia or sodium bicarbonate to create rocks that can be smoked.

Symptoms

- Hyperthermia, hypertension, cerebral haemorrhage.
- Myocardial infarction or cardiomyopathy, leading to heart failure.
- Seizures, tremors, delirium.
- Renal failure.

Ecstacy (MDMA)

A stimulant and hallucinogenic. Adverse effects are more likely with exercise in hot environments (e.g. dancing in clubs). Encouragement to drink lots of water has led to cases of death from severe hyponatraemia.

Symptoms

- tachycardia, hypertension, heart failure.
- hyperthermia and dehydration (sometimes severe).
- loss of consciousness, seizures, stroke, DIC.
- muscle cramps.
- rhabdomyolysis leading to compartment syndrome and renal failure.
- permanent brain damage (in areas of thought and memory).

Heroin (diamorphine)
An opiate synthesized from morphine.

Symptoms
- Slow, shallow and laboured breathing, respiratory arrest.
- Hypotension.
- Disorientation, delirium, drowsiness, coma.
- Pinpoint pupils, cold, clammy skin.
- Muscle cramps, gastro-intestinal spasms.

Benzodiazepines

Symptoms
- Respiratory depression.
- Confusion, drowsiness, coma.
- Blurred vision, slurred speech.

Gamma-hydroxybutyrate (GHB)
A synthetic depressant, which can be snorted, smoked, or mixed into drinks.

Symptoms
- Nausea, dizziness, amnesia.
- Drowsiness, visual disturbances.
- Respiratory distress.
- Seizures, coma.

Amphetamines
Potent psycho-stimulators causing release of the neurotransmitters dopamine and noradrenaline (norepinephrine).

Symptoms
- Tachypnoea, tachycardia.
- Confusion, hallucinations, psychosis.
- Arrhythmias, hypertension.
- Hyperthermia.
- Stroke, seizures, coma.

Specific treatment
- Acidification of the urine can increase excretion.
- iv phentolamine for severe hypertension.

Barbiturates
Depress the activity of the CNS, respiratory, and cardiovascular systems.

Symptoms
- Severe weakness.
- Confusion, extreme drowsiness.
- Shortness of breath.
- Bradycardia.
- Hypotension.

Specific management
Alkalinization of the urine increases the elimination of phenobarbital.

Evaluating the effects of critical care

Evidence-based care

Evidence-based practice is the use of the best available critically-evaluated research to guide the choice of interventions, management, and care of the patient. The gold standard is the randomized, controlled trial (RCT). However, caution should be exercised in terms of validity and applicability when extrapolating results from the RCT with various inclusion and exclusion criteria to the ICU population as a whole.

Unfortunately, many aspects of nursing care have not been or cannot be captured by RCT or other quantitative methodology testing. Much nursing research has depended on qualitative methodology that can be subjective in nature.

Qualitative research

Qualitative research is rigorous, detailed, simultaneous collection and analysis of data. The aim of which, is an in-depth understanding of a situation, society, individual or culture. Examples are case studies, grounded theory and phenomenology.

Quantitative research

Quantitative research is the systematic, scientific investigation of quantifiable properties and phenomena, and their relationships. Measurement is central to quantitative research because it provides the ability to describe with a statistical level of certainty the connection and relationships between interventions and outcome. Examples are experimental research like the randomized controlled trial.

Levels of evidence

Evidence to support a particular intervention or method of care delivery can be graded based on the reliability of the research available to support it.

Grading of evidence (grading system used by Scottish Intercollegiate Guideline Network - SIGN). Reproduced with permission.

1++ High-quality meta-analyses, systematic reviews of RCTs, or RCTs with a very low risk of bias

1+ Well-conducted meta-analyses, systematic reviews of RCTs, or RCTs with a low risk of bias

1– Meta-analyses, systematic reviews of RCTs, or RCTs with a high risk of bias*

2++ High-quality systematic reviews of case–control or cohort studies,

High-quality case–control or cohort studies with a very low risk of confounding, bias or chance and a high probability that the relationship is causal

2+ Well-conducted case–control or cohort studies with a low risk of confounding, bias or chance and a moderate probability that the relationship is causal

2– Case–control or cohort studies with a high risk of confounding, bias, or chance and a significant risk that the relationship is not causal

3 Non-analytic studies (for example, case reports, case series)

4 Expert opinion, formal consensus

Grading of recommendations.

A: At least one meta-analysis, systematic review, or RCT rated as 1++, and directly applicable to the target population; or a body of evidence consisting principally of studies rated as 1+, directly applicable to the target population, and demonstrating overall consistency of results.

B: A body of evidence including studies rated as 2++, directly applicable to the target population, and demonstrating overall consistency of results; or extrapolated evidence from studies rated as 1++ or 1+.

C: A body of evidence including studies rated as 2+, directly applicable to the target population and demonstrating overall consistency of results; or extrapolated evidence from studies rated as 2++.

D: Evidence level 3 or 4; or extrapolated evidence from studies rated as 2+.

Further information

National Institute for Health and Clinical Excellence (2006) *Guideline Handbook, Reviewing and Grading the Evidence*, 48. Available at: http://www.nice.org.uk/niceMedia/pdf/2006GuidelinesManualChapter7.pdf

Scottish Intercollegiate Guidelines Network. (2008) *SIGN 50: A Guideline Developer's Handbook*. Available at: http://www.sign.ac.uk/guidelines/fulltext/50/index.html

Monitoring the impact of critical care

There are many possible outcomes from critical care, ranging from simple survival to function, life quality, and health and well being. Evaluating the effects of critical care requires monitoring of these outcomes using a range of measurement tools and monitoring techniques. This is a complex process as high-quality critical care must meet every aspect of the patient's (and their family's) needs, both in the critical care unit and beyond.

Outcomes require review from a number of perspectives:
• The patient (and family).
• The staff working in critical care (and the rest of the hospital).
• The healthcare system and society as a whole.

The patient's perspective

Assessing the patient's perspective of the impact of critical care can take place from their discharge from the unit, through to discharge home and for years afterwards. Most recovery of function is seen in the first year.

Mortality rates

The easiest to monitor is survival to discharge from critical care. However, as 23–31% of ICU patients who die, do so following discharge from critical care, it is more appropriate to look at survival to discharge home and, in some cases, to up to 1 year later.

Functional status

This is physical and mental capability measured by a wide range of different factors, e.g. washing and dressing, being able to socialize, etc. Individual capability can be assessed by others.

Health-related quality of life

This is the level of well-being and satisfaction that the individual attributes to their life following an episode in critical care. It is a subjective measure, which only the individual themselves can rate. A variety of tools have been developed to assess this, such as sickness impact profile (SIP), Short Form (SF-36) and EuroQol. These measure aspects of the patient's life, based on the patient's perceptions, physical function, disability, etc., and can be repeated at intervals to assess ongoing recovery. They cover health-related domains, such as pain and impairment, functional status, and mobility, social role, satisfaction, and perceptions.

Quality of life years

Quality of life years is also a measure used to compare the ongoing effects of illness and the impact of treatment. It is defined as the equivalent of a completely healthy year of life or a year of life that is free of symptoms or health-related disabilities. 'QALY's' provide a standard to allow the effect of technology and treatment to be compared.

Impairment
This is an objective measurement of the individual's anatomical, physiological, or biochemical status following critical care e.g. vital capacity or glomerular filtration rate. These are the underlying features of altered function that can be assessed or measured against normal ranges, rather than the symptoms or problems that patients report.

Further information

Black N, Jenkinson C, Hayes J, et al. (2001) Review of outcome measures used in adult critical care. *Crit Care Med* **29**, 2119–24.

Evaluating cost and outcome in critical care

Critical care is an expensive and limited resource, and the outcome and quality of life of patients who become critically ill should be balanced against this, as well as the likelihood of survival.

In most critical care units, the highest costs are associated with a small group of patients (approximately 10% of the total) who remain in critical care over long periods. These patients are usually in the middle range of illness severity, but have an ICU mortality rate of 30–45%.

Factors associated with poor outcome from critical care include age, poor previous health status, severity of the acute illness, and the underlying cause.

Mortality rates in patients who are ventilated for >48h in the United States are high, with only 44% surviving at 1 year post-ICU stay. Of these, 57% require caregiver assistance for some aspect of daily living activities.

However, overall outcome from critical care for all ventilated patients has improved slightly with mortality reducing from 26 to 23% between 1993 and 2003 in New Zealand and Australia, suggesting that improvements in care may be having an impact.

While cost is a limiting factor, there is an ongoing need to be able to:
• Identify those patients who are likely to benefit from critical care.
  A variety of severity scoring systems, e.g. those based on SAPS and or APACHE II, have been used, but do not provide a definitive means of deciding which patient should and should not receive critical care, or of prognosticating individual, rather than population survival.
• Increase the efficiency of the service offered.
• Reduce the impact of factors likely to prolong length of stay, such as adverse incidents or unnecessarily prolonged sedation.

Best practice factors, such as the presence of an intensive care specialist to lead the critical care unit, or the use of the evidence-based care and care bundles can improve some outcomes.

Factors thought to influence cost in critical care

- **Size of ICU:** numbers of beds and economy of scale.
- **Case-mix of patients:** severity of illness and level of organ support.
- **Ratio of emergency to elective patients.**
- **Length of stay.**
- **Organizational structure:** availability of high dependency beds or step-down units.
- **Grade mix of nurses and seniority of medical staff.**
- **Hospital type:** university or non-university.

Further information

Chelluri L, Kyung I, Belle S. (2004) Long-term mortality and quality of life after prolonged mechanical ventilation. **32**, 61–9.

Edbrooke D, Ridley S, Hibbert C. (2001) Variations in expenditure between adult general intensive care units. *Anaesthesia*, **56**, 208–16.

Moran JL, Bristow P, Solomon PJ, et al. (2008) Mortality and length-of-stay outcomes, 1993–2003, in the binational Australian and New Zealand intensive care adult patient database. *Crit Care Med* **36**, 46–61.

Ethical issues in critical care

Ethics are the rules and principles that govern behaviour and conduct. In the critical care unit, this applies to all healthcare professionals, and is underpinned by expectations of society and by codes of conduct from professional bodies, such as the Nursing and Midwifery Council in the UK.

Ethics are an important issue in critical care due to the many dilemmas facing staff around extending life or prolonging death, the frequent inability to consult the patient directly, and the limited availability of resources.

Ethical principles

Two approaches tend to dominate the philosophy of ethics.

Consequentialist or utilitarian

The overall good of an expected outcome should be weighed against any harm involved, i.e. bringing about the best outcome for all concerned.

Deontology

The action itself should be considered against principles of duty, right, and justice. Thus, the act itself is judged right or wrong, and any consequences are not considered.

These two approaches are unified within four principles that should form the basis of any discussion around the ethical issues in critical care:
- **Autonomy:** the principle of self-determination or freedom to choose.
- **Non-malfeasance:** first do no harm – avoid inflicting harm.
- **Beneficence:** always aim to benefit the patient – prevent harm and promote good.
- **Justice:** fair and equitable distribution (delivery) of healthcare .

Common dilemmas facing critical care staff include:
- Determining when critical care treatment is futile.
- Withholding resuscitation measures.
- Determining when the burden of treatment outweighs the benefits.

Resolving ethical dilemmas in critical care

Providing they are mentally competent, any treatment decision should be discussed with the patient and their views respected.

Although the medical consultant in charge of the patient's care will be responsible for the final decision, all staff involved in care should be offered the opportunity to express an opinion. In addition, the family should be approached for their view of the patient's known wishes if the patient is unable to express them for themselves.

Mental capacity and advanced directives

The principle of autonomy is central to ensuring that patients can make healthcare decisions for themselves. However, it is common for critically ill patients to be unable to communicate their wishes. The patient must have the capacity to take the decision required at the time the decision must be made.

The patient is considered unable to make a decision if they cannot:
- Understand information about the decision to be made.
- Retain that information in their mind.
- Use or weigh that information as part of the decision-making process.
- Communicate their decision (by talking, sign language or other means).

Lack of capacity must be determined by the healthcare professionals caring for the patient. Where there is lack of capacity, all care and treatment decisions must be made in the patient's best interest, notwithstanding the sometimes opposing views of the family.

Decisions regarding withdrawing or withholding life-sustaining treatment

All reasonable steps that are in the patient's best interests should be taken to prolong their life. Where treatment is futile, overly burdensome to the patient, or where there is no prospect of recovery, an assessment of best interests may lead to the conclusion to withdraw or withhold life-sustaining treatment. This decision should be made having consulted, wherever possible, with staff, family and those who know the patient as to what the patient's wishes would likely be, and what would constitute their best interests. However, the accuracy of surrogates in determining the patients' wishes is not guaranteed, with only 66% matching in one study.

Advanced directives (Living Will)

An advance directive enables an individual (age >18 years), while still capable, to refuse specified medical treatment at a time in the future when they may lack the capacity to consent to or refuse that treatment. In the UK, the directive must be written, signed, witnessed, and dated, and the signatory must be competent and understand the implications of the document at the time of signing.

Doctors cannot ignore a written statement that is a valid advance decision to refuse treatment.

Further information

Booth M. (2002) Ethics issues in critical care outcome. In: Ridley, S. (ed.) *Outcomes in Critical Care*. Oxford: Butterworth-Heinemann, pp. 223–45.

Department for Constitutional Affairs (2007) *Mental Capacity Act 2005 Code Of Practice*. London: Stationary Office.

Hare J, Pratt C, Nelson C. (1992) Agreement between patients and their self-selected surrogates on difficult medical decisions. *Arch Intern Med* **152**, 1049–54.

Follow-up and long-term problems

Critical care has a long-term impact on many patients, often leaving them with physical and/or psychological problems.

Post-critical care follow-up clinics

- Specific follow-up clinics are part of some critical care services within the UK. Patients are seen between 2 and 6 months after discharge from hospital to assess their physical and mental state. This gives an opportunity for evaluating responses to their critical care stay and to identify any ongoing problems.
- Assessment techniques vary, but the Short Form (SF 36) questionnaire addressing both physical and psychological issues is commonly used.
- Ideally, the patient should have access to a range of healthcare professionals during the consultation, such as dietician, psychologist, and physiotherapist, as well as a clinical nurse specialist and/or intensivist.
- The appointment can also act as an opportunity to gain feedback from the patient about the way the critical care service is delivered.

Interventions to aid recovery

Many patients are unable to fully recall their critical care stay. They often find it difficult to understand why they are so weak and recovery is taking so long. Diaries recording their experience in critical care have been shown to help some patients with this.

A rehabilitation programme covering both physical and psychological issues will significantly improve function in patients after critical care. Interventions include a workbook of exercises and advice, as well as telephone follow-up and clinic visits.

Common problems during recovery from critical care

- **Muscle weakness and fatigue:** muscle wasting may take up to a year to rebuild.
- **Complications of intubation/tracheostomy:** tracheal stenosis and skin tethering.
- **Swallowing difficulties/taste alterations:** contribute to poor nutritional intake and delay recovery.
- **Breathlessness on mild exertion.**
- **Altered sleeping patterns.**
- **Poor memory and lack of concentration.**
- **Nightmares, hallucinations, delusional memories.**
- **Post-traumatic stress disorder:** the incidence is high amongst patients recovering from critical care. If identified, appropriate referral can be made for treatment and ongoing support.
- **Social isolation and conflict** between couples is also commonplace.

Delusional memory: definitions

- A dream, nightmare, or hallucination experienced by the patient during their critical care stay.
- A belief or memory of critical care that has been rejected as false by the patient.
- A belief or memory of events in critical care that is not shared by medical/nursing staff or family members present during the patient's stay.

Post-traumatic Stress Disorder (PTSD): definition

Post-traumatic stress disorder is the development of characteristic symptoms (e.g. intrusive recollections, difficulties sleeping, feelings of constant danger, irritability, etc.) after one or more traumatic events. Events that trigger PTSD involve experiencing a serious threat to one's own physical integrity, which is experienced with intense fear, horror, and helplessness.

Further information

Griffiths RD, Jones C. (2002) Practical aspects after intensive care. In: Ridley S. (ed.) *Outcomes in Critical Care*. Oxford: Butterworth-Heinemann, pp.169–80.

Jones C, Skirrow P, Griffiths R. (2003) Rehabilitation after critical illness: a randomized, controlled trial. *Crit Care Med* **31**, 2456–61.

Index

gut function
  assessment 375
  infective causes 360–1
  management 360–1
  non-infective
    causes 360–1
  prevention 360
diazepam 58–9
digoxin 512
dihydrocodeine 312
diltiazem 512
discharge guidelines 20
disorientation see sensory
  imbalance
diuretics 336–7
dobutamine 277
Doppler ultrasound 114
  blood velocity profile 115
  contraindications 114
  oesophageal probe
    insertion 114
  transcranial 133
  waveform response 115
drowning see near drowning
drug overdose see illicit
  drug overdose
dying patients
  family and loved ones,
    supporting 68, 70–1
  nursing interventions 70
  priorities of 69
  treatment withdrawal
    decision 68

E

eclampsia 506
ecstasy 530
electrical cardioversion 280
  biphasic defibrillator 280
  indications for use 280
  monophasic
    defibrillator 280
  synchronized
    defibrillation, method
    for 280
electrocardiogram 92, 100
  analysis of 100
    ischaemic heart
      disease 100
    other diseases 101
    pericardial heart
      disease 101
    ventricular and atrial
      hypertrophy 101
  basic principles 92
  chest lead positions 100
  electrode placement 100,
    92–3
  monitor adjustment 92
  QRS complex 92–3, 96,
    98, 100
  rhythm strip analysis 93

timing of 92
electroencephalogram
  (EEG) 54, 133
electrolytes 136
  aneurysmal subarachnoid
    haemorrhage
    (SAH) 312
  anion gap 137
  blood transfusions 466
  chloride and
    bicarbonate 137
  enteral nutrition 379
  hyperkalaemia, causes
    of 136
  hypernatraemia, causes
    of 136
  hypokalaemia, causes
    of 136
  hyponatraemia, causes
    of 136
  metabolic acidosis 137
  pancreatitis 372
  parenteral nutrition 386
  plasma ranges,
    normal 137
electronic foetal
  monitoring (EFM) 513
Emergency Response
  Team call criteria
  (UCL) 8
enalapril 279
encephalitis 320, 322
endotracheal tubes 202
  complications 203
  cuff management 202
  intubation, indications
    for 202
  tube, securing 202
  tubes, size of 203
  tubes, types of 202
enoxaparin 236
enteral nutrition 374, 376,
  378, 380
  advantages 377
  complications 378
    abdominal
      distension 378
    aspiration 378
    constipation 379
    cramping 379
    diarrhoea 378
    electrolyte/
      trace element
      abnormality 379
    hypercapnia 379
    mechanical 378
  disadvantages 377
  enteral feeding 382
  patient care 376
    feed tolerance,
      checking 376
    tube obstruction,
      preventing 376

tube placement,
  monitoring 376
prokinetic agents 377
tube types 380
  fine-bore nasogastric
    tubes 380
  nasojejunal tube 380
  percutaneous
    gastrostomy tube
    (PEG) 380
  percutaneous
    jejunostomy tube
    (PEJ) 380
  wide-bore nasogastric
    tubes 380
epidemics, infectious 439,
  442
epinephrine 276, 284, 489
equipment checks 75, 327,
  379, 407
erythrocyte disorders 448
  polycythaemia 448
  sickle cell anaemia 448
esmolol 279, 512
ethanol 519
ethical issues 540
  ethical dilemmas 540
  ethical principles 540
evidence-based care 534
  evidence levels 534–5
  qualitative research 534
  quantitative research 534
  randomized controlled
    trials (RCTs) 534
extubation 212
  complications 212
  patient preparation 212
  principles of 212
  short tem ventilation:
    indications for
    extubation 212
eye care 84
  dry eyes 84
  exposure
    keratopathy 84
  eye assessment 85
  eye infections 84
  neurological care 304
  tear film 84

F

fentanyl 51, 297, 311
fluids, and neurological
  care 298
  electrolytes 298
  fluid regulation 298
  fluid therapy 298
  hypernatraemia 293
    brain stem dead 293
    dehydration 293
    diabetus insipidus
      (DI) 293